Child Behavioral and Parenting Challenges for Advanced Practice Nurses

Mary Muscari, PhD, MSCr, CPNP, PMHCNS-BC, AFN-BC, is a pediatric nurse practitioner (NP), psychiatric clinical specialist, forensic nursing clinical specialist, and a criminologist, who combines her unique educational background with over 40 years of experience working with a wide variety of children and adolescents. She has authored and coauthored numerous books and articles.

Dr. Muscari has been a pediatric NP since 1980, when she earned her MSN/PNP from Columbia University, New York, New York. She earned a master's degree in pediatric nursing (1980) from Columbia University; a post-master's certificate in psychiatric nursing (1988) and a PhD (1992), both from Adelphi University, Garden City, New York; a post-master's certificate in forensic nursing (2003) from Duquesne University, Pittsburgh, Pennsylvania; and a master's degree in criminology (2012) from Regis University, Denver, Colorado. She attended the Infant Death Investigation Academy (2007) through the Centers for Disease Control and Prevention. She has taught nursing since 1988, at Luzerne Community College, Nanticoke, Pennsylvania (1988–1992), the University of Scranton, Scranton, Pennsylvania (1992–2007), and Binghamton University–The State University of New York (2007–present), where she established a forensic health program. Dr. Muscari has worked clinically as a pediatric NP in a variety of environments and currently practices with the Pennsylvania Sex Offender Assessment Board (2005–present), conducting offender assessments, as well as acting as a private consultant on child health/mental health, parenting, and forensic issues.

Dr. Muscari has published several nursing books, including *Pediatric Nursing Review* (the fourth edition of which was published in 2015), *Quick Reference to Child and Adolescent Forensics* (2010), and *Advanced Pediatric Clinical Assessment* (2001). She has also published seven consumer books, including *Everything Parents Guide to Raising Adolescent Girls* (2008), *Everything Parents Guide to Raising Adolescent Boys* (2008), *Let Kids Be Kids: Rescuing Childhood* (2006), *Not My Kid: 21 Steps to Raising a Non-Violent Kid* (2002), and *Not My Kid 2: Protecting Your Children From the 21 Threats of the 21st Century* (2004).

Child Behavioral and Parenting Challenges for Advanced Practice Nurses

A Reference for Frontline Health Care Providers

Mary Muscari, PhD, MSCr, CPNP, PMHCNS-BC, AFN-BC

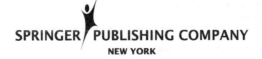

SPRINGER PUBLISHING COMPANY

NEW YORK

Springer Publishing Company, LLC
11 West 42nd Street
New York, NY 10036
www.springerpub.com

Acquisitions Editor: Elizabeth Nieginski
Senior Production Editor: Kris Parrish
Composition: S4Carlisle Publishing Services

ISBN: 978-0-8261-2058-8
e-book ISBN: 978-0-8261-2059-5
Instructor's Manual ISBN: 978-0-8261-2024-3
Instructor's PowerPoints ISBN: 978-0-8261-2019-9
Parent Teaching Guide ISBN: 978-0-8261-2013-7

Instructor's materials are available to qualified adopters by contacting textbook@springerpub.com.
A parent teaching guide is available from www.springerpub.com/muscari.

16 17 18 19 20 / 5 4 3 2 1

The author and the publisher of this Work have made every effort to use sources believed to be reliable to provide information that is accurate and compatible with the standards generally accepted at the time of publication. Because medical science is continually advancing, our knowledge base continues to expand. Therefore, as new information becomes available, changes in procedures become necessary. We recommend that the reader always consult current research and specific institutional policies before performing any clinical procedure. The author and publisher shall not be liable for any special, consequential, or exemplary damages resulting, in whole or in part, from the readers' use of, or reliance on, the information contained in this book. The publisher has no responsibility for the persistence or accuracy of URLs for external or third-party Internet websites referred to in this publication and does not guarantee that any content on such websites is, or will remain, accurate or appropriate.

Library of Congress Cataloging-in-Publication Data
Names: Muscari, Mary E., author.
Title: Child behavioral and parenting challenges for advanced practice nurses:
  a reference for front-line health care providers / Mary Muscari.
Description: New York, NY : Springer Publishing Company, LLC, [2016] |
  Includes bibliographical references and index.
Identifiers: LCCN 2016007629| ISBN 9780826120588 | ISBN 9780826120243
  (instructor's manual) | ISBN 9780826120199 (instructor's PowerPoints) |
  ISBN 9780826120595 (eBook)
Subjects: | MESH: Mental Disorders | Child | Adolescent | Parent-Child
  Relations | Mental Disorders--nursing | Nursing Assessment
Classification: LCC RJ499 | NLM WS 350.6 | DDC 618.92/89—dc23 LC record available at http://lccn.loc.gov/2016007629

Special discounts on bulk quantities of our books are available to corporations, professional associations, pharmaceutical companies, health care organizations, and other qualifying groups. If you are interested in a custom book, including chapters from more than one of our titles, we can provide that service as well.

For details, please contact:
Special Sales Department, Springer Publishing Company, LLC
11 West 42nd Street, 15th Floor, New York, NY 10036-8002
Phone: 877-687-7476 or 212-431-4370; Fax: 212-941-7842
E-mail: sales@springerpub.com

This book is dedicated to all primary care providers who work with families who experience child behavioral and parenting challenges.

CONTENTS

Appendices

CONTRIBUTORS

Sonya Sariego
PMHNP Student Class of 2016
Binghamton University—The State University of New York
Binghamton, New York
Appendix E—Cognitive Behavioral Therapy Mini-Guide

Jean Van Kinglsey
PMHNP Student, Class of 2016
Binghamton University—The State University of New York
Binghamton, New York
Appendix D—Motivational Interviewing

Christy Williams
PMHNP Student, Class of 2016
Binghamton University—The State University of New York
Binghamton, New York
Appendix C—Crisis Intervention: A Quick Guide for Health Care Professionals

PREFACE

Behavioral health integration results from a team of primary care and behavioral health clinicians working together with patients and families, using a systematic and cost-effective approach to provide patient-centered care for a defined population. This mode of care can address mental health and substance abuse conditions, health behaviors, life stressors and crises, stress-related physical symptoms, and unproductive patterns of health care utilization (Peek & the National Integration Academy Council, 2013).

Primary care providers have been integrating behavioral health care into their practices for decades, and have often experienced frustration with the health care system and the lack of training in behavioral health problems. Behavioral health integration, however, is now finally being recognized as a necessity to practice, with policy papers emerging from numerous government agencies and national organizations. The Substance Abuse and Mental Health Services Association (SAMHSA; Hoge, Morris, Laraia, Pomerantz, & Farley, 2014) core competencies for integrated care are as follows:

- Interpersonal Communication: The ability to establish rapport quickly and to communicate effectively with consumers of health care, their family members, and other providers

- Collaboration and Teamwork: The ability to function effectively as a member of an interprofessional team that includes behavioral health and primary care providers, consumers, and family members

- Screening and Assessment: The ability to conduct brief, evidence-based, and developmentally appropriate screening and to conduct or arrange for more detailed assessments when indicated

- Care Planning and Care Coordination: The ability to create and implement integrated care plans, ensuring access to an array of linked services, and the exchange of information among consumers, family members, and providers

- Intervention: The ability to provide a range of brief, focused prevention, treatment and recovery services, as well as longer term treatment and support for consumers with persistent illnesses

- Cultural Competence and Adaptation: The ability to provide services that are relevant to the culture of consumers and their families

- Systems-Oriented Practice: The ability to function effectively within the organizational and financial structures of the local system of health care
- Practice-Based Learning and Quality Improvement: The ability to assess and continually improve the services delivered as an individual provider and as an interprofessional team
- Informatics: The ability to use information technology to support and improve integrated health care

These core competencies are compatible with those already in place, such as the American Association of Colleges of Nursing's Essentials of Master's Education in Nursing 2011 (www.aacn.nche.edu/education-resources/MastersEssentials11.pdf) and the National Organization of Nurse Practitioner Faculties Nurse Practitioner Core Competencies 2012 (c.ymcdn.com/sites/www.nonpf.org/resource/resmgr/competencies/npcorecompeten-ciesfinal2012.pdf), and the American Academy of Physician Assistants Competencies for the Physician Assistant Profession 2012 (www.aapa.org/WorkArea/DownloadAsset .aspx?id=2178).

Today's parents face more problems with fewer means of support, while health care providers struggle with decreased client contact time and minimal parenting-oriented education to assist parents and their children. Most parents and providers are prepared to manage potty training and the first day of school, but many have difficulty with issues such as anxiety and aggression, let alone gambling, cutting, and hoarding.

The purpose of this book is to provide health care providers and students with the information they need to intervene with child behavioral problems and to assist parents with today's challenges in a quick and easy-to-read format. The objectives of this book are:

- To provide practitioners with the basic foundations needed to understand, identify, and manage the behavioral problems and challenges faced by today's parents
- To discuss the primary health care professional's role in working with these issues
- To identify the description, assessment strategies, and prevention/intervention strategies for today's childhood challenges, from abductions through weapons

Challenges and behavioral issues are presented in an A-to-Z format that includes the description, assessment, diagnosis, levels of prevention/intervention, parenting tips, and resources for the primary care management of 30 childhood challenges. These challenges include adolescent angst, aggression and violence, bullying, cyberdelinquency and victimization, depression and suicide, gambling, mood dysregulation, nonsuicidal self-injury, sexual aggression and victimization, substance abuse, technology dependence, and traumatic stress. Lesbian, gay, bisexual, transgender, questioning, intersex, and two-spirit (LGBTQI2) youth and transition age youth are also included because of the unique needs of these populations and the challenges they need to manage because of societal issues.

The appendices provide additional resources. There is a developmental chart that provides social/cognitive, language, and fine and gross motor milestones for ages that coincide with wellness visits. The Pediatric Symptom Checklist (PSC)-17 and the Youth Pediatric

Symptom Checklist-17 are included with scoring instructions, providing comprehensive tools that can screen for, not diagnose, many of the challenges noted throughout the book, in an easy-to-administer format. The author thanks the PSC developers for allowing their inclusion. Lastly, there are guides for motivational interviewing, basic cognitive behavioral therapy skills, and the essentials of crisis intervention. These techniques are easy to learn and use for a number of behavioral challenges.

This book is not a text; it is not designed to teach behavioral health or treatment of psychiatric disorders. Health care providers still need to know their state's practice acts and other relevant statutes, issues of insurance reimbursement, and their own limitations with regard to their educational and experiential background when caring for youths and their families. The main focus of this book is on identification for early intervention, as many of these challenges go unrecognized, even though they often carry over from youth into adulthood, creating lifelong burdens for individuals, families, and communities, as well as society in general, especially in terms of the cost of care, missed work, and the aftermath the destructive behaviors can cause.

The book is designed to be used as an ancillary for health care professionals working with youths up through age 21. There will be many instances where referral to an appropriate psychiatric professional will be the best intervention, but the book will provide primary care providers with critical information and resources on their role while awaiting referral and in maintaining their primary care role with the child and family during the psychiatric intervention process. It will also provide primary care providers with information needed for problem identification, which is the first step in intervention. *Qualified instructors may obtain access to ancillary materials, including an instructor's manual and PowerPoints, by contacting textbook@springerpub.com. A parent teaching guide is available at www .springerpub.com/muscari.*

We can make a difference when tens of thousands of primary health care providers each help one family at a time.

References

Hoge, M. A., Morris, J. A., Laraia, M., Pomerantz, A., & Farley, T. (2014). *Core competencies for integrated behavioral health and primary care*. Washington, DC: SAMHSA—HRSA Center for Integrated Health Solutions.

Peek, C. J., & the National Integration Academy Council. (2013). *Lexicon for behavioral health and primary care integration: Concepts and definitions developed by expert consensus* (AHRQ Publication No.13-IP001-EF). Rockville, MD: Agency for Healthcare Research and Quality. Retrieved from http:// integrationacademy.ahrq.gov/sites/default/files/Lexicon.pdf

ACKNOWLEDGMENTS

The author acknowledges the efforts of Elizabeth Nieginski, Rachel Landes, Kris Parrish, Joanne Jay, and Dennis Anderson from Springer Publishing Company, and Vinolia Benedict Fernando at S4Carlisle Publishing Services, for their editorial and production guidance and assistance on this book. The author is especially grateful to Ms. Nieginski, who strongly believed in the need for this book and helped nurture it from idea to completion.

CHAPTER 1

Adolescent Angst

A. Description

Webster's defines *angst* as a strong feeling of apprehension or insecurity about one's life or situation ("Angst," 2016). Adolescent angst is an acute feeling of anxiety or apprehension that is often accompanied by depression; it is a frustrating, painful, and occasionally frightening problem for teens and parents alike.

> a. Hormonal changes, development of the amygdala, peer pressure, and other social influences combine to create episodic angst. Temporal differences in adolescent brain development probably add to the behavioral disinhibition and affective dysregulation that are characteristic of adolescence, as well as psychopathology (Wetherill & Tapert, 2013).

B. Assessment

> a. Risk factors: Consider monitoring for risks associated with aggression, anxiety, and depression, as discussed in those chapters.

> b. Obtain specific history about the behavior, including the length of time the child has been engaging in this behavior and whether the behavior is interfering with the child's activities of daily living.

> c. Signs that signify a problem other than adolescent angst include:
> - Lack of peer group or best friend (confidant)
> - Extreme identification with exclusive group
> - Sudden disengagement from favorite activities
> - Spending prolonged periods of time in their rooms or withdrawing from social contacts

- Moodiness that persists for more than a couple of days or extreme mood swings
- Feeling of worthlessness or hopelessness
- Constant complaints of boredom
- Prolonged periods of time alone
- Lack of interest in appearance, decreased energy levels, or fatigue
- Persistent defiance and lying
- Delinquent behaviors, such as animal cruelty, stealing, or truancy; gang membership
- Diminished ability to think clearly and make decisions
- Self-destructive behaviors or self-inflicted injuries (cutting, self-embedding)
- Preoccupation with music, movies, or TV shows that focus on death
- Signs of substance abuse, including possession of drug paraphernalia, school failure or absence, secretive peers, sudden aggression, or apathy
- Preoccupation with violence or death themes (thoughts, music, art, movies, television shows, video/computer games)
- Reliance on violence space to solve problems or fascination with weaponry or explosives

d. If concerned about a specific more serious problem, use a problem-specific screening tool, such as:

- Mood and Feelings Questionnaire (MCFQ), available at devepi.duhs.duke .edu/mfq.html
- Generalized Anxiety Disorder 7-Item (GAD-7) scale, available at www .integration.samhsa.gov/clinical-practice/GAD708.19.08Cartwright.pdf
- Alcohol Screening and Brief Intervention for Youth: A Practitioner's Guide, available at www.integration.samhsa.gov/Alcohol_Screening_and_Brief_ Intervention_for_Youth_Guide_and_Medscape_Promotion.pdf

Further information on these problems can be found in their topic-specific chapters.

e. If not sure, utilize a generalized screening tool, such as GAPS, HEEASSS, or the Pediatric Symptom Checklist (see Appendix B).

C. Diagnosis

Differentiate angst from more serious problems, particularly mood and anxiety disorders, and substance abuse. Angst is temporary, related to developmental and situational crisis, such as the transition into each adolescent stage, final exams, and relationship break-ups.

D. Levels of Prevention/Intervention

a. Primary

Angst is normal through the course of adolescence, particularly in the early and middle stages. Teach parents about the stages of adolescent development to better prepare them to understand behavioral norms (Elkind, 1967; Muscari, 2004; Spano, 2004).

- Early adolescence (females: 11–13 years; males: 12–14 years) begins with the remnants of concrete thinking, with teens seeing the world in terms of black and white, all good or all bad. They are rooted in the present and have difficulty seeing the long-term consequences of their behaviors. Great daydreamers, early adolescents frequent fantasy worlds, daydreaming about unrealistic goals, wanting to be a supermodel one day, a lawyer the next. They look to celebrities as heroes and imagined mates. This interest, as well as their preoccupation with peers, may result in a temporary drop in academic performance during junior high or middle school. During this stage teens are intensely preoccupied with privacy and "being normal." Young teens scrutinize their appearance and habitually groom. Pubertal changes cause them to become extremely body conscious, creating angst about acne, menstruation, nocturnal emissions, and body size. They compare themselves to friends and the unrealistic images portrayed in the media, sometimes creating unrealistic expectations and intense self-criticism. Emotional reactions may overwhelm the early adolescent's ability to understand and cope as the adolescent can easily become confused and frightened by the changes he or she is experiencing. Young teens experience wide mood swings that can move them from exhilaration to melancholy in a matter of minutes without obvious predisposing factors. The transient nature of these mood swings and their relationship to normal developmental processes differentiate them from the unremitting, long-standing mood and behavior changes of serious depression. They may argue and disrespect rules to challenge parental authority, assert their independence, and try different value systems. Same-sex best friends are crucial, and some may engage in transient homosexual experimentation. Sexual feelings develop in general, creating interest in sexually explicit movies, television shows or magazines, sex-related jokes, and foul language.

- Middle adolescents (females: 13–16 years; males: 14–20 years) challenge authority and attempt to renegotiate rules. They conform to peer group norms, such as designer gear, unusual hairstyles, and body art. The peer group promotes their own communication style and conduct, and peer pressure climaxes. Sexual drives lead them into dating and sexual experimentation, with intercourse starting at earlier ages. Risk-taking behaviors such as experimentation with drugs and dangerous activities occur more often at this stage of adolescence than the others, and these behaviors result from feelings of omnipotence and infallibility. Middle adolescents are egotistic and have their own personal fable—feeling invincible, they believe that their thoughts and actions are special or unique; thus, "no one understands them." This adds to their mirror time, the need for privacy, frequent embarrassment, and arrogant behavior. Middle adolescents demonstrate increased thinking ability and creativity; however, they can also demonstrate "pseudostupidity" by overthinking. Overthinking can lead to lack of decisiveness and the assigning of complicated explanations to simple situations. They may even distort a parental suggestion into an intention to undermine their independence or competence.

- Late adolescents (both sexes: 17–25 years) are on the verge of adulthood; thus their reasoning skills are at an adult level, allowing them to understand the consequences of their actions, make sophisticated judgments, and comprehend inner motivations. They are future oriented; some enter careers and/or marriages; some enter the military; others enter college to complete their developmental tasks in a supportive, structured environment. The level of peer relationships changes, and late adolescents rekindle their relationships with parents in a more adult-like manner. Many establish their sexual identity and commit to an intimate relationship.

b. Secondary

Help parents cope with adolescent angst. Explain that most mood swings are temporary and best managed by being supportive. Advise parents to stay calm, offer more praise than criticism, and to learn to ignore small mistakes. Adolescence is a period of trial and error, and sometimes teens will make decisions that do not always seem logical.

- Make communication a priority, and recognize that positive communication is the sharing of ideas, feelings, thoughts, information, opinions, and explanations.
- Set clear expectations and rules that are consistently reinforced.
- Utilize effective disciplinary measures. Effective discipline takes place all the time, not just when children misbehave. It is a system of attitudes, instructions, models, rewards, and punishments designed to help children learn how to control their behavior. Discipline relies on good relationships and praise; therefore, discipline children with empathy and nurturing. Oppositional behaviors may relate to egocentrism and independence seeking, but they are not socially acceptable. Despite protest, most adolescents recognize discipline as a sign of caring.
- Encourage interaction with peers, and get to know their teens' friends and their parents. Tolerate peer-imitating behaviors within reason. Behaviors should be

safe and permissible under family/house rules. Spend time with their teens. Engage in mutually enjoyable activities. Have frequent heart-to-heart talks, letting their teens know that they are always there when needed.

- Respect privacy needs, especially their teens' things and space. But respecting privacy does not mean abdicating responsibility; parents still need to check on their teens both in the real world and in cyberspace.
- Take their teens' concerns seriously, no matter how inconsequential they may sound.
- Nurture independence and self-esteem by encouraging responsibilities, such as chores and volunteering. While arguing or refusing to do chores may relate to normal adolescent egocentrism and independence seeking, they are not socially acceptable.
- Most importantly, encourage parents to spend time with their adolescent, to listen and to engage in mutually enjoyable activities. Heart-to-heart talks let teens know that their parents will always be available when needed.

c. Tertiary

Adolescence has periodic roadblocks, but the route is generally smooth and successful. When the behaviors move beyond angst, utilize interventions appropriate for the actual problem (e.g., depression, substance abuse).

E. Parenting Tips

a. Realize that most mood swings are temporary and are best dealt with by being supportive.

b. Offer more praise than criticism and learn to overlook little mistakes. Adolescence is a period of trial and error, and your teen may make decisions that do not seem logical. When discussing points of dispute, use "I" statements instead of accusatory "you" statements. For example, say, "I feel angry when you. . . ."

c. Listen carefully to your teen's opinions, and foster decision-making skills by providing opportunities and choices, but set limits.

d. Behaviors such as arguing or refusing to do chores may relate to normal adolescent egocentrism and independence seeking; however, they are not socially acceptable. Know that, despite protests, most adolescents recognize discipline as a sign of caring.

e. Respect your child's need for privacy, and take adolescent concerns seriously.

f. Encourage peer interaction, but get to know your child's friends. It is okay to tolerate peer-imitating behaviors—within reason. These behaviors, however, should be safe and permissible under family and house rules.

g. Nurture independence and self-esteem by encouraging your teen to take on responsibilities, such as household chores and volunteer work.

h. Most of all, spend time with your adolescent to listen and to engage in mutually enjoyable activities. Frequent heart-to-heart talks let your teen know that you will always be available when needed.

Resources

American Academy of Child & Adolescent Psychiatry Preparing for Adolescence: www.aacap.org/ AACAP/Families_and_Youth/Facts_for_Families/Facts_for_Families_Pages/Parenting_Preparing_ For_Adolescence_56.aspx

Centers for Disease Control and Prevention Adolescent and School Health: www.cdc.gov/ healthyyouth/

MedlinePlus Adolescent Development: www.nlm.nih.gov/medlineplus/ency/article/002003.htm

References

Angst. (2016). *Merriam-Webster's dictionary online.* Retrieved from www.merriam-webster.com/ dictionary/angst

Elkind, D. (1967). Egocentrism in adolescence. *Child Development, 38,* 1025–1034.

Muscari, M. (2004). *Not my kid 2: Protecting your children from the 21 threats of the 21st century.* Scranton, PA: University of Scranton Press.

Spano, S. (2004). Stages of adolescent development. *ACT for Youth Upstate Center for Excellence: Research Facts and Findings.* Retrieved from www.actforyouth.net/resources/rf/rf_stages_0504.pdf

Wetherill, R., & Tapert, S. (2013). Adolescent brain development, substance use, and psychotherapeutic change. *Psychology of Addictive Behavior, 27*(2), 393–402.

CHAPTER 2

Adolescent Relationship Abuse

A. Description

The U.S. Department of Justice (2014) defines dating violence thus: "Violence committed by a person who is or has been in a social relationship of a romantic or intimate nature with the victim is dating violence. The existence of such a relationship shall be determined based on a consideration of the following factors: length of the relationship; type of relationship; and frequency of interaction between the persons involved in the relationship." The term *adolescent relationship abuse* (ARA) is preferred because many romantic relationships are fleeting; hence the terms hanging out, hooking up, going out, and others. ARA provides a broader definition (Miller & Levenson, 2012). While the term "adolescent" is utilized here, this material is still appropriate for transition age youth.

a. ARA can be: physical (threatening with a weapon, hurting the victim's pet, hitting, choking); emotional (name calling, spreading rumors, criticizing victim's friends and family, threatening to commit suicide if the victim tries to break up); financial (controlling what partner can and cannot purchase); sexual (forced sex acts, birth control sabotage, forcing victim to get pregnant); social (monitoring victim's phone calls, getting angry if victim talks to someone else, monitoring victim's whereabouts); or any combination of these. ARA is prevalent and can have major health consequences.

b. Adolescent female victims of ARA have an elevated risk of: alcohol, tobacco, and cocaine use; engagement in unhealthy weight control; negative body image; engagement in sexual health risk behavior, including first intercourse before the age of 15 years and multiple partnering; becoming pregnant or having sexually transmitted infection; becoming overly dependent on others; and seriously considering or attempting suicide. Many of these risks are associated with experiences of either physical or sexual ARA; however, it is not clear whether ARA increases the risk of these problems, whether these problem behaviors make girls more vulnerable to ARA, or whether other factors place them at greater risk for ARA and these other concerns. What is clear is that, regardless of directionality or mechanism, adolescent females who experience ARA engage in a number of problem behaviors that put them at risk for negative outcomes ranging from contracting HIV to pregnancy and suicide.

c.   Females are also perpetrators, and males, victims. While reports vary, it appears that males and females abuse at an equal rate, although females do suffer more severe harm. Female perpetrators tend to be more emotionally abusive, although they can also be physically and sexually abusive. Males need to hear the same message as females.

d.   While the incidence, types, purpose, and cycle of abuse are similar to those of the heterosexual population, there are some key differences related to LGBTQI2 (lesbian, gay, bisexual, transgender, questioning, intersex, two-spirit) intimate partner violence: very limited services for LGBTQI2 youth; homophobic/biphobic/transphobic culture; shelters may not be sensitive to the needs of this population. There are also additional abuse mechanisms, including threats to out (reveal) the victim partner's sexual orientation, gender identity, or HIV status.

e.   Cyberdating abuse is abuse using technology and new media. Research is new and sparse in this area; however, there are some data showing ways in which technology is used in ARA: emotional aggression; monitoring partner's whereabouts and controlling his or her activities; using partner's social networking site without permission; hacking partner's social media account to read e-mails and demanding explanations of them; unwanted sexual messages and requests for naked photos of partner; threats; and creating a "hate website on former partners and allowing others to post insults" (Daucker & Martsolf, 2010; Zwieg, Dank, Yahner, & Lachman, 2013).

f.   All 50 states and the District of Columbia have laws against ARA behaviors such as sexual assault, domestic violence, and stalking, but the term "dating violence" is almost never used in these laws. Many states and the District of Columbia allow victims of ARA to apply for protective orders against the perpetrator.

B. Assessment

a.   Risk factors: frequency and severity of teen ARA increase with age; living in poverty, coming from disadvantaged homes, or receiving child protective services; being exposed to community or neighborhood violence; participation in risky behaviors (e.g., substance abuse, alcohol use, violence); beginning dating at an early age; participation in sexual activity prior to age 16; having problem behaviors in other areas; having a friend involved in ARA; participation in peer violence or having violent friends; believing that ARA is acceptable or more accepting of rape myths and violence against women; beginning menstruating at an early age (for women); having been exposed to harsh parenting; inconsistent discipline; lack of supervision, monitoring, and warmth; low self-esteem, anger, or depressed mood; use of emotional disengagement and confrontational blaming as coping mechanisms; exhibition of maladaptive or antisocial behaviors; having aggressive conflict-management styles; and/or having low help-seeking proclivities.

b.   Risk factors for teen ARA perpetration: Factors that are developmentally normal in youth, such as little to no relationship experience, vulnerability to peer pressure, and unsophisticated communication skills; believing that it is acceptable to use threats or violence to get one's way or to express frustration or anger; problems managing anger or frustration; association with violent peers; low self-esteem and depression; not having parental supervision and support; and/or witnessing violence at home or in the community. Early adolescent aggressive/oppositional problems at home and aggressive/oppositional problems at school may be risk factors for dating violence in late adolescence (Makin-Byrd & Bierman, 2013).

c.   The National Youth Violence Prevention Resource Center notes that teens rarely report ARA and may even view it as a normal part of a relationship; thus, health care professionals need to use an active approach and screen all adolescents for ARA. This is best performed during wellness visits, as well as episodic exams when presenting manifestations suggest the possibility of assault. One approach to screening begins with an open-ended question about relationships with peers, narrows the focus by asking how they resolve conflicts with peers, followed by direct questions about specific behaviors, such as pushing, hitting, being afraid, being hurt, or being forced to have sexual contact. Practitioners should avoid using emotionally loaded terms such as abuse, rape, or violence.

d.   Assess the dangerousness of the situation to determine immediate risk of harm. Ask about threats, physical violence, presence of weapons, and forced sex.

e.   Assess for general signs and symptoms of distress that may or may not be related to ARA, such as depression, anxiety, mood swings, abdominal pain, pelvic pain, sudden changes in relationships with family and friends or in functioning at school, and drug and alcohol abuse. Other possible indicators include school failure, truancy, dropping out of school, substance abuse, pregnancy, isolation, and withdrawal.

- Signs and symptoms that are more specific to intentional injury, including ARA, such as contusions; abrasions; lacerations to the torso, breasts, face, and genital or anal area; fractures, burns, multiple sites of injury, and a pattern of injury over time. Suspect abuse if the stated explanation for injury is inconsistent with the apparent mechanism of injury.
- Signs that the individual is afraid of his or her boyfriend or girlfriend
- The boyfriend or girlfriend seems to try to control the individual's behavior, making all of the decisions, checking on his or her behavior, demanding to know who the individual has been with, and acting jealous and possessive.
- The boyfriend or girlfriend lashes out, criticizes, or insults the individual.

- The individual apologizes for the boyfriend's or girlfriend's behavior to you and others.
- The individual casually mentioned the boyfriend's or girlfriend's temper or violent behavior, but then laughed it off as a joke.
- The boyfriend or girlfriend is observed acting abusive towards other people or things.

f.   Health care providers should also monitor for signs of ARA perpetration as noted by the Alabama Coalition Against Domestic Violence (ACADV), including: extreme jealousy; controlling behavior; quick involvement; unpredictable mood swings; alcohol and drug use; explosive anger; attempts to isolate you from friends and family; use of force during an argument; hypersensitivity; belief in rigid sex roles; blaming others for his or her problems or feelings; cruelty to animals or children; verbal abusiveness; abuse of former partners; and threats of violence.

g.   As previously noted regarding cyberviolence, cell phones can become "leashes" in ARA situations, whereby the perpetrator keeps tabs on the victim with constant phone calls and/or text messages. Asking about cell phone usage, particularly how often they speak to their partner, may be a clue to a controlling situation. Signs of sleep deprivation may also be red flags since abusers may call often during the night.

h.   Consider using screening tools, such as RED FLAGS, a user-friendly tool that allows for early identification of ARA, and provides safety resources. It is for use with adolescents aged 12 to 19 (cyfd.org/docs/red_flags.pdf).

C. Diagnosis

When assessing violence, make sure to rule out self-injury and child abuse. Also, assess the youth for associated problems, including depression, substance abuse, and pregnancy. When assessing youth who are perpetrators of ARA, differentiate immaturity and inexperience from underlying psychiatric disorders.

D. Levels of Prevention/Intervention

a.   Primary

- A 2013 Cochrane Review of 38 studies to examine educational and skills-based interventions for preventing relationship abuse and ARA in adolescents and young adults found no evidence of effectiveness of interventions for relationship violence or on attitudes, behaviors, and skills related to it (Fellmeth, Heffernan, Nurse, Habibula, & Sethi, 2013). However, one review noted that effective prevention programs may be ones that target youth who have experienced adverse childhood events, have particular mental health problems, behave aggressively, have aggressive attitudes, use substances, and are in hostile or unhealthy dating relationships (Vagi et al., 2013).

- Health care providers can also teach about healthy relationships, as well as safe dating. A safe dating teaching plan can include the recommendation to adopt the following strategies when dating:

  - Double-date or "mall" date for the first few dates
  - Know exact plans before leaving for a date, and make sure parents know these plans, as well as the time the teen is expected home
  - Avoid drugs and alcohol, which decrease reaction abilities
  - Carry a cell phone with a charged battery
  - Do not leave a party alone with someone you do not know
  - Assert yourself when necessary
  - Be straightforward in relationships
  - Trust your instincts
  - If a situation arises, remain calm, and remove yourself from the situation

b. Secondary

Secondary prevention promotes early identification and intervention of teens at risk. Projects should target young people involved in a violent relationship so that they do not repeat the observed pattern.

c. Tertiary

- Interventions are warranted when clients are victims or perpetrators of dating violence. Victims should receive support, as well as care for injuries, and should be referred to an appropriate therapist and community support group. Most counties have women's or victims' resource centers. Victims may need assistance to end the relationship because of dependence and/or fear, and some may benefit from the interventions suggested in the chapter on stalking, such as keeping diaries; others may need to obtain an order of protection. Perpetrators should also be referred for counseling, as well as to programs for juvenile batterers. In some jurisdictions, health care providers may also be required to report dating violence to law enforcement.

- Safety first. Provide the youth with the phone number for the National Teen Dating Abuse Helpline: 866-331-9474 or text "loveis" to 77054, as well as contact information for appropriate victim resource agencies in your area. Ensure that the youth have a safe place to stay, as well as plans to stay safe in school/work. Altering or ending the relationship requires counseling to increase self-esteem and planning to end or alter the relationship. It is of importance that the health care provider who recognizes ARA does not recommend that the young person "just leave" the relationship. Further evaluation before making any recommendation is necessary. Leaving a violent dating relationship can be very dangerous to the victim. Interpersonal violence offenders have been known to attack their victims when they attempt to leave the relationship. Breaking up should be done in a public place and in the company of another trusted person.

- Health care providers should also provide safety tips for victims of ARA (Family Violence Prevention Fund, n.d.):
  - Keep a journal describing your partner's behavior.
  - Keep your parents or another trustworthy adult informed of what is happening.
  - Create a code word to use discreetly with persons you trust when you are in danger.
  - Consider changing your school locker or lock.
  - Consider changing your route to/from school.
  - Use a buddy system for going to school, classes, and after school activities.
  - Have a back-up plan whenever getting a ride home in case you are stranded.
  - Get rid of or change the number to any beepers, pagers, or cell phones the abuser gave you.
  - Keep spare change, calling cards, number of the local shelter, number of someone who could help you, and restraining orders with you at all times.
  - Have safe places to go to, such as on your route from home to school, and a safe place for family to pick you up.
  - Keep a cell phone handy in case you need to call your parents or 911.
- Additional tips for transition-age youth living on their own or who lived with abusive partner: create a safety pack or easy access to critical items (birth certificate, social security card, driver's license, additional photo identification, car information [title/loan papers, registration, insurance]); cash/ATM/credit cards; keys; cell phone (not on the same plan as the abuser); medications; spare clothes; and keepsakes. If the victim is a parent, also have quick access to child's birth certificate, bottles/formula/food; diapers; medications; medical records; clothes and favorite toy/blanket. If the victim owns a pet, work with the local shelter to create a plan for the pet, since pets can be used as pawns in violent relationships. Have quick access to pet's food, bowls, bed, toy, and medications.
- If needed, discuss the possibility of the youth obtaining an order of protection, especially transition age youth living alone or with the abusive partner. Several states and the District of Columbia allow victims of ARA to obtain an order of protection. This is a legally binding court order that restrains an individual who has committed an act of violence against a person from further acts against that person. Protective orders vary from state to state and are called by

various names (e.g., restraining orders, protection from abuse orders [PFAs], etc.). Most are used to protect against family/intimate partner violence; some jurisdictions use them for strangers. Health care providers can contact the police, district attorney's office, or victim advocate center to learn how victims may obtain protective orders in their areas. However, it is best they do this before a situation occurs and keep the information readily available for emergencies. The protection order can prohibit the abuser from committing acts of violence; exclude the abuser from the residence shared by the petitioner and abuser; prohibit the abuser from harassing or contacting the petitioner by mail, telephone, or in person; award temporary custody of minor children; establish temporary visitation, and restrain the abuser from interfering with custody; prohibit the abuser from removing the children from the jurisdiction of the court; and order the abuser to participate in treatment or counseling. Some states, including New York, include pets in the protective orders. Although seemingly powerful, protective orders are nothing more than pieces of paper—they are not bullet proof. They seem to work best on those abusers who have something to lose if they disobey them, and in some cases, may aggravate the situation. Therefore, victims still need to take precautions to keep themselves safe.

E. Parenting Tips

a. The American Academy of Pediatrics (2000) recommends that parents:

- Understand that teens: do not often tell their parents that they are being abused; may not know it is abuse and confuse jealousy with love; feel that being in a relationship is critical; and feel afraid that they will be forced to break up or be punished.
- Know the signs of abuse: school problems; changes in personality; crying jags; bruises and other injuries; sudden changes in make-up or clothes; avoiding friends; sleeping and eating changes; substance use; and thinking that having a baby will make things better.
- Know the signs of abusive behavior: wanting the relationship to become serious quickly and refusing to take no for an answer; jealousy and possessiveness; controlling and bossy behaviors, threatening and verbally abusive; trying to create guilt; blaming partner for wrongs; giving excuses or apologizing for negative behavior (may also give gifts after violent/negative episodes).
- Talk about healthy relationships.

b. Youth.gov recommends that parents teach teens about the characteristics of healthy relationships: mutual respect, trust, honesty, compromise, individuality, good communication, anger control, fighting fair, problem solving, understanding, self-confidence, being a role model, and healthy sexual relationships.

Resources

Adolescent Relationship Abuse & Sexual Assault: www.idvsa.org/focus/adolescent-relationship-abuse

Campus Dating Violence Fact Sheet: http://ncfy.acf.hhs.gov/sites/default/files/docs/16444-Campus_Dating_Violence-Fact_Sheet.pdf

Community United Against Violence (CUAV): www.cuav.org

Dating Matters Initiative: www.cdc.gov/violenceprevention/datingmatters/index.html

Dating Violence Resource Center: http://victimsofcrime.org/help-for-crime-victims/get-help-bulletins-for-crime-victims/bulletins-for-teens/dating-violence

References

American Academy of Pediatrics. (2000). *Teen dating violence: Tips for parents.* Elk Grove Village, IL: Author. Retrieved from www.healthychildren.org/English/ages-stages/teen/dating-sex/Pages/Dating-Violence-Tips-for-Parents.aspx

Daucker, C., & Martsolf, D. (2010). The role of electronic communication technology in adolescent dating violence. *Journal of Child and Adolescent Psychiatric Nursing, 23*(3), 133–142.

Family Violence Prevention Fund. (n.d.). *Create a teen safety plan.* Retrieved from www.futureswithoutviolence.org/userfiles/file/PublicCommunications/Create%20a%20Teen%20Safety%20Plan.pdf

Fellmeth, G., Heffernan, C., Nurse, J., Habibula, S., & Sethi, D. (2013). Educational and skills-based interventions for preventing relationship and dating violence in adolescents and young adults. *Cochrane Database of Systematic Reviews, 2013*(6). doi:10.1002/14651858.CD004534.pub3

Makin-Byrd, K., & Bierman, K. (2013). Individual and family predictors of the perpetration of dating violence and victimization in late adolescence. *Journal of Youth and Adolescence, 42,* 536–550.

Miller, E., & Levenson, R. (2012). *Hanging out or hooking up: Clinical guidelines on responding to adolescent relationship abuse: An integrated approach to prevention and intervention.* San Francisco, CA: Futures Without Violence. Retrieved from www.futureswithoutviolence.org/userfiles/file/HealthCare/hanging%20out%20guidelines_46797.pdf

U.S. Department of Justice. (2014). *Dating violence.* Retrieved from www.justice.gov/ovw/dating-violence

Vagi, K., Rothman, E., Latzman, N., Tharp, A., Hall, D., & Breiding, M. (2013). Beyond correlates: A review of risk and protective factors for adolescent dating violence perpetration. *Journal of Youth and Adolescence, 42,* 633–649.

Zwieg, J., Dank, M., Yahner, J., & Lachman, P. (2013). The rate of cyber dating abuse among teens and how it relates to other forms of teen dating violence. *Journal of Youth and Adolescence, 42,* 1063–1077. doi:10.1007/s10964-013-9922-8

CHAPTER 3

Aggression and Violence

A. Description

Aggression is hostile, destructive, or violent attitudes or behavior toward oneself, others, animals, or objects. However, aggression can also be constructive, when self-protective or self-assertive. Interpersonal violence has been defined as "the intentional use of physical force or power, threatened or actual, against another person or against a group or community that results in or has a high likelihood of resulting in injury, death, psychological harm, maldevelopment, or deprivation" (Dahlberg & Krug, 2002). Examples of aggression and violence include verbal threats, property destruction, animal cruelty, and self-harming behaviors. Early violence is a risk marker for serious criminality, as well as social and mental health problems in youth and adulthood (Lösel & Farrington, 2012). Thus, childhood aggression should be taken seriously at every age.

    a.   Aggressive behaviors arise from attempts to control, act upon, and master ourselves and our environment, including the people in it. Problematic aggressive behaviors occur when children show disregard for the feelings, physical safety, rights, or property of others. This hostile destructiveness presents in angry, nasty, hurtful behaviors such as threatening, bullying, torturing, and vengefulness. Violence is the outcome of destructive aggressive behavior that results in physical injury or property damage. Violence does not occur in a vacuum. It involves multiple factors, and feelings of anger, shame, poor self-esteem, and powerlessness underlie violent behaviors.

    b.   The strongest predictor of aggression in late adolescence and adulthood is the level of aggression shown during childhood. However, no single risk factor leads to aggression. Watson, Fischer, Andreas, and Smith (2004) found evidence to support two pathways to aggression in children, which they labeled severe risks approach and cumulative effects approach. The severe risks approach focuses on the most detrimental or severe risk factors and how they relate to each other. In this approach, children who share certain characteristics (such as high-conflict, low-cohesion families, high levels of harsh parental discipline, high levels of victimization by peers, and high behavioral inhibition) are at risk for developing defensive, reactive aggressive behaviors.

The cumulative effects approach focuses on the amassed effects of several risk factors in leading to aggressive behavior, irrespective of the particular risk factors involved. It assumes that normal child development can be undermined when overwhelmed with too many challenges. Neither approach takes protective factors into account.

c.   Lösel and Farrington (2012) noted that direct protective factors predict a low probability of violence and buffering protective factors predict a low probability of violence when occurring in the presence of risk factors. More than half of the children in high-risk groups develop relatively normally, and the majority of serious offenders stop over time.

B. Assessment

a.   Risk factors: Identify both risk and protective factors. The National Center for Injury Prevention and Control (NCIPC, 2015), the American Academy of Child & Adolescent Psychiatry (AACAP, 2011), and the New York State Office of Mental Health (NYSOMH, 2012) identify several factors that place youth at risk for violence, and categorize these factors into four clusters: individual (personal), family, peer/ social (school), and community (environmental):

- Individual (personal) risk factors: genetic factors, history of violent victimization; attention deficits, hyperactivity, or learning disorders; history of early aggressive behavior; involvement with drugs, alcohol, or tobacco; low IQ; poor behavioral control; deficits in social-cognitive or information-processing abilities; brain damage (prenatal drug exposure; traumatic brain injury [TBI], lead poisoning); high emotional distress; history of treatment for emotional problems; history of tantrums or uncontrollable anger outbursts; habitual name-calling or cursing; bullying; cruelty to animals; fire setting; past suicide attempts; frequent depression or chronic mood swings; blames others for own problems; recent humiliation, loss, or rejection; antisocial beliefs and attitudes; preoccupation with weapons; unstructured time; and exposure to violence and conflict in the family.
- Family risk factors: authoritarian child-rearing attitudes; harsh, lax, or inconsistent disciplinary practices; absence of clear expectations for behavior; low parental involvement; low emotional attachment to parents or caregivers; low parental education and income; parental substance abuse or criminality; poor family functioning; history of family violence or weapons use by family members; and poor monitoring and supervision of children.
- Peer and social risk (school) factors: aggression in grades K to 3; association with delinquent peers; social isolation; involvement in gangs; social rejection by peers; lack of involvement in conventional activities; poor academic

performance; serious disciplinary problems; getting into fights or misbehaving in class; truancy, suspension, or expulsion; low commitment to school and school failure; and anger/frustration noted in essays or artwork.

- Community and environmental risk factors: diminished economic opportunities; high concentrations of poor residents; high level of transiency; high level of family disruption; low levels of community participation; socially disorganized neighborhoods; few organized activities for youths; past destruction of property or vandalism; and exposure to violent media.

b. Protective factors: Safeguard young people from becoming violent. These factors exist at various levels and have not yet been studied as extensively or rigorously as risk factors. However, identifying and understanding protective factors are equally as important as researching risk factors. Most research is preliminary; however, studies propose the following protective factors (NCIPC, 2015):

- Individual protective factors: intolerant attitude toward deviance; high IQ; high grade point average (as an indicator of high academic achievement); positive social orientation; highly developed social skills/competencies; highly developed skills for realistic planning; and religiosity.

- Family protective factors: connectedness to family or adults outside the family; ability to discuss problems with parents; perceived parental expectations about school performance are high; frequent shared activities with parents; consistent presence of parent during at least one of the following: when awakening, when arriving home from school, at evening mealtime, or going to bed; involvement in social activities; and parental/family use of constructive strategies for coping with problems (provision of models of constructive coping).

- Peer and social protective factors: possession of affective relationships with those at school that are strong, close, and prosocially oriented; commitment to school (an investment in school and in doing well at school); close relationships with nondeviant peers; membership in peer groups that do not condone antisocial behavior; involvement in prosocial activities; exposure to school climates that are characterized by: intensive supervision, clear behavior rules, consistent negative reinforcement of aggression, and engagement of parents and teachers.

c. Assess for aggression early; aggression that begins at a young age continues throughout development (Reebye, 2005).

d. Conduct a thorough history and physical examination to determine potential underlying problems, such as neurological insult.

e. As with all pediatric behaviors, developmental and cultural norms are considered. Some aggression is part of the normal path to autonomy and independence.

Toddlers have tantrums, siblings fight, adolescents break rules, and the roughhousing of sports such as football and lacrosse are socially sanctioned. But typical developmental deviations do not result in serious harm or destruction, nor do they occur persistently. When assessing aggression and violence, key factors are intensity, frequency, and context—how severe is the behavior and damage caused by it, how often does it occur, why did it occur, where did it occur, and who was involved. The health care provider should also ascertain whether aggressive/violent acts are affective (more spur of the moment) or predatory (planned; McEllistrem, 2004).

f.   Assess for the different types of aggression: verbal (name-calling, threats); physical (spitting, biting, hitting, punching, shoving, fighting, animal cruelty, property destruction, weapons use), and relational (shunning peers).

g.   Assess for warning signs of violence: For some children, combinations of behaviors and events may lead to violence. Signs include: gradual withdrawal from social contacts, and eventually complete withdrawal; expression of feelings of isolation and being alone; expression of feelings of being rejected; irrational beliefs and ideas; fascination with weaponry or explosives; unreciprocated romantic obsession; drastic change in belief system; family or fellow students feel fear because of the child; violence toward inanimate objects; sabotages projects or equipment; when doing school projects, displays "dark side" that shows anger or frustration; inappropriate access to firearms; brings weapon to school; and increased risk-taking behaviors. Health care providers can assume that these warning signs, especially when they are presented in combination, indicate a need for further analysis to determine an appropriate intervention. But there is a real danger that early warning signs will be misinterpreted, and therefore, health care providers need to understand basic principles:

- Do no harm: The intent should be to get early intervention for the child. Early warning signs should not be used to exclude, isolate, or punish a child, nor should they be used as a checklist for formally identifying, mislabeling, or stereotyping children. Formal disability identification under federal law requires individualized evaluation by qualified professionals, and all referrals to outside agencies based on the early warning signs must be kept confidential and must be done with parental consent (except referrals for suspected child abuse or neglect).

- View warning signs within a developmental context: Children at different levels of development have varying social and emotional capabilities. They may express their needs differently at each stage. Know developmentally typical behavior, so that behaviors are not misinterpreted.

- Understand that violence and aggression occur within context: Violent and aggressive behavior is an expression of emotion with antecedent factors that exist within the school, the home, and the larger social environment. Certain environments or situations can even trigger violence in at-risk children. Some children may act out if stress becomes too great, if they lack positive coping skills, and/or if they have learned to react with aggression.

- Avoid stereotyping: Stereotypes interfere with and can even harm the ability to identify and help children. It is important to be aware of false cues, including race, socioeconomic status, cognitive or academic ability, or physical appearance. Stereotypes can unfairly harm children, especially when the school community acts upon them.

- Understand that children typically exhibit multiple warning signs: It is common for troubled children to exhibit multiple signs. Research confirms that most children who are at risk for aggression exhibit more than one warning sign, repeatedly, and with increasing intensity over time. Do not overreact to single signs, words, or actions.

h. Assess for warning signs of imminent violence: These signs indicate that a child is dangerously close to behaving violently and require immediate action. The safest action would be to contact police immediately. Signs include: serious physical fighting with peers or a family member, severe property destruction, severe rage for apparently minor reasons, possession or use of firearms or other weapons, and having a detailed plan (time, place, method) to harm others.

i. Consider using screening tools for aggression/violence:

- The Pediatric Symptom Checklist (PSC-17; www.massgeneral.org/psychiatry/services/psc_home.aspx) is a brief, validated, psychosocial screening instrument developed to facilitate recognition and referral of child psychosocial problems by primary care providers. The PSC-17 Externalizing Problems Subscale screens for: fights with others, does not listen to rules, does not understand other people's feelings, teases others, blames others for his or her troubles, takes things that do not belong to him or her, and refuses to share. Children with scores of 7 or higher on this subscale usually have significant problems with conduct.

- Structured Assessment of Violence Risk in Youth (SAVRY): The SAVRY is composed of 24 items in three risk domains (Historical Risk Factors, Social/Contextual Risk Factors, and Individual/Clinical Factors), drawn from existing research and the professional literature on adolescent development, and violence and aggression in youth. Each risk item has a three-level rating structure with specific rating guidelines (low, moderate, or high). The tool also contains six protective factor items that are rated as either present or absent. The SAVRY is useful in the assessment of adolescents between the ages of 12 and 18, and may be used by professionals in a variety of disciplines who conduct assessments and/or make intervention or supervision plans concerning violence risk in youth. The SAVRY is not a formal test or scale; there are no assigned numerical values, nor are there any specified cutoff scores. Instead, it helps in structuring an assessment so that the important factors will not be missed, and, thus, will be emphasized when formulating a final professional judgment about a youth's level of risk. Further information on the SAVRY can be found at www.fmhi.usf.edu/mhlp/savry/statement.htm.

- The FiGHTS screen is used to identify adolescents attending school who are at risk for carrying firearms. One point is assigned for each positive response to five questions, and a score of 2 or more is considered positive for carrying firearms (Hayes & Sege, 2003).

  - Fighting: During the past 12 months, have you been in a physical fight?
  - Gender: Male?
  - Hurt: During the past 12 months, have you been in a fight in which you were injured and had to be treated by a doctor or nurse?
  - Threatened: During the past 12 months, have you been threatened with a weapon such as a knife or gun on school property?
  - Smoker: Have you ever smoked cigarettes regularly, that is, at least one cigarette per day for 30 days?

C. Diagnosis

a.   Aggressive behaviors can be noted in children with developmental disorders, including autistic spectrum disorder. Differential diagnosis should also include co-morbidities, as aggressive children often have more than one mental health issue, including substance abuse, depression or bipolar disorder, anxiety, posttraumatic stress disorder, learning disorders, and attention deficit hyperactivity disorder (ADHD).

b.   Biting typically occurs in very young children who are teething or exploring. Infants explore with their mouths and are impulsive. Some babies bite because they are excited or overstimulated, because they want to touch or smell something, or simply because there is something there to bite. They most likely do not understand that biting others causes pain. Toddlers ages 12 to 36 months may use biting to communicate frustration as they learn language and social and self-control skills. They do not have the language skills to control a situation, nor can they plan ahead, so biting can become a powerful communication tool. Biting shows autonomy and acts as a fast way to get a desired object or attention. Information and sensory overload can lead to frustration and biting in the toddler, as can stress, lack of routine, or inadequate adult interaction. Biting is rare after the toddler stage; however, some preschoolers may bite when regressed to exert control or express frustration. But biting after age 3 years tends to indicate a behavioral problem, developmental disorder, autistic spectrum disorder, or sensory integration dysfunction (Banks & Yi, 2002). Biting at any age requires correction.

c.   Young children have minimal self-control, so pushing and hitting are common during early childhood. These and other forms of physical aggression may be natural ways of solving conflicts and expressing negative emotions, and they may be part of the normal processes of developing self-identity, self-control, and the understanding of social relations. The development of physical aggression is nonlinear, peaks at about age 20 to 22 months, and declines around 26 months (Nærde, Ogden, Janson, & Zachrisson, 2014). While this, like biting, is a developmental norm, it also is not socially acceptable behavior, and thus requires correction.

d.   Conduct disorder (CD) is a common and difficult to manage mental health problem in children and adolescents that is characterized by a persistent pattern of violating rules and/or the rights of others. These youths usually do not perceive their behavior as a problem; on the contrary, they view others as threatening or the cause of their troubles. The *Diagnostic and Statistical Manual of Mental Disorders, 5th Edition* (*DSM-5*), published by the American Psychiatric Association (APA, 2013), identifies several behaviors as indicative of conduct disorder. These behaviors are categorized as aggression toward people or animals, destruction of property, deceitfulness or theft, and serious violations of rules. Examples include bullying, threatening, deliberate fire setting, stealing with (violent crime) or without (property crime) confronting the victim, and truancy. CD can range from mild to severe, and those children with the severe form have no remorse about the consequences of their behaviors, blame others for their actions, and can appear superficially sincere or manipulative (APA, 2013). Childhood-onset CD begins before age 10 years and has a poorer prognosis when untreated. This type may be noted in children as young as 2 years old and who demonstrate poor attachment, irritable temperament, poor compliance, inattentiveness, and impulsivity (Bernstein, 2014). These children may also have parents who are antisocial and involved in the criminal justice system. Children without symptoms prior to age 10 years have adolescent-onset CD. Left untreated, those with child-onset CD are at risk for substance abuse, risky sexual behaviors, unintentional injuries, involvement with the juvenile justice system, and the development of antisocial personality disorder as an adult. The prognosis is better for those with adolescent onset.

e.   Children with oppositional defiant disorder (ODD) have a 6-month or more pattern of uncooperative, defiant, disobedient, and often hostile behavior toward authority figures to the point where their behaviors seriously interfere with their day-to-day functioning. Left untreated, ODD can progress to CD, usually in childhood. The *DSM-5* (APA, 2013) identifies several behaviors as indicative of ODD. These behaviors are characterized as angry or irritable mood, argumentative or defiant behavior, and vindictiveness. Examples include frequent loss of temper, arguing with authority figures, being annoying on purpose, blaming others for their own negative actions, and spitefulness.

f.   Intermittent explosive disorder is characterized by unprovoked, sudden aggressive outbursts that can be correctly diagnosed only when the child's behavior does not meet the criteria for CD. The outbursts are grossly out of proportion to the precipitating stressor or provocation. The aggression is affective, not predatory, and is due to the child's inability to control aggressive impulses. These children deny plans to harm anyone and report that they "snapped" and assaulted another person. These episodes are the only signs of behavior disturbance, and these children do not engage in repeated violations of other rules or in illegal behavior (Searight, Rottnek, & Abby, 2001).

D. Levels of Prevention/Intervention

a. Primary

The American Academy of Pediatrics (AAP) developed its Connected Kids (www. aap.org/ConnectedKids) program to address violence prevention. Designed with input from clinicians, parents, and adolescents from across the country, Connected Kids is a systematic method for enhancing the violence prevention anticipatory guidance that is made up of four elements:

- Clinical guide: The clinical guide provides an overview to the entire program. It also describes some details of its development and its rationale.
- Counseling schedule: The color-coded counseling schedule is designed for three separate age groups: green for infancy to early childhood, blue for middle childhood, and red for adolescence. The schedule recommends topics to be introduced, topics to be reinforced, and brochures to be distributed for each health supervision visit. Examples of introductory anticipatory guidance topics include parental frustration for the 2-day to 4-week visit, bullying for 6 years, and conflict resolution for early adolescence.
- Educational brochures: Twenty-one educational brochures have been designed for parents and children to reinforce each of the 44 topics covered in Connected Kids. The color codes from the counseling schedule are also incorporated into the brochures to facilitate distribution. Topics include Pulling the Plug on TV Violence and Dating Violence: Tips for Parents.
- PowerPoint presentation: The PowerPoint presentation offers an alternative presentation of the material in the clinical guide. This presentation may be helpful for personnel in-service training before implementing Connected Kids.

b. Secondary

While violence is only one aspect of delinquency, it is probably the most troublesome. Therefore, health care providers can also participate in prevention strategies such as the National Center for Injury Prevention and Control of the Centers for Disease Control and Prevention's (CDC) Best Practices for Violence Prevention, and the Office of Juvenile Justice and Delinquency Prevention's (OJJDP, n.d.) The National Juvenile

Justice Action Plan. The CDC's Best Practices for Violence Prevention identifies four strategies for combating the problem of youth violence, and offers specific suggestions for implementation. These strategies include:

- Family-based strategies that combine training in parenting skills, education about child development, and exercises to help parents develop skills for communicating with their children and resolving conflict nonviolently.

- A home visiting strategy that brings community resources to at-risk families in their homes, especially for pregnant and first-time parents.

- A social-cognitive strategy that helps children develop the skills they need to deal effectively with difficult situations by teaching nonviolent methods for resolving conflict and establishing (and strengthening) nonviolent beliefs in young people.

- A mentoring strategy that emphasizes the importance of a positive adult role model in reducing risk for violence and delinquent behavior.

The OJJDP has developed The National Juvenile Justice Action Plan, which is a comprehensive approach to reducing youth violence that combines violence prevention with graduated sanctions for youth offenders. The Action Plan emphasizes five key areas of best practice for communities developing a response to violence. The five key best practices recommend:

- Mobilizing communities
- Strengthening the juvenile justice system
- Decreasing gangs, guns, and drugs
- Creating opportunities for youth
- Breaking the cycle of violence through family strengthening and parent education

c. Tertiary

The University of Arkansas Psychiatric Research Institute (Gathright & Tyler, 2014) recommends the following for primary care management of disruptive behaviors: support and nurture parents; assist parents in understanding developmentally normal versus concerning behaviors; emphasize parenting styles that acknowledge the child's strengths, use positive reinforcement, actively ignore benign behaviors, and provide effective limit-setting and nonpunitive punishment; promote the power of positive parental attention; ask parents to show you or tell you what they do and say; promote parental role modeling; refer parents to programs that are fiscally accessible and convenient; and teach skills and techniques to help parents cope.

- There is no U.S. Food and Drug Administration (FDA) medication approved for use with children and adolescents who have disruptive behavior disorders.

- Left untreated, CD can result in substance abuse and other risk behaviors, as well as the development of antisocial personality disorder in adulthood. Treatment of

CD, and its comorbidities, is multifaceted and dependent on the severity. Treatment needs to be highly structured with specific goals and established behavioral techniques. Parental involvement is critical, but may be difficult when parents have their own psychopathologies. Parent management training (PMT) has been demonstrated to have the greatest effect on children's coercive patterns of behavior (Bernstein, 2014). Primary care providers can encourage parents to maintain open lines of communication, provide appropriate monitoring, encourage involvement in supervised and structured peer activities (e.g., sports, scouting, after-school programs), enforce clear and specific rules including curfews, follow through on consequences for negative behaviors, and develop a reward system for positive behaviors. Individual psychotherapy has not been shown to be effective for CD; however, sessions can help facilitate compliance with the overall treatment regimen, which should also address comorbidities, including affective and anxiety disorders, substance abuse, cognitive and academic deficits, and ADHD. Because of the similarity between CD and ADHD characteristics, health care providers should evaluate for ADHD. If ADHD is present, pharmacological treatment is indicated for the ADHD. There are FDA-approved drugs for aggression in children and adolescents, with the exception of irritability-associated aggression in children with autism, and psychotropic drugs have not yet shown specific effectiveness in the treatment of CD. However, improving attention and increasing the child's inhibitory activity may improve the child's ability to benefit from psychotherapies. Therefore, primary care providers should consult with mental health specialists before prescribing medications for aggression. They should also consider referral to a subspecialist, especially when symptoms are severe, yet avoid recommendations for more extreme treatments, such as boot camp, which may have immediate benefits but tend to have worsening problems in the long term, including higher arrest rates (Bernstein, 2014; Searight et al., 2001).

- There are no specific medications for ODD. Treatment includes educating parents to develop more positive parenting skills, cognitive problem solving therapy, and social skills training. Parent–child interaction therapy emphasizes parent-directed interaction to empower the parent with behavioral techniques.

E. Parenting Tips

Teach parents to observe for atypical behaviors (Muscari, 2002 ; National Center for Injury Prevention and Control of the Centers for Disease Control and Prevention, 2002):

a.   Your Toddler or Preschooler

Occasional and controllable outbursts are typical of very young children, and isolated instances of aggressive behavior, regardless of the degree of physical injury or property damage, may be part of the normal growth process. But when your preschooler becomes overly aggressive and difficult to handle, be concerned. Researchers now know that children who have behavior problems in preschool do not outgrow them. Most continue to have problems in grade school, and they are subsequently less competent and more likely to have significant problems in adolescence and adulthood.

The following circumstances warrant professional evaluation:

- Chronic anger or anxiety: Your angry child may not feel good about himself or herself and may displace those feelings on others. Aggressive children may actually be depressed since chronic sadness and depression are frequently masked by hostile behavior in children.
- Serious aggressive behavior (behavior that results in bodily harm or property damage)
- Frequent or recurring aggressive behaviors
- Biting beyond the age of 2.5 years: This indicates considerable anger, high frustration levels, or a language delay.
- Aggressive behavior that occurs in multiple settings (home, school, playground)
- Your child is expelled from preschool.
- Multiple temper tantrums in a single day or several that last for more than 15 minutes when the child often cannot be quieted
- Persistent breath holding or head banging, or tantrums with deliberate injury are not normal, and may be early signs of aggressive behavior as well as other behavioral problems.
- Extreme activity level, impulsiveness, and fearlessness
- Constant refusal to listen and follow directions
- Your child does not appear to be attached to you. Unattached children do not touch parents or look for them in strange places.
- Your child frequently engages in play with violent themes, watches violent television shows, or is cruel to other children.
- Your child intentionally causes harm to animals.
- Intentional destruction of objects
- Anger and aggression *may* be disguised under the following behaviors:
  - Soiling pants with stool
  - Smearing stool
  - Intentional self-injury (biting self, head banging)
  - Frequent unintentional injuries ("accident-prone child")

b.   Your School-Age Child

During the school years, playful behavior becomes more intense, purposeful, and consequential. Rough play is not unusual, but when it persists in the pursuit of domination, it becomes bullying, a precursor to aggressive behavior. Bullying occurs frequently in children who lack appropriate social or academic skills and usually represents an attempt to act out resentment for poor peer relationships.

A key factor to watch for is the intent to do harm. School-age children begin to understand the consequences of injury and the finality of death. They know they can hurt and even kill someone. Considering this knowledge level, planned aggressive acts (carrying a weapon, deliberately destroying property) are very worrisome.

The following behaviors warrant professional attention:

- Ages 6 to 8 years
  - Problems making and keeping friends: Making friends is an important step at this age. It is so important that by age 7, some children care more about the opinion of their friends than their parents.
  - Prefers to stay home alone: School-age children tend to enjoy the company of other children, so it is very unusual for them to want to stay home alone.
  - Unable to say something special about self: Poor self-esteem plays an important role in the development of many childhood problems, including violence.
- Ages 8 to 10 years
  - Lack of hobbies or interests: "Doing things," such as sports, clubs, music, and collections (cards, dolls, the latest fad), is critical in this age group. Idle hands really are the devil's workshop.
  - Lack of best friend: Children normally begin to develop best friends by age 8, and they start to dress and act like their friends.
- Ages 10 to 12 years
  - Lack of participation in extracurricular activities or team sports: Many children of this age select an activity that they want to excel in. Participation boosts self-esteem and promotes peer interaction.
  - Lacks understanding of rules: Children become aware of rules and the difference between right and wrong well before this age. At this point, they face variation in rules between the family and the outside world, and they may even have trouble making decisions. However, they should understand the basic rules.
  - Poor peer influence, interest in gangs: Gang violence is no longer isolated in inner cities. Children who feel the need for a "family," as well as those

who feel alienated from the mainstream, may seek camaraderie through gang membership.

- Entire school-age period
  - Frequently disrupts classroom activities
  - Frequently gets into fights
  - Reacts with revenge or extreme anger or blame to criticism, disappointments, or teasing
  - Prefers violent TV shows, movies, and video games
  - Actively and consistently refuses to listen to adults, or shows consistent defiance
  - Does not care about the feelings of others
  - Abuses animals
  - Makes friends with children known to be aggressive
  - Is labeled a bully by the other children
  - Creates drawings with teeth, strong force lines, or uses extensive forceful coloring-in
  - "Sneaky" behavior in girls (may be a covert aggressive behavior)
  - Threats
  - Lying, cheating, and overt stealing
  - Destruction of property
  - Interest in fires or fire setting
  - Temper tantrums and a high rate of annoying behaviors such as yelling and whining
  - Consistently blames others for own mistakes
- The following *may* precipitate or accompany aggressive behaviors, and thus also warrant professional attention:
  - Difficulty paying attention and concentrating
  - Does poorly in school
  - Has few friends
  - Is easily frustrated

c. Your Adolescent

Some degree of teen–parent friction is expected, but disruptive family conflict is not normal. Neither is persistent defiance, fighting, or property destruction. This turmoil represents pathology, and it will not be outgrown. The early appearance of antisocial behavior is associated with more serious problems later in the adolescent period and on into adulthood.

The following behaviors warrant professional attention:

- Early adolescence (12–14 years)
    - Early experimentation with alcohol or drugs, including tobacco
    - Persistent refusal to participate in household chores
    - No close or best friends
- Middle adolescence (15–17 years)
    - Recurrent experimentation or frequent use of drugs or alcohol, or blackouts
    - Excessively oppositional, defiant of all authority
    - Abusive dating relationships
    - No identified peer group
    - No life goals
    - Poor judgment
- Late adolescence (18–21 years)
    - Substance abuse; drinking and driving
    - Lacks intimate relationships
    - Abusive dating relationships
    - Unable to keep a job
    - Does not dream about adult career
    - Poor judgment
- Entire adolescent period
    - Negative feelings of self-worth
    - No identified peer group, extreme isolation, and withdrawal from the family
    - Deterioration in physical appearance or personal hygiene
    - Pervasive sad or depressed mood
    - School fights
    - Secretive and defensive behavior regarding actions
    - Stealing money or objects from family, friends, or relatives (may be using the money for drugs)
    - Disruptive behavior
    - Poor grades, chronic absenteeism, class skipping, suspension, drop out
    - Unable to control own behavior (anger, impulsivity)
    - Consistently does not listen to authority figures
    - Does not pay attention to the rights or feelings of others

- Mistreats people and seems to rely on threats or physical violence to solve problems
- Believes that others or life have treated him or her unfairly
- Preoccupation with TV shows, movies, video games, TV games, Internet sites, or books with violent themes
- Themes of violence and death appear in conversations, writings, or art work
- Steals or destroys property
- Indulges in fire setting or is fascinated with fire
- Joins a gang or cult
- Carries weapons, brings them to school

Some children and teens make threats, most of which are not carried out. The threats are usually the child's way of getting attention or acting tough, or they are reactions to perceived hurts or rejections. Potential danger exists if your child threatens to hurt or kill himself or herself or someone else, damage or destroy property, or run away from home. It is difficult at best to predict future behavior with compete accuracy. However, your child's past behavior is one of the best predictors of future behavior, and children with a past history of violence, carrying weapons, refusing to accept responsibility, or bullying are at higher risk for carrying out threats. Do not dismiss serious threats, including those made in a joking manner. In other words, if your child kids about bringing his or her father's gun to school to shoot classmates, take it seriously. If your child makes a serious threat, talk to him or her immediately. If your child is at risk, refuses to talk, is argumentative or defensive, or continues to express violent thoughts, make arrangements for immediate evaluation by a mental health professional. If your child refuses to go, you may need to contact the local police.

Resources

American Academy of Child and Adolescent Psychiatrists Conduct Disorder Resource Center: www.aacap.org/AACAP/Families_and_Youth/Resource_Centers/Conduct_Disorder_Resource_Center/Home.aspx

American Academy of Pediatrics Connected Kids: Safe, Strong, Secure Clinical Guide: www2.aap.org/connectedkids/ClinicalGuide.pdf

Bernstein, B. (2014). Conduct disorder. *Medscape Emedicine*. Retrieved from http://emedicine.medscape.com/article/918213-overview

Conduct Disorder—Johns Hopkins Medicine: www.hopkinsmedicine.org/healthlibrary/conditions/mental_health_disorders/conduct_disorder_90,P02560

Centers for Disease Control and Prevention Youth Violence: www.cdc.gov/ViolencePrevention/ youthviolence/index.html

National Criminal Justice Reference Service Youth Violence: www.ncjrs.gov/yviolence/

World Health Organization Youth Violence: www.who.int/mediacentre/factsheets/fs356/en/

References

American Academy of Child & Adolescent Psychiatry. (2011). Understanding violent behavior in children and adolescents. *Facts for Families Guide* (No. 55). Retrieved from www.aacap.org/AACAP/ Families_and_Youth/Facts_for_Families/FFF-Guide/Understanding-Violent-Behavior-In-Children-and-Adolescents-055.aspx

American Psychiatric Association. (2013). *Diagnostic and statistical manual of mental disorders* (5th ed.). Washington, DC: Author.

Banks, R., & Yi, S. (2002). *Dealing with biting behaviors in children.* Champaign, IL: The Early Childhood and Parenting (ECAP) Collaborative, Department of Special Education, University of Illinois at Urbana-Champaign. Retrieved from http://ecap.crc.illinois.edu/poptopics/biting.html

Dahlberg, L., & Krug, E. (2002). Violence: A global public health problem. In E. G. Krug, L. L. Dahlberg, J. A. Mercy, A. B. Zwi, & R. Lozano (Eds.), *World report on violence and health* (pp. 1–21). Geneva, Switzerland: World Health Organization.

Gathright, M., & Tyler, L. (2014). *Disruptive behaviors in children and adolescents.* Little Rock, AR: University of Arkansas Psychiatric Research Institute. Retrieved from http://psychiatry.uams.edu/ fildisobedient and often hostile behavior es/2015/02/disruptive.pdf

Hayes, D., & Sege, R. (2003). FiGHTS: A preliminary tool for adolescent firearms-carrying. *Annals of Emergency Medicine, 42*(6), 798–807.

Lösel, F., & Farrington, D. (2012). Direct protective and buffering protective factors in the development of youth violence. *American Journal of Preventative Medicine, 43*(251), S8–S23.

McEllistrem, J. (2004). Affective and predatory violence: A bimodal classification system of human aggression and violence. *Aggression and Violent Behavior, 10*(1), 1–30.

Muscari, M. (2002). *Not my kid: 21 steps to raising a nonviolent child.* Scranton, PA: University of Scranton Press.

Nærde, A., Ogden, T., Janson, H., & Zachrisson, H. (2014). Normative development of physical aggression from 8 to 26 months. *Developmental Psychology, 50*(6), 1710–1720.

National Center for Injury Prevention and Control. (2015). *Youth violence: Risk and protective factors.* Atlanta, GA: Centers for Disease Control and Prevention. Retrieved from www.cdc.gov/violenceprevention/youthviolence/riskprotectivefactors.html

National Center for Injury Prevention and Control of the Centers for Disease Control and Prevention. (2002). *Best practices of youth violence prevention.* Retrieved from www.cdc.gov/violenceprevention/pdf/introduction-a.pdf

New York State Office of Mental Health. (2012). *Violence prevention: Risk factors.* Retrieved from www.omh.ny.gov/omhweb/sv/risk.htm

Office of Juvenile Justice and Delinquency Prevention. (n.d.). *The national juvenile justice action plan.* Washington, DC: Author.

Reebye, P. (2005). Aggression during early years—Infancy and preschool. *Canadian Child Adolescent Psychiatric Review, 14*(2), 16–20.

Searight, H., Rottnek, F., & Abby, S. (2001). Conduct disorder: Diagnosis and treatment in primary care. *American Family Physician, 63*(8), 1579–1589.

Watson, M., Fischer, K., Andreas, J., & Smith, K. (2004). Pathways to aggression in children and adolescents. *Harvard Educational Review, 74*(4), 404–430.

CHAPTER 4

Animal Cruelty

A. Description

Animal abuse or cruelty is socially unacceptable behavior that intentionally causes unnecessary distress, suffering or pain, and/or death of an animal. Children who are exposed to violence may in turn abuse animals, and children who abuse animals may become violent toward other humans.

a. Animal cruelty is typically classified as follows:

- *Neglect* occurs when a person deprives an animal of food, water, shelter and/or veterinary care. Neglect cases are acts of omission rather than commission and do not give satisfaction to the person whose animals are neglected; thus, neglect is not a typical form of juvenile animal cruelty. However, household animal neglect may indicate human neglect or inappropriate parental expectations if the animal was neglected by a child charged with the animal's care.

- *Physical abuse* results from malicious torturing, maiming, mutilation, or killing. These acts of intentional cruelty are often shocking and usually indicative of a serious human behavioral problem. Juveniles who commit these intentional acts of cruelty may derive satisfaction in causing harm.

- *Animal sexual abuse*, or *bestiality*, is the sexual molestation of animals by humans and includes a wide range of behaviors, including: fondling, vaginal, anal, or oral penetration; oral–genital contact; penetration with an object; and injuring or killing an animal for sexual gratification. Like rape, this is an eroticization of violence, control, and exploitation. Fleming, Jory, and Burton (2002) found that 96% of their juvenile subjects who had engaged in sex with nonhuman animals also admitted to sex offenses against humans and reported more offenses against humans than other sex offenders their same age and race. They also had histories of more emotional abuse, neglect, and victimization events than other offenders. Thus, sex with animals may be an important indicator of potential or co-occurring sex offenses against humans, and may be a sign of severe family dysfunction.

- *Hoarding*, which is similar to neglect, occurs when a person accumulates a large number of animals, provides minimal standards of nutrition, sanitation, and veterinary care, and fails to act on the deteriorating condition of the animals and/or the environment. The majority of hoarders are adult; however, a child may be living in a household with an animal hoarder, exposing the child to health and safety concerns.

- *Organized criminal enterprise* involves the deliberate fighting of animals for the purpose of monetary profit. *Cockfighting* is the term used when two or more specialty birds, or gamecocks, are placed in an enclosure to fight to the death, sometimes of both birds; it is illegal in all 50 states. Organized *dog fighting* is illegal in the United States and is a felony in all 50 states. Dog fighting is a contest between two specifically bred, conditioned and trained to fight dogs that are placed in a pit to fight. Usually the loser dies, is left to die, or is killed by the owner. Both cockfighting and dog fighting are intended for gambling or entertainment, and both, particularly dog fighting, may be associated with other criminal activity. During a *hog–dog fight* ("hog–dog rodeo") a trained dog attacks a trapped feral hog inside an enclosed pit from which there is no escape. Fight organizers give the advantage to the dog by either cutting off the hog's tusks or outfitting the dog in a Kevlar vest. The dog is timed to see how quickly it can pin down the hog by tearing into the hog's snout, ears, and eyes. Hog–dog fight promoters often bill these fights as "family entertainment"; however, they are closely connected to other crimes and forms of violence in addition to cruelty to animals. In some cases, the operator encourages children into a game of "catch the pig." The handler tapes the hog's snout closed and encourages children to chase the terrified animal around the pen.

- Crush videos, and their underlying crush fetish, are a subset of the sadomasochistic culture (Phillips & Lockwood, 2013). These are typically videos depicting the feet (usually bare or in stiletto heels) crushing small animals.

b.   Children may abuse animals for several reasons: curiosity, imitation, posttraumatic play/reenactment, peer pressure, control the animal or people, retaliation against the animal or people, breed/species prejudice, fear of animal, channeling aggression, mood enhancement, shock, amusement, sexual gratification, and sadism. Children may abuse animals because they identify with an abuser or because an abuser orders the child to harm the animal. They may also rehearse on an animal before committing a violent act on another human or themselves.

c.   Animal cruelty has been associated with child abuse, intimate partner violence, elder abuse, assault, and sexual assault. Animal fighting crimes, now listed as racketeering offenses (Racketeer Influenced and Corrupt Organization Act [RICO]) in some states, are related to other crimes, including gambling, weapons offenses, drug offenses, sexual assault, assault, and human trafficking.

d.   All 50 states and the District of Columbia have anticruelty laws (www.aspca.org/ fight-cruelty/advocacy-center/state-animal-cruelty-laws), and most currently have felony statutes for certain types of animal cruelty. Some felony statutes require psychiatric counseling for convicted abusers.

B. Assessment

a.   Risk factors: Parental interpersonal violence (IPV) perpetration, but not victimization, is predictive of their children's history of animal cruelty (Knight, Ellis, & Simmons, 2014). Interestingly, a study by Vaughn et al. (2011) showed that the cumulative effects of childhood adversities did not have a strong effect on the increased likelihood of animal cruelty. Peers may influence teenage boys to engage in cruelty to gain approval or prove their masculinity—at least half of juvenile cruelty perpetrators act as part of a group. Negative role modeling, particularly behaviors that create chaotic and abusive households, can lead to cruelty. Children mimic these abusive behaviors on others they have some power over, typically animals and/or other children, and some later perpetuate the cycle by continuing to be violent into adulthood. Thus, juvenile animal cruelty can reveal information about the family as well as the child, and therefore may be a marker for family violence—corporal punishment, child abuse, and domestic violence.

b.   Assessing for animal cruelty should be part of all routine child health visits and episodic visits for children who present with behavioral problems or signs of child abuse. Children as young as 4 years old may harm animals, but such behavior is most common during adolescence. Cruelty is often associated with poor academic performance, low self-esteem, few friendships, bullying, truancy, vandalism, and other antisocial behaviors. Ascione (2001) provides a typology of juvenile animal abusers:

- *Exploratory/curious animal abusers* are likely to be preschoolers or very early school-age children who are poorly supervised and lack training on the physical care and humane treatment of animals. These children abuse animals out of innocent exploration and do not intend to cause harm. Developmentally delayed children may also fit into this category.
- *Pathological animal abusers* are more likely to be older (but not necessarily). These children may be symptomatic of psychological disturbances of varying severity, and/or may have a history of physical abuse, sexual abuse, or exposure to domestic violence. These children intend to cause harm.
- *Delinquent animal abusers* are typically adolescents with other antisocial behaviors, sometimes gang or cult related. Substance abuse may be involved with the cruelty. These children intend to cause harm and may derive pleasure from the animal's suffering.

c. The Society & Animal's Forum's *AniCare Child: An Approach for the Assessment and Treatment of Childhood Animal Abuse* recommends four steps in assessing juvenile animal cruelty:

- Ask about the child's relationship with animals.
- Obtain data from multiple sources (parents and other family members, teachers, guidance counselors, medical and court records, psychological evaluations, principal, previously attended schools, social worker, neighborhood friends, veterinarian).
- If the child has committed animal cruelty, assess the extent, nature, and motivation.
- If the child has witnessed cruelty, assess the effects.

d. To assess extent, nature, and motivation of child animal abuse, assess for the following factors:

- Severity: degree of injury frequency and duration; prolonged or immediate injury; number and kind of species, including level of sentience (degree to which the animal is capable of feeling or sensation); intimacy of injury infliction (shot at a distance or stabbed).
- Culpability: developmental level (whether consequences are understood); degree of planning; obstacles that were overcome to commit act; solitary or group activity (if group, leader or follower); coerced or dominant individual; videoed or photographed incident.
- Psychodynamics/motivation: curiosity; reaction to fear of the animal; retaliation against human; peer pressure; other antisocial behavior; rehearsing other delinquent behavior; rage; mood enhancement; pleasure from suffering (sadism); sexual arousal; ritualistic features.
- Attitudes/beliefs: level of awareness of physical or psychological needs of the animal: has little thought as to role of animals in society; prejudice against specific species; cruelty as a way to control or discipline an animal; cultural practice/acceptance.
- Emotional intelligence: capacity for empathy; capable of reciprocal relationships; understanding of relationships; capable of forming attachments.
- Family history: domestic violence; child abuse; neglect; animal cruelty; harsh and inconsistent discipline; spanking and other physical punishment.
- Mitigating circumstances: accepts responsibility; expresses remorse, shame, or guilt; seeks to make restitution; assists law enforcement; capable of forming bond with an animal.

e. It is not possible to predict dangerousness. However, there are aggravating factors that suggest an animal abuser has been or will be involved in violence against people. Lockwood (Phillips & Lockwood, 2013) suggests that exhibiting multiple factors should cause serious concern that a person may be at risk for perpetrating human violence. These factors include, but are not limited to the following: victim vulnerability (small size, age extremes); the victim is a companion animal of the perpetrator; multiple animal victims during the same incident or multiple incidents over a brief period of time; severe, direct contact, or multiple forms of injury; use of fire as a weapon; torture; predatory/planned abuse as opposed to reactive abuse; abuse associated with other criminal behavior; the act involves sexual violence or symbolism; the perpetrator records the incident; the perpetrator lacks remorse or derives pleasure from the incident; and the perpetrator leaves threatening notes (Phillips & Lockwood, 2013).

f.   Assess the parents: Research demonstrates that parent/family characteristics are essentially related to the development of antisocial behavior in children. Parental stress, psychopathology, social isolation, poor parental relations, child-rearing practices, depression, and substance abuse contribute to aggressive behavior in children.

Observe the child's skin for bites, lacerations, cuts, and scratches that may indicate injuries from an animal that may have fought back.

g.   Consider using the Children and Animals Inventory (CAI; www.neacha.org/resources/cruelty%20paper.Inventory.pdf), a brief self- and parent-report measure of Ascione's nine parameters of cruelty: severity (based on degree of intentional pain and injury caused to an animal), frequency (the number of separate acts of cruelty), duration (period of time over which the cruel acts occurred), recency (the most recent acts), diversity across and within categories (number of animals abused from different categories and the number of animals harmed from any one category), sentience (level of concern for the abused animal), covertness (child's attempts to conceal the behavior), isolation (whether the cruelty occurred alone or with other children/adults), and empathy (the degree of the child's remorse for the cruel acts; Dadds et al., 2004).

C. Diagnosis

Possible diagnoses include attention-deficit and disruptive behavior disorders, including conduct disorder. But other underlying problems are possible, including depression and attachment difficulties. Please refer to the sections on those challenges.

D. Levels of Prevention/Intervention

a.   Primary

Teach parents and children humane education:

- Teach by example; use real-life situations to instill a sense of respect for all life. Encourage children to help feed the birds or rescue a bug. With older children, discuss animal-cruelty cases publicized in the news.
- Encourage children to speak up for animals.

- Report animal cruelty. Ignoring it communicates the sense that it is acceptable behavior. Do not engage in physical confrontation, but when appropriate, report the incident to the proper authorities.
- Practice responsible pet guardianship:
  - Obtain annual veterinarian examinations and proper immunizations.
  - Provide the best pet food you can afford.
  - Ensure they get proper love, attention, exercise, and rest.
  - Spay and neuter them.
- Show respect for wildlife.
- Volunteer at a local shelter or rescue group.

b. Secondary

Early identification and prevention of child abuse and parental IPV minimizes family dysfunction and decreases the risk of juvenile animal cruelty.

c. Tertiary

- Animal cruelty is not part of normal development. All episodes of abuse, even those done out of curiosity, warrant intervention. Interventions can be based on typology:
  - Exploratory/curious animal abusers: Humane education is likely to be sufficient intervention; however, age should not be the only determining factor as animal cruelty is one of the earliest signs of conduct disorder.
  - Pathological animal abusers: Professional counseling is warranted.
  - Delinquent animal abusers: Both psychiatric and judicial interventions may be required.
- Many states recommend or require psychological counseling for persons convicted of animal cruelty. The Doris Day Animal Foundation notes that:
  - A thorough evaluation of the convicted abuser must be conducted before a treatment is recommended.
  - Prescribing the wrong treatment can do harm, as well as be a missed opportunity.
  - Psychological counseling for animal abuse should have the same high standards as other types of counseling.
  - Practitioners should not rely on a "one size fits all" approach.
- Treatment of juvenile animal cruelty resembles other psychological treatments for children with other problems, and thus, the basic theoretical and clinical models of diagnosis and interventions will also apply to children who abuse animals. However, there are some distinguishing features that focus on animal abuse, whether it is central to the treatment, or one component of it.

Animals—and the child's relationship with them, attitudes toward them, beliefs about them, learned behavior around them—will be a central feature in the treatment. Children will learn skills such as problem solving, empathy, or self-management (Shapiro, Randour, Krinsk, & Wolf, 2014).

E. Parenting Tips

Children who spend most of their lives indoors have minimal contact with nature and wild animals, which may result in their developing fear or aversion to even simple creatures such as spiders, snakes, and skunks. This can cause them to treat wildlife with minimal respect (Rule & Zhbanova, 2012). Foster children's compassion toward all animals (American Humane Society, 2013; PETA, n.d.; Rule & Zhbanova, 2012):

a. Live by the rule "Do unto others as you would have them do unto you."

b. Teach children to respect and protect even the smallest and most despised.

c. Foster empathy development.

d. Teach by example.

e. Include animals in your life.

f. When little creatures make their way into your home, help them out nonviolently.

g. Keep your pets healthy and safe.

h. Watch animal-friendly movies, and read animal-friendly books with your children to help them understand that animals have feelings.

i. Use art, poetry, drawings, and other types of play to help young children develop greater understanding of animals and to develop greater compassion and empathy.

j. Create a space in your garden to attract butterflies and hummingbirds.

k. When wildlife gets too close to home, handle the situation humanely, and find ways to coexist with animals.

Resources

American Humane Society: www.americanhumane.org

American Society for the Prevention of Cruelty to Animals: www.aspca.org

Humane Society of the United States First Strike Program: www.hsus.org/firststrike

Latham Foundation: www.latham.org

National Association for Human and Environmental Education: http://nahee.org/

People for the Ethical Treatment of Animals: www.peta.com

Society and Animal Forum: www.psyeta.org

References

American Humane Society. (2013). *Be kind to animals week*. Retrieved from http://behumane.org/component/content/article/2-uncategorised/82-be-kind-to-animals#.Vruk8PkrJD8

Ascione, F. (2001). Animal abuse and youth violence. *OJJDP Juvenile Justice Bulletin* (NCJ 188677). Retrieved from www.ncjrs.org/html/ojjdp/jjbul2001_9_2/contents.html

Dadds, M. R., Whiting, C., Bunn, P., Fraser, J. A., Charlson, J. H., & Pirola-Merlo, A. (2004). Measurement of cruelty in children: The cruelty to animals inventory. *Journal of Abnormal Child Psychology, 32*(3), 321–334.

Fleming, W. M., Jory, B., & Burton, D. L. (2002). Characteristics of juvenile offenders admitting to sexual activity with nonhuman animals. *Society & Animals: Journal of Human-Animal Studies, 10*(1), 31–45.

Knight, K. E., Ellis, C., & Simmons, S. B. (2014). Parental predictors of children's animal abuse: Findings from a national and intergenerational sample. *Journal of Interpersonal Violence, 29*(16), 3014–3034. doi:10.1177/0886260514527825

People for the Ethical Treatment of Animals. (n.d.). Teaching kids compassion toward animals. Retrieved from www.petakids.com/parents/teaching-compassion/

Phillips, A., & Lockwood, R. (2013). *A guidebook on safer communities, safer families and being an effective voice for animal victims*. Alexandria, VA: National District Attorneys Association, National Center for Prosecution of Animal Abuse. Retrieved from www.ndaa.org/pdf/NDAA%20Animal%20Abuse%20monograph%20150dpi%20complete.pdf

Rule, A., & Zhbanova, K. (2012). Changing perceptions of unpopular animals through facts, poetry, crafts, and puppet plays. *Early Childhood Education Journal, 40*, 223–230. doi:10.1007/s10643-012-0520-2

Shapiro, K., Randour, M., Krinsk, S., & Wolf, J. (2014). *The assessment and treatment of children who abuse animals*. Cham, Switzerland: Springer.

Vaughn, M., Fu, Q., Beaver, K., DeLisi, M., Perron, B., & Howard, M. (2011). Effects of childhood adversity on bullying and cruelty to animals in the United States: Findings from a national sample. *Journal of Interpersonal Violence, 26*(17), 3509–3525. doi:10.1177/0886260511403763

CHAPTER 5

Anxiety and Fear

A. Description

Anxiety is a feeling of general uneasiness and differs from fear. Fear is a specific response to a real or perceived immediate threat, while anxiety is more diffuse. Anxiety is also anticipatory; one foresees whatever it is that bothers one, and becomes anxious in anticipation of it. Anxiety, a normal reaction to stress, can help children cope, but it can become disabling when excessive.

a. Anxiety may be acute (state) or chronic (trait). Acute or state anxiety is triggered by a change or imminent loss that threatens your sense of security. One's sense of security is critical to one's well-being; as Maslow (1968) noted, the need for safety and security is second only to our need for oxygen, food, and water. Chronic or trait anxiety is a characteristic of one's personality that exists in a person for a long time. People can have low or high levels of either type.

b. *Anxiety disorder* is a term used for a group of disorders characterized by intense and/or persistent anxiety. These disorders include separation anxiety disorder, selective mutism, generalized anxiety disorder (GAD), social anxiety disorder (formerly called social phobia), specific phobia, panic disorder, agoraphobia, anxiety secondary to medical condition, and substance-induced anxiety disorder. Acute stress and post-traumatic stress disorders were once labeled anxiety disorders, but are not considered trauma-induced disorders, and are discussed elsewhere in this book. Anxiety disorders are some of the most common psychiatric illnesses affecting children and adults.

c. Test anxiety, a type of performance anxiety, is usually caused by fear of failure, previous problems with testing, or lack of preparation.

B. Assessment

a. Risk factors for anxiety disorders include family history of anxiety disorders, female sex, trauma, chronic illness, chronic stress, emotional dysregulation, having other mental health disorders, and substance abuse.

b. Anxiety may be mild, moderate, severe, or panic.

- *Mild anxiety* is part of day-to-day life. The ability to perceive reality is brought into sharp focus. People see, hear, and grasp more information, and their problem-solving skills surface. However, even good anxiety has its discomforts, or it would not be anxiety. Mild anxiety still causes people to feel uneasy, restless, tense, fidgety, or even irritable. But these sensations can be worthwhile, as mild anxiety can be very motivating.

- When people escalate to *moderate anxiety*, their perception narrows and they begin to miss details. Instead of senses being heightened, they decrease, and people see, hear, and understand less information. People may develop selective inattention, noticing only certain things around them or those things pointed out by others. They cannot think as clearly as they would normally. They can still problem solve, but are not at their best and may have to ask questions repeatedly before making sense of the answer. They feel the symptoms of anxiety. Moderate anxiety signals that something needs attention, yet it is still a normal fact of life.

- *Severe anxiety* decreases people's ability to focus to the point where they may get stuck on one tiny detail or many scattered ones. They feel lost in their own space and cannot notice what is going on around them, even if someone points it out. When people are this dazed and confused, problem solving no longer functions, and their behavior becomes automatic in an attempt to relieve or reduce the marked symptoms of anxiety. They may feel a sense of dread or impending doom or may become demanding and threatening.

- *Panic* is anxiety at its extreme. The individual cannot process. Speech can become unintelligible or even nonexistent, and the individual can become extremely hyperactive, aggressive, or psychotic, experiencing hallucinations (faulty sensory perceptions, such as hearing voices that are not there) or delusions (false beliefs, such as thinking someone is trying to kill you). Panic can lead to exhaustion and warrants immediate attention because people can hurt themselves or others.

c. Anxious children may present with somatic symptoms (such as headaches or stomachaches, palpitations, dizziness, and chest pain), crying, withdrawal, mood swings, sleep problems, school problems or refusal, rumination, hyperactivity, verbal or physical aggression, and substance abuse. Very young children may be irritable or clingy; they may have changes in their feeding patterns or regress to an earlier stage of behavior (toilet-trained children soiling their pants).

d. A thorough history and physical are warranted when anxiety begins to interfere with normal activities. When somatic symptoms are caused by anxiety, few findings are noted on the physical exam. The history should include ascertaining all drugs and substances, including caffeine, taken by the child and a family history of anxiety disorders. It is important that the provider ascertain the nature, degree, and consequences of the anxiety in order to properly intervene.

e.   Test for physiological problems, as appropriate.

f.   Screen for anxiety

- The Pediatric Symptom Checklist 17 (www.massgeneral.org/psychiatry/ services/psc_home.aspx) Internalizing Subscale screens for: feeling sad, unhappy; feeling hopeless; being down on oneself; worrying a lot; and seeming to have less fun. Children who have scores of 5 or higher on this subscale usually have significant impairments with anxiety and/or depression. Further discussion with the parent and child regarding the questions is warranted (Borowsky, Mozayeny, & Ireland, 2003).

- The Revised Children's Anxiety and Depression Scale (RCADS; www .childfirst.ucla.edu/RCADSGuide20110202.pdf) is a youth self-report, 47-item questionnaire that yields a Total Anxiety Scale and a Total Internalizing Scale. It also includes subscales for: separation anxiety disorder (SAD), social phobia (SP), GAD, panic disorder (PD), obsessive-compulsive disorder (OCD), and major depressive disorder (MDD).

- The Spence Children's Anxiety Scale (SCAS; scaswebsite.com/) is a 44-item measure that assesses six domains of anxiety including generalized anxiety, panic/agoraphobia, social phobia, separation anxiety, OCD, and physical injury fears.

- The Screen for Child Anxiety Related Disorders (SCARED), which targets children ages 8 through 18, is a child and parent self-report screen that is available at no cost at www.pediatricbipolar.pitt.edu.

C. Diagnosis

a.   Differentiate anxiety from normal developmental fears, which are transient and do not interfere with normal function. Anxiety disorders, on the other hand, cause significant distress or impairment in social, academic, occupational, or other important areas of functioning, such as school.

- Infants: Loud noises, sudden movements, and changes in the home can induce fear. Stranger anxiety typically begins around age 6 months. An infant commonly seeks comfort from a security object (e.g., blanket, favorite toy) during times of uncertainty or stress.

- Toddlers: Common fears of toddlers include: loss of parents (known as separation anxiety), stranger anxiety, loud noises, going to sleep, large animals, Santa Claus, and their health care provider. Separation anxiety is developmentally normal until approximately 3 to 4 years of age and is characterized by mild distress and clinging behavior when children are separated from their attachment figures.

- Emotional support, comfort, and simple explanations may allay a toddler's fears.

- Preschoolers: Children usually experience more fears during the preschool period than at any other time. Common fears include: the dark; being left alone, especially at bedtime; animals, particularly large dogs; ghosts and monsters; and body mutilation, pain, and objects and people associated with painful experiences. The preschooler is prone to induced fears that stem from parental remarks and actions, and parents are typically unaware that their behavior or words instill fear in the child. Allowing preschoolers to have a night-light and encouraging them to play out fears with dolls or other toys may help them develop a sense of control over the fear. Exposing the child to a feared object in a controlled setting may provide an opportunity for desensitization and reduction of fear.

- School-age children: During the school-age years, many fears of earlier childhood resolve or decrease; however, school-age children may hide fears to avoid being labeled "chicken" or a "baby." Common fears include: being a failure at school, bullies, intimidating teachers, spiders and snakes, being home alone, bad storms, illness, scary television shows and movies, and something bad happening to their parents. Parents and other caregivers can help reduce a child's fears by communicating empathy and concern without being overprotective. Children need to know that people will listen to them and that they will be understood.

- Adolescents: Common fears and stressors of adolescents include: relationships, ability to assume adult roles, terrorist attacks/other violence, being alone, failure, animals, and the unknown. Listening to an adolescent's concerns and encouraging open communication help the adolescent develop increased confidence in his or her ability to cope.

b.   Differentiate anxiety from a physiological disorder, such as peptic ulcer disease, asthma, obstructive sleep apnea syndrome, hypoglycemia, thyroid disease and other endocrine disorders including pheochromocytoma, and cardiac disorders. Ensure that the anxiety is not due to medications or substances, or alcohol withdrawal.

c.   Differentiate normal, transient anxiety from anxiety disorder. Anxiety disorders are persistent, cause distress, and interfere with the child's functioning, and their symptoms are not explained by another disorder. Changes in the *Diagnostic and Statistical Manual of Mental Disorders*, *5th Edition (DSM-5*; American Psychiatric Association [APA], 2013) from the fourth edition-text revision include: separation anxiety disorder and selective mutism reclassified as anxiety disorders; agoraphobia classified

as a stand-alone diagnosis, and obsessive-compulsive disorder grouped under obsessive-compulsive and related disorders; and post-traumatic and acute stress disorders
listed as trauma-related and stressor-related disorders. A significant change in the
DSM-5 in this area is the inclusion of a developmental approach and examination of
disorders across the life span.

- Separation anxiety is a relatively common anxiety disorder in children.
  These children experience intense anxiety, sometimes to the point of panic,
  when separated from a parent or other loved one. The *DSM-5* (APA, 2013)
  identifies several behaviors as indicative of separation anxiety. These include
  excessive and persistent worry about losing attachment figures, worrying
  about events that may lead to being removed from attachment figures, and
  refusal to go away from home. These symptoms may be manifested in different ways, such as sleep refusal when not near the primary caregiver, excessive
  distress or tantrums when separation is looming, nightmares with separation
  themes, homesickness, or frequent somatic complaints (Bernstein, 2014b).
  Separation anxiety can give way to school phobia, whereby the child will refuse
  to go to school, fearing separation from the parent.

- Selective mutism usually occurs by age 5 years, but may not be noted until the
  child attends school. Children with this disorder are unable to speak aloud in
  certain situations when conversation is expected. This is typically a child who
  barely whispers in school or other social settings, but who speaks comfort-
  ably at home; however, some may be completely mute. These children fear
  speaking and social interactions where communication is expected. Selective
  mutism may also cause school refusal with or without social anxiety disorder,
  although most children with selective mutism do have social anxiety disorder.
  Language is usually intact, although selective mutism can co-occur with communication and language disorders (Bernstein, 2014a). Some children have
  sensory processing disorder (SPD) and may be sensitive to lights, sounds,
  touch, odors, and tastes. SPD can lead to misinterpretation of the environment
  and social cues, leading to more anxiety and frustration.

- Children with social anxiety disorder (SAD) tend to be fearful of being rejected by peers or publicly failing when performing school tasks. They are not
  just shy; their fear and anxiety are out of proportion and disabling. They avoid
  social or performance situations, and may cry, throw tantrums, cling, or freeze
  when in a social situation. Older children may realize that their fear is not
  reasonable (APA, 2013).

- Specific phobias (SP) involve an extreme and persistent fear of specific objects
  or situations that present little to no actual threat. This fear is recognized as
  unreasonable and is triggered by a specific object: snakes, spiders, computers, close spaces, heights, flying, and getting injured. Exposure to the object

immediately provokes anxiety. The distress is so severe that it interferes with the child's functioning or routine. Fears of objects or situations are common during childhood, especially during the preschool period, but they do not interfere with the child's daily functioning. Common childhood fears need to be differentiated from SP, as the latter is irrational, interferes with daily routines, and leads to maladaptive behaviors. Children with SP may have symptoms similar to those of adults, or the child may present with crying, tantrums, clinging, freezing, psychomotor agitation, or immobilization. The blood-injection-injury type of SP is specified if the fear is precipitated by seeing blood or an injury or by receiving an injection or other invasive medical procedure. The anxiety response is often characterized by a strong vasovagal response (Muscari, 2007).

- Children who seem to worry excessively about almost everything may have general anxiety disorder (GAD). The *DSM-5* (APA, 2013) identifies several behaviors as indicative of GAD. These include worrying excessively about multiple issues, including family, friends, school, sports, their health, past actions, upcoming events, and world news. This anxiety expresses itself in physiological symptoms of cognitive vigilance, autonomic hyperreactivity, and motor tension. Cognitive vigilance creates difficulty in concentrating, irritability, and an increased startle response. Motor tension symptoms most commonly include shakiness, restlessness, and headaches. Other symptoms are having an unrealistic view of problems, nausea, needing to go to the bathroom frequently, and sleep problems. Children can also be restless, easily fatigued, or irritable.

- Panic disorder (PD) creates feelings of terror that strike abruptly and repeatedly, sometimes with no warning. The attacks are unexpected, and thus they have no known trigger. Children cannot name the source of the fear, which creates confusion and difficulty concentrating. They may experience extreme fearfulness, a sense of unreality, lightheadedness, difficulty breathing, sense of choking or smothering, nausea, stomach or chest pain, palpitations, shaking, trembling, a fear of dying, or a feeling of losing their mind. Children may begin to avoid situations or places that they associated with panic, with some becoming so fearful they develop agoraphobia; others can develop substance abuse or depression and may be at risk for suicidal ideation (APA, 2013; Queen, Ehrenreich-May, & Hershorin, 2012).

- Although OCD is categorized separately from anxiety disorders in the *DSM-5*, it will be discussed here. Once thought to occur only in adults, this disorder is now more frequently diagnosed in children. OCD is characterized by persistent obsessions (intrusive, unwanted thoughts, images, or urges) and compulsions (intensive, uncontrollable, and repetitive behaviors or mental acts related to the obsessions) that cause distress and consume a vast amount of the child's time. The most common obsessions involve dirtiness and contamination, repeated doubts, and the need to have things a specific way. Frequent compulsions include repetitive handwashing, using tissues or gloved hands to touch things, touching and counting things, counting rituals, repeating actions, and requesting reassurance. Children with OCD become trapped in the cycle of repetitive thoughts and actions. Even though older children realize that their thoughts and behaviors appear senseless and distressing, the behaviors are very hard to stop. Comorbidities include depression, anxiety, ADHD, and autistic spectrum disorder (APA, 2013; Weidle, Ivarsson, Thomas, Lydersen, & Jozefiak, 2015).

- Adjustment disorder with anxiety occurs within 3 months of a specific stressor, such as a move, change of school, or parental divorce. The child experiences feelings of anxiety, nervousness, and worry that cause considerable distress in excess of what would be expected from the situation and that could seriously impair his or her social or school performance. The problem usually dissipates 6 months after the initiating stressor ceases (APA, 2013).

d. Anxiety can also be found in other behavioral disorders, warranting both the ruling out of differential diagnoses and the inclusion of comorbidities. These include: depression, substance abuse, autistic spectrum disorder, anorexia nervosa, trichotillomania, trauma exposure, somatic disorders, and disruptive behavior disorders.

e. When children refuse to go to school, differentiate social anxiety disorder from bullying, victimization, and other traumas at school, as well as learning disorders.

D. Levels of Prevention/Intervention

a. Primary

- Anxiety is inevitable, and some anxiety is needed for self-preservation and development. However, children can function at a more optimal level when they are aware of life stressors and have the ability to cope with them.

b. Secondary

- Children whose parents have anxiety disorders are more likely to develop them too. Family-based intervention may prevent the onset of anxiety disorders in the offspring of parents with anxiety disorders. This secondary prevention aims to modify parental behaviors of overprotection, excessive criticism, and excessive expression of fear and anxiety in front of their children (Ginsburg, Drake, Tein, Teetsel, & Riddle, 2015). Commenting on this study, Yager (2015) noted that longer follow-up is required to determine whether this intervention averts anxiety disorders or merely delays their onset. Also, nonintervention controls are required to determine whether information-only control conditions might unintentionally generate anxiety. Nonetheless, the study strongly suggests that this brief intervention can at least delay the onset of anxiety disorders among children at high risk for them.

- Intervene before anxiety symptoms reach the disorder level, before there is impairment. The Bi-Ped Project of the Maryland Chapter of the American Academy of Pediatrics recommends the following to minimize anxiety (Grossman, n.d.):

  - Acknowledge the discomfort of the child's anxiety.

  - Do not advise the child to avoid the scenarios that make them anxious.

  - Support the child in developing a plan that allows him or her to master anxiety-provoking scenarios through incremental steps just at or beyond the child's comfort zone.

  - Give the child tools that help handle anxiety: positive self-talk, visual imagery, deep breathing, and progressive relaxation.

  - Encourage proper nutrition, rest, and exercise.

c. Tertiary

- Agency for Healthcare Research and Quality (AHRQ, 2010) treatment considerations: enlisting family's help with plan; setting treatment goals and monitoring management (avoid pitfalls, such as avoidance of feared situations); nonpharmacological treatment (counseling, cognitive behavioral therapy [CBT], specialist referral); pharmacological therapy (fluoxetine, fluvoxamine, or sertraline); combination pharmacological and nonpharmacological treatment; monitoring medication and follow-up.

- A 2015 Cochrane Review found that CBT is an effective treatment for child and adolescent anxiety disorders, although evidence suggesting that it is more effective than non-CBT therapies or medication is limited (James, James, Cowdrey, Soler, & Choke, 2015). Children learn how to identify anxious feelings, their reactions to them, and how to develop a plan to cope with the anxiety-producing situations.

- Motivational interviewing (MI) is defined by its originators, Miller and Rollnick (2002), as "a client-centered, directive approach designed to enhance intrinsic motivation for change through understanding and resolving ambivalence about change." The four central principles of MI are: express empathy, develop discrepancy (differentiate where the person is now and where the person wants to be) between the undesirable behaviors and values that are inconsistent with those behaviors, roll with resistance rather than confronting it directly, and support self-efficacy. The relational context, or MI spirit, consists of collaboration, evocation, and preserving client autonomy.

The client, not the counselor, acts as a change advocate (Westra, Arkowitz, & Dozois, 2009).

- Play therapy can help younger children understand the reasons behind their feelings.

- Behavior therapy, including CBT and exposure therapy, is the first line of treatment for specific phobia.

- Selective serotonin reuptake inhibitors (SSRIs) are the medications of choice for the treatment of childhood anxiety disorders. However, the U.S. Food and Drug Administration (FDA) has approved the use of only some SSRIs (sertraline and fluvoxamine) for the treatment of pediatric OCD (clomipramine is also FDA approved). Creswell, Waite, and Cooper (2014) note that although there is evidence of effectiveness of pharmacological treatments for children and youth with anxiety disorders, routine prescription is not recommended due to concerns about possible harm.

E. Parenting Tips

a. Everyone gets anxious from time to time, and we all have our fears. However, signs of excessive anxiety mean that your child should be evaluated by a professional. Talk to your health care provider if your child exhibits any of the following:

- Shows difficulty concentrating
- Becomes more or less active than usual
- Eats a lot more or less than usual
- Regresses to earlier behavior (starts sucking his or her thumb again)
- Has trouble sleeping
- Complains of stomachaches or headaches
- Wets or soils his or her pants

b. Take care of yourself first. Kids detect parental anxiety in a heartbeat, and it becomes contagious.

c. Realize that fears do not go away overnight.

d. Do not belittle your child's fears, but do not cater to them either.

e. Be matter-of-fact when you talk to your child about his or her fears to avoid increasing anxiety. But do not force your child to face his or her fears. This can make the situation worse and frighten your child even more. Let your child face them at his or her own pace.

f. Tell your child it is okay to be afraid and not to feel guilty or embarrassed by such fears.

g. Praise success, but do not tell children that they are big boys or girls when they overcome their fears. This places too much pressure on them.

h.   Sit down and talk with older kids and teens, but do so while assuring them that you are there for them and that they are safe. Younger children may do better with puppet play, coloring, painting, or play-acting. And make sure to listen to what they have to say.

i.   Help your child understand his or her fears: play shadow puppets to help the child deal with fear of the dark; explain that dogs bark because that is how they talk.

j.   Take the time to point out what is right with the world, including school. Yes, there are a lot of drugs and bullies, but there are a lot of positive people and role models, too. Use positive talk about one's self and situation.

k.   Minimize the amount of time your kids spend watching the news on TV and the Internet. Kids under 6 years old should not watch the news at all.

l.   Encourage your kids to talk about what is bothering them as well as what they are happy with. If they are hesitant, ask them to draw their feelings.

m.   Let your kids be kids. Childhood should be a journey, not a race. Do not push them to grow up too fast. Instead, allow them to tackle developmentally appropriate challenges on their own, even if they stumble, so that they can become independent and self-assured.

n.   Get them a pet (as long as they are old enough and responsible)! Cuddling up with a bundle of unconditional love can help decrease anxiety.

o.   Encourage quick return to school, if your child is refusing to go, and encourage him or her to participate in all normal/routine activities.

Resources

American Academy of Child and Adolescent Psychiatry: www.aacap.org

Child and Adolescent Anxiety Disorders: www.adaa.org/living-with-anxiety/children

Selective Mutism Anxiety Research & Treatment Center: www.selectivemutismcenter.org

Separation Anxiety Support: www.helpguide.org/articles/anxiety/separation-anxiety-in-children.htm

References

Agency for Healthcare Research and Quality. (2010). Anxiety and depression in children and youth—Diagnosis and treatment. In: *National Guideline Clearinghouse*. Retrieved from www.guideline.gov/content.aspx?id=38904&search=anxiety

American Academy of Child & Adolescent Psychiatry. (2012). Practice parameter for the assessment and treatment of children and adolescents with obsessive-compulsive disorder. *Journal of the American Academy of Child and Adolescent Psychiatry, 51*(1), 98–113.

American Psychiatric Association. (2013). *Diagnostic and statistical manual of mental disorders* (5th ed.). Washington, DC: Author.

Bernstein, B. (2014a). Pediatrics social phobia and selective mutism. In: *Medscape Emedicine.* Retrieved from http://emedicine.medscape.com/article/917147-overview

Bernstein, B. (2014b). Separation anxiety and school refusal. In: *Medscape Emedicine.* Retrieved from http://emedicine.medscape.com/article/916737-overview

Borowsky, I., Mozayeny, S., & Ireland, M. (2003). Brief psychosocial screening at health supervision and acute care visits. *Pediatrics, 112*(1, Pt. 1), 129–133.

Cresswell, C., Waite, P., & Cooper, P. (2014). Assessment and management of anxiety disorders in children and adolescents. *Archives of Disease in Childhood, 99*(7), 674–678.

Ginsburg, G., Drake, K., Tein, J., Teetsel, R., & Riddle, M. (2015). Preventing onset of anxiety disorders in offspring of anxious parents: A randomized controlled trial of a family-based intervention. *American Journal of Psychiatry, 172*(12), 1207–1214. doi:10.1176/appi.ajp.2015.14091178

Grossman, L. (n.d.). Brief interventions: Anxiety (non-pharmacological approaches). *Bi-Ped Project of the Maryland Chapter of the American Academy of Pediatrics.* Retrieved from www.mdaap.org/Bi_Ped_Brief_Interv_Anxiety.pdf

James, A., James, G., Cowdrey, F., Soler, A., & Choke, A. (2015). Cognitive behavioural therapy for anxiety disorders in children and adolescents. *Cochrane Database of Systematic Reviews, 2015*(2). doi:10.1002/14651858.CD004690.pub4

Maslow, A. H. (1968). *Toward a psychology of being.* New York, NY: D. Van Nostrand.

Miller, W. R., & Rollnick, S. (2002). *Motivational interviewing: Preparing people for change.* New York, NY: Guilford Press.

Muscari, M. (2007, April). What can I do to help patients with belonephobia (fear of needles)? In: *Medscape.* Retrieved from www.medscape.com/viewarticle/555513

Queen, A., Ehrenreich-May, J., & Hershorin, E. (2012). Preliminary validation of a screening tool for adolescent panic disorder in pediatric primary care clinics. *Child Psychiatry & Human Development, 43*, 171–183. doi:10.1007/s10578-011-0256-z

Weidle, B., Ivarsson, T., Thomas, P., Lydersen, S., & Jozefiak, T. (2015). Quality of life in children with OCD before and after treatment. *European Child & Adolescent Psychiatry, 24*, 1061–1074. doi:10.1007/s00787-014-0659-z

Westra, H. A., Arkowitz, H., & Dozois, D. J. A. (2009). Adding a motivational interviewing pretreatment to cognitive behavioral therapy for generalized anxiety disorder: A preliminary randomized controlled trial. *Journal of Anxiety Disorders, 23*(8), 1106–1117.

Yager, J. (2015). An effective way to prevent childhood anxiety disorders? *New England Journal of Medicine Journal Watch*. Retrieved from www.jwatch.org/na39186/2015/10/01/effective-way-prevent-childhood-anxiety-disorders

CHAPTER 6

Asphyxial Games

A. Description

Asphyxial games, including the choking game and autoerotic asphyxia, are activities that involve attempts to get high or increase sexual pleasure by temporarily depriving the brain of oxygen. These activities are not new phenomena, dating back at least to primitive Celtic culture; however, there has been an increase in lethality as a result of the increased use of ligatures and playing the game alone.

    a.   Various techniques are used to obtain the desired effect, but the general goals are strangulation and self-induced hypoxia.

    b.   *Strangulation* restricts the blood flow to the brain through compression of the carotid arteries. The participant achieves this by either pressing the thumbs against the arteries on both sides of the neck simultaneously or by using a ligature or constricting band.

    c.   *Self-induced hypocapnia* requires hyperventilation, causing light-headedness or dizziness, followed by a breath-hold. This alone causes a blackout, but often a number of other actions are used for enhancement, such as a bear hug given from behind or pressure applied to the chest by another person.

    d.   Strangulation results in a dizzy sensation ("cool") that results from the obstruction of cerebral blood flow and an increased carbon dioxide tension. This brief euphoric ("high") feeling comes before possible loss of consciousness, and is followed by the surge of blood flow when the constraint is removed ("rush," "second high"). If loss of consciousness occurs, it can result in injury from subsequent falling (concussions, broken bones), as well as hypoxic injuries that include altered mental status, severe headache, visual impairments, bloodshot eyes, marks on neck, recurrent syncope, behavioral changes, seizures, and coma. As already noted, it can also result in death.

    e.   The *choking game* or *self-asphyxial risk-taking behavior* (SAB), refers to self-strangulation or strangulation by another person by hand or noose to achieve short-term cerebral hypoxia-induced euphoria that is not sexual in nature. Thus, the name "choking game" is a misnomer as choking refers to obstruction of the inner airway, and it is certainly not a harmless game. Some children participate to see who can go the longest without passing out or to see who is the toughest, whereas others do it on a dare or as part of bullying activity. It is performed alone, in pairs, or in groups, and most commonly in children aged 7 through 21, with a peak age around 13. The hands or a ligature are used to produce a euphoric state caused by cerebral hypoxia. Some versions of this "game" involve breath holding and/or compression of the abdomen or thorax. The object is to release the pressure just before loss of consciousness. Unfortunately, failure to do so can result in death, particularly when the activity is performed alone using ligatures. There are numerous other names for this activity. Terms usually depend on geographical location and age of the children. Alternate names include: airplaning, American dream, blacking out/blackout/black hole, breath play, California choke, cloud nine, dream game, fainting game, flat liner, funky chicken, hang-man, knockout, pass-out game, purple dragon, purple hazing, scarf game, something dreaming game, rush, space cowboy, space monkey, suffocation roulette, snuff, and tap-out. Both sexes engage in this activity, with a male:female ratio of 2:1. According to the Centers for Disease Control and Prevention's Injury Center (Deevska, Gagnon, Cannon, Thamboo, & Macnab, 2008), at least 82 children and adolescents have died as a result of playing the "choking game" since 1995. These children were ages 6 through 19, with a peak at 13.3 years. Eighty-seven percent were male, and the majority of these deaths occurred when the children were playing alone. Macnab, Deevska, Gagnon, Cannon, and Andrew (2009) noted that 6.6% of adolescents ages 9 through 18 engaged in this activity and that 94% of them participated while someone else was present. Yet Andrew and Fallon (2007) stated that this behavior is usually acted out alone. Ramowski, Nystrom, Rosenberg, Gilchrist, and Chaumeton (2012) used data from the 2009 Oregon Healthy Teens survey and found a lifetime prevalence of the choking game participation at 6.1% for eighth graders, with 64% of them engaging in the activity more than once. The choking game is not sexual in nature, but some consider it an early manifestation of autoerotic asphyxiation.

f.   *Autoerotic asphyxia* (AEA) involves choking oneself during sexual stimulation to heighten sexual pleasure. Also referred to as scarfing, bagging, or breath play, autoerotic asphyxia may involve elaborate bindings, sophisticated escape mechanisms, sexual images, or cross-dressing, although these are said to be more common in adults than in adolescents. The motivation for the activity is said to be more the sexual arousal from the restriction of breathing than the effects of oxygen deprivation. Death can occur if loss of consciousness leads to inability to reverse or stop the means of strangulation. Autoerotic death is usually associated with a constrictive cervical ligature tied to other parts of the victim's body or to an inanimate object such as a door. Other modalities include ligature around the thorax or abdomen, plastic bags covering the face, electrical current, inhalation of a toxic gas or chemicals, or partial or total submersion, known as *aquaerotic asphyxiation.* Sexual asphyxia can also be practiced as part of a consensual sadomasochistic activity between two or more people, and can still result in fatality. Participants in asphyxial activities are at risk for short-term memory loss, hemorrhage and retinal damage, as well as head injuries from falling when unconscious, stroke, seizures, permanent brain damage, coma, and death. Death can be caused by prolonged asphyxia or nerve pressure that causes the heart to stop. Most participants are older adolescent and adult males under age 30; however, troubled youth may engage in this activity for sexual experimentation. The number of deaths from autoerotic asphyxia is unknown since it is most often practiced in secrecy and solitude. Most cases become apparent when the results are fatal. However, approximately 500 to 1,000 autoerotic fatalities are reported each year in the United States and Canada. Adolescents are especially vulnerable to a fatal outcome because they often do not understand the risks associated with this behavior.

B. Assessment

a.   Risk factors: Children involved in asphyxial activities may be well-adjusted youths with positive family and peer relationships, while others may engage in other risk-taking behaviors or have histories of mental illness or substance abuse. Health care providers should be cognizant of these activities and discuss it at wellness visits. Asphyxial activities should also be added to the differential diagnosis when assessing headaches, behavior changes, head injuries, or abnormal marks around the neck or neck area in youth. Busse and colleagues (2015) found that those who engage in SAB are persons who engage in other risk behaviors.

b.   Assess children as young as 6 years old, and continue through the transition-age period (through age 26). The majority of children involved in this activity are 9 to 16 years old, but younger children have engaged in the activity, as have college students. This should be part of a routine wellness exam, as well as episodic exams when associated symptoms (e.g., bloodshot eyes) present.

c.   The following signs indicate that a child may be involved in asphyxial activities:

- Discussion of the game or its aliases (for the choking game)
- Bloodshot eyes
- Marks on the neck
- Wearing high-necked shirts, even in warm weather
- Frequent, severe headaches
- Disorientation after spending time alone

- Increased and uncharacteristic irritability or hostility
- Ropes, scarves, and belts tied to bedroom furniture or doorknobs or found knotted on the floor
- Wear marks on furniture (bunk beds, curtain rods) from previous incidents
- The unexplained presence of dog leashes, choke collars, bungee cords, and so on
- Petechiae under the skin of the face, especially the eyelids, or the conjunctiva

   d.   In cases where AEA is suspect, also assess for (Cowell, 2009):

- Tangential or hesitant responses to the sexual history, which may warrant additional questioning, such as "Have you experienced sexual gratification by temporarily depriving yourself of oxygen?" and "Do you participate in risk-taking behaviors related to sexual activity or stimulation?"
- Unusual oral, vaginal, or anal injuries, such as signs that orifices may have been repeatedly subjected to foreign-body insertion
- Abrasions that suggest bondage
- Ornamental piercing of intimate body parts
- Erythema or ligature marks on the penis or scrotum

   e.   Assess for substance abuse, as an association has been noted between the two (Dake, Price, Kolm-Valdivia, & Wielinski, 2010)

C. Diagnosis, Including Differential Diagnoses, When Appropriate

   a.   Mood and/or anxiety disorders may underlie or be comorbid with asphyxial games.

   b.   Self-injurious behavior

   c.   The choking game should be considered in the differential diagnosis of a syncopal episode in children and adolescents.

   d.   *Persistent autoerotic asphyxia* can be classified, as in the *Diagnostic and Statistical Manual of Mental Disorders, 5th Edition (DSM-5;* American Psychiatric Association [APA], 2013) as a specifier of sexual masochism disorder. *Hypoxyphilia, asphyiophillia,* or *asphyxiaphilia* is a form of sexual masochism that involves sexual arousal by oxygen deprivation via ligature, noose, chest compression, plastic bag, mask, or chemicals. A paraphilia is a persistent, intense sexual interest in something other than fondling and genital stimulation with phenotypically normal consenting human partners; it becomes a paraphilic disorder when it creates distress or impairment to self or others. Persons with sexual masochism become sexually aroused by being humiliated or being made to suffer (Brannon, 2015).

D. Levels of Prevention/Intervention

a. Primary

Deevska et al. (2008) noted that 40% of youth saw no risk associated with asphyxial activities, which stresses the importance of primary prevention to dispel the myth of harmlessness. Include discussion of the choking game and its consequences in anticipatory guidance, beginning in the early school age. Since many children see this as a "safe" alternative to drugs and alcohol, consider including it with substance abuse teaching.

b. Secondary

Identify children at risk, and ensure they receive preventive teaching.

c. Tertiary

If a child is already participating in asphyxial games, determine: frequency, how the youth is "choking" himself or herself, whether the youth is doing it alone and/or with peers; and why the youth is engaging in this activity. Assess siblings to see whether they are also participating in the activity. A complete psychosocial evaluation is warranted. Refer to a counselor if the child exhibits signs of mood or other psychiatric disorder. Paraphilias can be transient during the adolescent years; however, they can also become lifelong and be associated with other paraphilias. Since disability and death are potential outcomes of AEA, adolescents and transition-age youth who engage in this practice should be evaluated by a therapist skilled in working with sexual disorders.

E. Parenting Tips

Talk to your child about the dangers of this activity. Explain that a person can become unconscious in seconds, making it impossible for them to stop the choking. Talk about the consequences, including the effects of brain damage and that brain damage can occur in as little as 3 minutes.

Be observant for signs that your child may be playing the choking game (NYS Department of Health, 2010):

a. Belts, ropes, scarves, computer cables, shoelaces, and anything else that can be made into a noose tied to doorknobs or bedroom furniture

b. Presence of unexplained dog leashes, choke collars, or bungee cords

c. Acting "out of it" after spending time alone

d. Signs of increased or uncharacteristic irritability or hostility

e.   Frequently wearing high neck shirts or scarves

f.   Physical signs: bloodshot eyes, headaches, marks on neck, pinpoint blood spots on face, eyes, and eyelids

If you think your child is playing the choking game (NYS Department of Health, 2010):

a.   Talk to them and discuss the dangers.

b.   Increase supervision.

c.   Remove items that can be used to hurt themselves.

d.   Talk to your health care provider about injuries that may have occurred because of the game, and discuss the possibility of the child having a mental health evaluation.

e.   Contact the school because other children may be involved.

Resources

Centers for Disease Control and Prevention Choking Game Podcast (archived): www2c.cdc.gov/podcasts/player.asp?f=8057

Games Adolescents Shouldn't Play: www.gaspinfo.com

Oregon Health Authority–The Choking Game: Facts for Parents and Teachers: https://public.health.oregon.gov/HealthyPeopleFamilies/Youth/Pages/ChokingGame.aspx

References

American Psychiatric Association. (2013). *Diagnostic and statistical manual of mental disorders* (5th ed.). Washington, DC: Author.

Andrew, T. A., & Fallon, K. K. (2007). Asphyxial games in children and adolescents. *American Journal of Forensic Medical Pathology, 28*(4), 303–307.

Brannon, G. (2015). Paraphilic disorders. *Medscape Emedicine*. Retrieved from http://emedicine.medscape.com/article/291419-overview

Busse. H., Harrop, T. Gunnell, D., & Kipping, R. (2015). Prevalence and associated harm of engagement in self-asphyxial behaviours ("Choking game") in young people: A systematic review. *Archives of Diseases in Children, 100*, 1106–1114.

Cowell, D. (2009). Autoerotic asphyxiation: Secret pleasure—Lethal outcome? *Pediatrics, 124*(5), 1319–1324. doi:10.1542/peds.2009-0730

Dake, J., Price, J., Kolm-Valdivia, N., & Wielinski, M. (2010). Association of adolescent choking game with selected risk behaviors. *Academy of Pediatrics, 10*(6), 410–416. doi:10.1016/j.acap.2010.09.006

Deevska, M., Gagnon, F., Cannon, W. G., Thamboo, A., & Macnab, A. J. (2008). An adolescent risk-taking behavior: "The choking game." *Paediatric Child Health, 13*(Suppl. A), 52. Retrieved from www.health.ny.gov/prevention/injury_prevention/children/fact_sheets/6-19_years/choking_game_prevention_6-19_years.htm

Macnab, A. J., Deevska, M., Gagnon, F., Cannon, W. G., & Andrew, T. (2009). Asphyxial games or "the choking game": A potential fatal risk behaviour. *Injury Prevention, 15*(1), 45–49. doi:10.1136/ip.2008.018523

NYS Department of Health. (2010). *Choking game prevention, children ages six to 19 years.* Retrieved from www.health.ny.gov/prevention/injury_prevention/children/fact_sheets/6-19_years/choking_game_prevention_6-19_years.htm

Ramowski, S., Nystrom, M., Rosenberg, K., Gilchrist, J., & Chaumeton, N. (2012). Health risks of Oregon eighth-grade participants in the "choking game": Results from a population-based survey. *Pediatrics, 129*(5), 846–851. doi:10.1542/peds.2011-2482

CHAPTER 7

Bullying

A. Description

The Centers for Disease Control and Prevention (CDC) defines bullying as "any unwanted aggressive behavior(s) by another youth or group of youths, who are not siblings or current dating partners, involving an observed or perceived power imbalance and is repeated multiple times or is highly likely to be repeated" (CDC, 2015). The American Academy of Pediatrics (2009) defines bullying as a form of aggression in which one or more children repeatedly and intentionally intimidate, harass, or physically harm a victim who is perceived as unable to defend himself or herself. Others note that bullying invokes an imbalance of physical and psychological power between the persons involved. Attacks are unprovoked, systematic, and purposely harmful toward the same individual child. Regardless of the definition, the key factors in bullying are the imbalance of power (sheer size or strength, cognitive ability, or popularity) and the repeated pattern of abuse, as well as the critical point that bullying is not a developmental norm.

    a. Bullying behavior is purposeful and aimed at gaining control over another child. Bullying usually encompasses *direct behaviors,* such as taunting, threatening, hitting, kicking, stealing, and sexual harassment. However, bullying behaviors can also be *indirect (*also called *relational aggression),* such as gossiping or spreading cruel rumors that cause the victim to be socially isolated by intentional exclusion. Boys may tend to prefer direct methods, and girls, indirect methods. However, a meta-analysis on gender differences in direct and indirect (including relational, social, and indirect) aggression found a slight increase in girls over boys, but noted that the difference is very small (Card, Stucky, Sawalani, & Little, 2008).

    b. Bullying behaviors differ in form and severity. Forms include verbal, physical, and emotional intimidation, as well as racist and sexual bullying. Verbal bullying typically accompanies physical behavior, and includes name calling, spreading rumors, and persistent teasing. Physical bullying, the most obvious form, embodies punching, kicking, biting, hair pulling, pinching, and threatening. Emotional intimidation entails deliberate attacks on the victim's self-esteem, such as deliberate exclusion from a group activity or belittling. Racist bullying takes many forms, including mocking the victim's traditions, voicing racial slurs, and painting graffiti on a victim's locker. Sexual bullying encompasses unwanted physical contacts, such as "wedgies" or bra snapping, as well as derogatory comments. Bullying behaviors range in severity from mild (pushing, spitting, and spreading rumors) to moderate (stealing lunch money, making intimidating phone calls, and using racial slurs) to severe (inflicting bodily harm, threatening with a weapon, and spreading malicious rumors).

c.   Bully–victims are youths who both bully and are bullied by others. As examples, they may be bullied at home, and then bully at school; or they may be bullied as children and go on to bully as adolescents.

d.   Bystanders are children who are present when another child is bullied. They may be passive and do nothing, they may cheer on the bully, or they may support the victim.

B. Assessment

a.   Risk factors: No single risk factor puts a child at risk for bullying or being bullied. However, some groups, such as children with disabilities and LGBTQI2 (lesbian, gay, bisexual, transgender, questioning, intersex, two-spirit) youths, may be at increased risk for victimization.

- Risk factors for victimization include: internalizing symptoms, externalizing behavior; being perceived as different from peers, weak or unable to defend themselves; depression, anxiety, or low self-esteem; inadequate social skills; difficulty in solving social problems; having few friends or being less popular than others; not getting along with others; perceived as being annoying or antagonizing; rejected and socially isolated by peers; and having negative family, school, and community environments (National Institute of Child Health and Human Development, 2014).

- Bullies generally fall into two categories: the disconnected who may be depressed, anxious, less involved in school, and who have low self-esteem, are easily influenced by others, or who do not identify with the feelings of others; and the well-connected who have social power, like to be in charge or dominate, and who are overly concerned about popularity. Risk factors for becoming a bully include: externalizing behavior, internalizing symptoms; both social competence and academic challenges; views violence as positive; thinks poorly/negatively of others; has difficulty following the rules; has difficulty problem solving with others; is aggressive or easily frustrated; has friends who bully; perceives school as negative; and has problems at home and/or less parental involvement and monitoring (Cook, Williams, Guerra, Kim, & Sadek, 2010; U.S. Department of Health and Human Services, n.d.).

- Risk factors for bully–victims include: coexisting externalizing and internalizing problems; negative attitudes and beliefs about themselves and others; inadequate social problem-solving skills; poor academic performance; and both rejected/isolated by peers and negatively influenced by the peers with whom they interact (Cook et al., 2010).

b. Screen all school-aged and adolescent children during health maintenance examinations, and screen children who present with school phobia, mood and/or behavioral problems, or somatic complaints (trouble sleeping, headaches, enuresis, and stomachaches).

c. Victims: Children may not disclose bullying victimization for a number of reasons, including feeling helpless or humiliated, fear of retaliation from the bully, believing that no one cares, and fear of peer rejection (Robers, Kemp, & Truman, 2013). When asking children about school, monitor their demeanor to determine whether they behave in a shy or withdrawn manner, especially when discussing peer relationships and activities. Ask children about their route to and from school, because victims may be fearful of walking to and from school or riding the bus. Subtle signs, as well as obvious ones, may be present; however, realize that these signs can indicate other disorders, such as depression and substance abuse, which should be ruled out. Possible signs of victimization include the following: depression and/or suicidal ideation; anxiety; moodiness or sullenness, as well as withdrawal from family interaction; loss of interest in schoolwork; aggression; bullying siblings or other children; unexplained bruises or injuries; arrival at home with torn clothes or unexplained bruises; disappearance of personal belongings, asking for extra money or allowance for school lunch or supplies, or stealing money; waiting to use the bathroom at home or enuresis; crying during sleep or nightmares; stomachaches or mysterious illnesses invented to avoid going to school or outright refusal to go to school; drastic changes in sleep or eating patterns; desire to carry a weapon, such as a knife or gun, for protection; and unwillingness to discuss the situation at school or improbable excuses for the aforementioned signs.

d. Bullies: Detecting bullies is more difficult than detecting victims because bullies are adept at hiding their mistreatment of others. Parents may have no idea that their child is bullying until a teacher or another parent confronts them about it. Other parents may report that the child has little concern for others, is aggressive or manipulative, abuses animals, or possesses unexplained items or money. Bullies may act cocky, arrogant, and self-assured, and they may have difficulty accepting authority. When asked about bullying, they are apt to be condescending about responding to questions. Because most bullies lack empathy, they also tend to appear pleased or amused when providers ask them how they feel about other children getting hurt. Bullies may also exhibit many of the same signs as victims, especially depression, anxiety, and psychosomatic symptoms, and they may have substance abuse problems.

C. Diagnosis

a. Screen for psychiatric disorders, including depression, suicidal ideation, and anxiety (Klein, Myhre, & Ahrendt, 2013; Marvicsin, Boucher, & Eagle, 2013).

b. Repeated bullying may be a sign of conduct disorder. The primary diagnostic features of conduct disorder include aggression, theft, vandalism, violations of rules, and/or lying that have occurred for at least a 6-month period. Bullying has also been linked to other antisocial behaviors, including vandalism, fighting, theft, smoking, substance abuse, truancy, and dropping out of school (see Chapter 3).

D. Levels of Prevention/Intervention

a. Primary

Klein et al. (2013) recommend advocating for the use of evidence-based strategies in schools and the community to improve social–emotional learning and encourage bystander intervention.

b. Secondary

Secondary prevention involves early identification and management. All children should be screened at health maintenance visits and when exhibiting signs that may indicate bullying. However, special attention should be paid to those children who demonstrate risk factors, as delineated by earlier in this chapter.

c. Tertiary

Management of bullying should be multidisciplinary, involving the parents, primary health care provider, teachers, school administrators, school counselors, and other mental health professionals as needed. The health care professional can play a key role by acting as liaison between the affected family (bully or victim) and the school (Muscari, 2002).

- Victims: Encourage children and their parents to verbalize their feelings about the bullying. Victims and their parents need reassurance that the health care provider can help them find effective ways to respond to bullying and to change the children's behavior to prevent them from being bullied in the future.
    - Children are less likely to be bullied in a peer group. Because many victims have poor social skills and few friends, they need to practice socially acceptable behaviors.
    - Structured groups and activities, such as scouting, boys' and girls' clubs, sports, martial arts, and after-school activities help children develop these skills under adult supervision. Drama clubs teach children how to act in

a manner that does not show what they feel, a skill that can be used when bullied.

- In addition, health care providers can foster healthy self-esteem and teach problem-solving skills, and they can teach children to be assertive rather than submissive.

- Parents can make an appointment with their child's teacher, principal, and/ or counselor to discuss the problem and to ask about the school's antibullying policy. School personnel should take the problem seriously and investigate incidents of bullying.

• Bullies: Intervening with bullies can be a difficult undertaking because both the parent and the child may be reluctant to admit to bullying and/or not perceive it as a problem. Health care providers should avoid arguments and advise parents that this behavior will have negative consequences for their child's future. Like victims, bullies benefit from learning appropriate social skills. Thus, they, too, should be encouraged to participate in small group activities, preferably with older children, so that they can engage in cooperative tasks. Adult supervision is warranted during these groups, and bullies should receive positive reinforcement each time they engage in prosocial or caring behaviors, which enables them to learn more positive ways of gaining attention and affection.

- Health care providers can work with the parents to help them learn ways to demonstrate caring and affection toward their children, as well as ways to develop more consistent and appropriate disciplinary measures. Parents should be encouraged to become more involved with community activities and other parents. If the child demonstrates significant bullying behavior or signs of a conduct disorder, referral to a mental health professional is appropriate.

- Referral is warranted once children demonstrate the consequences of bullying. If resources are scarce, be creative and consider alternatives, such as developing an alliance with a university psychiatric nursing, psychology, social work, or counseling program, or investigate telepsychiatric services. Motivational interviewing (MI) can help build on the youth's strengths. This intervention's founders, Rollnick and Miller (1995), developed this strategy for people with alcohol and drug problems, who, like bullies, have behaviors that they find enjoyable and who do not seek help. Health care providers can use the Motivational Interviewing Guide in Appendix D and make it specific to bullying by encouraging self-exploration and explaining the potential risks and consequences associated with continuous bullying, assisting the youth with understanding his or her behavior and its effects, discouraging bullying behavior and encouraging socially acceptable behaviors, supporting the youth in implementing antibullying behavior, and fostering relapse prevention (Juhnke et al., 2013).

E. Parenting Tips (Muscari, 2002; Muscari & Brown, 2010; U.S. Department of Health and Human Services, n.d.)

a. For Parents Whose Child Is a Victim

- Look for signs that your child is being bullied: unexplained injuries; missing personal items; frequent aches and pains; changes in eating and/or sleeping habits; school problems (not wanting to go to school, dropping grades, loss of interest); withdrawing from activities; feelings of hopelessness; and self-destructive behaviors, including harming themselves.

- Do not overreact, and do not let your child see that you are upset. Your child may interpret that reaction to mean that you are disappointed with him or her.

- Talk to your child, and listen carefully to his or her concerns.

- Reinforce the idea that the incident was not your child's fault: "The bully has a problem, not you, and picked on you for no reason. You didn't do anything to cause it."

- Minimize bullying opportunities. Do not allow your child to take valuable possessions to school. Instruct your child to try to avoid places where the bully hangs out. Staying out of harm's way is sensible, not "chicken."

- Teach your child possible strategies to help handle the problem:

  - Instruct your child not to react by crying or becoming upset, because this is what the bully wants. Bullies get bored when they do not get the expected response.

  - Foster friendship, and tell your child to walk with a buddy.

  - Encourage your child not to do everything the bully says or wants and not to give any belongings to the bully. Your child needs to repair his or her self-esteem and recapture dignity, which will not be accomplished by giving in to the bully.

  - Persuade your child to stand tall, look the bully in the eye, and say something like "Stop it right now." Tell your child to then walk away and ignore any further comments from the bully.

  - Tell your child not to get angry or fight back. These reactions will not solve the problem; they actually make matters worse. It gives bullies what they want and encourages them to come back to taunt again. Fighting can also put your child at greater risk for physical injury.

  - Discourage your child from retaliating, because it only reinforces violence as a solution to problems.

  - Tell your child to find a teacher or other adult and report the incident.

  - Seek professional help if the bullying seems to have affected your child's self-esteem.

b. For Parents Whose Child Is a Bully

- Look for signs that your child is a bully: has friends who bully, gets into fights, is aggressive, has unexplained money or possessions, blames others for own negative behavior, is very competitive and worries about his or her popularity or reputation.

- Stay calm. Try to be objective, even though this may be difficult. Do not become angry or defensive. These reactions tend to make a bad situation even worse.

- Because your child most likely will not confess to the behavior, ask your child to tell you exactly what he or she has been doing. Talk to other parents and teachers to find out what has been happening.

- Explain how your child's behavior constitutes bullying, and ask why your child thinks he or she bullies and what might help your child to stop this behavior. But do not tolerate any excuses for the behavior.

- Because bullying often stems from unhappiness, try to find out what is bothering your child, and help him or her develop ways to cope with it.

- The following strategies will help modify your child's bullying behavior:

  - Take the problem very seriously. If your child is a bully, he or she is at risk for more severe problems later in life.

  - Supervise your child more closely, and stay nearby when your child plays with other children. If you cannot stay nearby, arrange for other adults to supervise the children, or ask that your child only participate in supervised activities.

  - Set limits. Tell your child that bullying will not be tolerated, and make sure your child understands you. Create consequences and follow through on them when needed. For example, limit or remove all media devices if the child engaged in cyberbullying.

  - Help your child to understand the rights and feelings of others. Ask how your child would feel if someone bullied him or her. Use examples from books, television, and movies.

  - Encourage your child to apologize to the victims.

  - Stop displays of aggression immediately, and help your child find nonviolent outlets to handle frustrations and problems.

  - Foster your child's participation in physical activities such as sports so that your child will have healthy ways to feel powerful and strong.

  - Praise your child for appropriate behaviors.

  - Teach your child to be assertive rather than aggressive.

- Talk to your child's school counselor and teacher, and explain that your child is trying to improve his or her behavior, and ask them for their assistance. Support the school if it institutes consequences for the child's bullying behavior.
- If older siblings tease your bullying child, instruct them to stop, and administer consequences as needed.
- Be a positive role model. Control your own aggression, including road rage.
- Seek professional help. Bullying behavior frequently requires outside assistance. Take advantage of the counseling services offered at your child's school or in your community.

c.   For All Parents Whose Child May be a Bystander (U.S. Department of Health and Human Services, n.d.)

- Do not give bullies an audience.
- Be a role model—set a good example.
- Tell a trusted adult.
- Be their friend, and let them know they are not alone.
- Help them get away without putting yourself in harm's way.
-

Resources

Bullying: It's Not OK, American Academy of Pediatrics: www.healthychildren.org/English/safety-prevention/at-play/Pages/Bullying-Its-Not-Ok.aspx

Bullying: MedlinePlus: www.nlm.nih.gov/medlineplus/bullying.html

Dealing With Bullying Kids Health: http://kidshealth.org/teen/your_mind/problems/bullies.html

Girl Bullying: www.girlshealth.gov/bullying/

Helping Kids Deal With Bullies: http://kidshealth.org/parent/emotions/behavior/bullies.html

It Gets Better Project: www.itgetsbetter.org/

National Bullying Prevention Center: www.pacer.org/bullying/resources/info-facts.asp

National Crime Prevention Council Bullying: www.ncpc.org/topics/bullying

Olweus Bullying Prevention Program: www.clemson.edu/olweus

Stop Bullying Now: stopbullyingnow.gov

References

American Academy of Pediatrics Committee on Injury, Violence, and Poison Prevention. (2009). Role of the pediatrician in youth violence prevention. *Pediatrics, 124*(1), 393–402.

Card, N., Stucky, B., Sawalani, G., & Little, T. (2008). Direct and indirect aggression during childhood and adolescence: A meta-analytic review of gender differences, intercorrelations, and relations to maladjustment. *Child Development, 79*, 1185–1229. doi:10.1111/j.1467-8624.2008.01184.x

Centers for Disease Control and Prevention. (2015). *Bullying research.* Retrieved from www.cdc.gov/violenceprevention/youthviolence/bullyingresearch/index.html

Cook, C., Williams, K., Guerra, N., Kim, T., & Sadek, S. (2010). Predictors of bullying and victimization in childhood and adolescence: A meta-analytic investigation. *School Psychology Quarterly, 25*(2), 65–83.

Juhnke, B. A., Juhnke, G. A., Curtis, R. C., Thompson, E. H., Coll, K. M., Yu, F., . . . Mullett, A. (2013). Using motivational interviewing with school-age bullies: A new use for a proven, evidence-based intervention. *Journal of School Counseling, 11*(14). Retrieved from http://files.eric.ed.gov/fulltext/EJ1034750.pdf

Klein, D., Myhre, K., & Ahrendt, D. (2013). Bullying among adolescents: A challenge in primary care. *American Family Physician, 88*(2), 87–92.

Marvicsin, D., Boucher, N., & Eagle, M. J. (2013). Youth bullying: Implications for primary care providers. *The Journal for Nurse Practitioners, 9*(8), 523–527.

Muscari, M. (2002). Sticks and stones: The NP's role with bullies and victims. *Journal of Pediatric Health Care, 16*, 22–28.

Muscari, M., & Brown, K. (2010). *Quick reference to child and adolescent forensics: A guide for nurses and other health care professionals.* New York, NY: Springer.

National Institute of Child Health and Human Development. (2014). What are risk factors for being bullied? Retrieved from www.nichd.nih.gov/health/topics/bullying/conditioninfo/Pages/risk-factors.aspx

Rollnick, S. & Miller, W. (1995). What is motivational interviewing? *Behavioural and Cognitive Psychotherapy, 23*(4), 325–334.

Robers, S., Kemp, J., & Truman, J. (2013). *Indicators of school crime and safety: 2012* (NCES 2013-036/NCJ 241446). Washington, DC: National Center for Education Statistics, U.S. Department of Education, and Bureau of Justice Statistics, Office of Justice Programs, U.S. Department of Justice.

U.S. Department of Health and Human Services. (n.d.). Risk factors [bullying]. Stop Bullying. Retrieved from www.stopbullying.gov/at-risk/factors/index.html

CHAPTER **8**

Cyberdelinquency

A. Description

Cyberdelinquency is a relatively new term that recognizes new deviances or crimes related to the online behavior of young people. The term *delinquency* has specific legal meaning; however, it is also a way to refer to juvenile antisocial behaviors that are not considered illegal. Behaviors can range from bullying to sharing music without regard for copyright to cyberstalking, as well as harassing via chat bots (programs designed to mimic human conversation) and hacking school computers to access forbidden sites, deface websites, or change grades. Bowker (1999) addressed cases where juveniles caused significant monetary damage to an Internet provider's system, downloaded child pornography, scanned real money to make counterfeit, and created a video shooting game featuring the photograph of another teen as the target. Interestingly, while delinquency is usually associated with poverty and disadvantage, many young Internet users come from more affluent backgrounds (Molesworth & Denegri-Knott, 2007). The neighborhood is no longer just the block; it is now the world.

a.   Cyberdelinquency has been explained as a facet of deindividuation, caused by a reduction in self-regulation, self-awareness, and conditions of anonymity that result in deviant behavior. Social cues, such as nonverbal communication, are removed, and individuals become self-absorbed, increasing their chance of behaving on impulse because they do not think they will get caught; cyberdelinquency can also be explained in terms of individual and group identity, salience, and identifiability; thus, sharing downloaded music with peers is acceptable because they do not identify with the copyright owners (Molesworth & Denegri-Knott, 2007). Low self-control can result in the inability to resist opportunistic temptation as when the perpetrator does not consider the long-term consequences of their behavior. These individuals are characterized as impulsive, insensitive, risk-taking, and attracted to tasks that require little thought or effort, as well as deviant peer groups both offline and online, and this may give rise to various types of cybercrime including digital piracy (Marcum, Higgins, & Ricketts, 2014).

b. Bowker (2000) presented four factors that contribute to cyberdelinquency in today's youth:

- Possession of more technical knowledge than previous generations
- Ethical deficit
- Interaction with a literally global peer group and access to websites that advocate negative behaviors and provide instructions on others
- The ease and anonymity of the Internet

Bowker (2000) also notes that some computer delinquents may be too young to understand the illegality of their actions, while others may go on to become adult cybercrime offenders. The latter get into a progression of computer crimes including "telecommunications fraud (making free long-distance calls), unauthorized access to other computers (hacking for fun and profit), and credit card fraud (obtaining cash advances, purchasing equipment through computers)" (Bowker, 2000). Thus, computer delinquency should not be ignored.

c. Like face-to-face aggression, online aggression can have negative consequences for both victims and perpetrators. Both have high levels of alcohol and substance abuse, and cyberaggression is linked to a higher prevalence of negative behaviors such as property damage and physical aggression (Mishna, Khoury-Kassabri, Gadalla, & Daciuk, 2012).

d. The U.S. Department of Justice Attorney's Office (2015) describes cybercrime as "unlawful acts wherein the computer is [used as] a tool, a target, or both." They list three categories of computer crimes:

- Crimes facilitated by a computer: The computer is used as a tool in criminal activity, such as storing records of fraud; perpetrating financial crimes via computers (creating counterfeit checks and money, credit card fraud, money laundering, etc.); manufacturing false identification; intellectual property crimes (software piracy, copyright infringement, trademark violations, theft of computer source code, etc.); collecting and distributing child pornography via the Internet; cyberstalking; and Internet fraud schemes (phishing and auction fraud, etc.).
- Crimes targeting a computer or computer system: This is an attack to commit crimes, such as unauthorized access to computer systems or networks; theft of information; denial of service attacks; virus/worm attacks; Trojan attacks; web jacking; and extortion.
- Crimes utilizing a computer as storage: The computer is used as an accessory, such as the storage of child pornography graphic files and copyright infringement by organized groups. Some juveniles may store images sexted from other minors, while others may store child pornographic images related to their deviant arousal.

e. Juvenile cyberdelinquent behaviors have included: hacking (intentional, unauthorized access of another's computer and network); swatting (making fake 911 calls to get significant police presence); trolling (intentionally causing online interpersonal conflict or controversy); cyberstalking (repeated electronic harassment); sexting (electronic sending/receiving of explicit sexual messages or images); and cyberbullying (electronic bullying). Gang members engage in Internet "banging," trading insults or threats that can lead to physical violence; they also brag about fights and murders (Patton, Eschmann, & Butler, 2013).

f. Cyberstalking may involve former intimate partners, acquaintances, or strangers. Technology makes for easier deception and anonymity, as well as the juvenile's sense of power over the victim. Cyberstalkers may use the victim's personal information to threaten or intimidate them; send repetitive unwanted emails, instant messages, or texts; or impersonate the victim online to gain access to their e-mail or social networking site. Cyberstalking can occur via phone, fax, global positioning system (GPS), cameras, computer software, or the Internet. It may be a precursor to stalking, and should be taken seriously (Marcum et al., 2014; National Institute of Justice, 2007). This is addressed further in Chapter 24.

g. Sexting is the sending, receiving, or forwarding of sexually explicit messages or images via cell phone, computer, or other digital device. It appears to be part of a cluster of risky sexual behaviors in adolescents (Rice et al., 2012), and in one study of middle-school children, sexting correlated with sexual activity and risk behavior, such as unprotected sex (Rice et al., 2014). However, a 6-year longitudinal study by Temple and Choi (2014) found that, while there is a temporal relationship between sexting and actual sexual behavior, there was not a link between sexting and risky sexual behavior over time, suggesting that sexting may be a new norm in adolescent development and not limited to just at-risk youth. This was echoed by Martinez-Rather and Vandiver (2014), who found that sexting is a component of romantic relationships or courting practices between youth, given that their study participants reported sexting images to boyfriends or someone they were interested in dating. They also found that youths said the ability to flirt with peers was a dominant motivation to engage in sexting, indicating that they perceive sexting as a normal means of communication. However, adolescent sexting can result in a number of difficulties, including legal ones. The sending or receiving of nude pictures of persons under the age of 18 risks charges of possession or distributing child pornography, carrying penalties that include being listed on a sex offender registry (Lewin, 2010). Sexted photos may also be distributed to others after romantic breakups ("revenge porn"). Sexted material can also be used to blackmail a youth into committing other acts. Images may also just be forwarded from one youth to another, adding to the psychosocial risks for the one pictured, and increasing the number of youths who can be affected legally (Strassberg, McKinnon, Sustaíta, & Rullo, 2013).

h. Cyberbullying is a form of electronic aggression that refers to bullying through technology via e-mail, texts, chat rooms, instant messaging, social media, online gaming, 3-D virtual worlds, interactive apps, or websites—essentially, anywhere youth can congregate in cyberspace (Hinduja & Patchin, 2014).

- Forms of cyberbullying include: flaming (sending angry, rude, or offensive messages); harassment (repeatedly sending a person offensive messages); denigration (sending or posting harmful, false, or cruel statements about a person to other people); outing (publishing embarrassing information about the victim); trickery (engaging in tricks to solicit embarrassing information about a person and then making that information public); trolling (using shock value to upset others); exclusion (actions that specifically and intentionally exclude a person from an online group, such as blocking a student from an instant messenger buddy list); impersonation (posing as another person, usually by breaking into his or her account); happy slapping (an unsuspected person is attacked, while an accomplice films the incident, typically with a cell phone, and then it is posted online); text wars (multiple people gang up on a victim); online polls (asking readers to answer very hurtful questions about a victim); malicious codes (intentionally spying on the victim or harming the victim's system); and griefing (causing a person chronic grief; NYS Division of Criminal Justice Services, n.d.).

- The traditional bullying paradigm does not readily translate into the cyber realm; here, bully–victims are common, and the criteria for power imbalance may not apply. Cyberbullying has other unique features that increase harm. Youths generally have technology access all day, meaning that cyberbullying can occur constantly, even in the safety of the victim's home. Bullies can say or write things that they would not say in a face-to-face situation and can attack anonymously, thinking that they cannot get caught. They can take unauthorized photos or video of unsuspecting peers and "upload them to the world to see, rate, tag and discuss" (Hinduja & Patchin, 2014, p. 2). Reproducibility, lack of emotional reactivity, perceived uncontrollability, relative permanence, and 24/7 accessibility increase the likelihood of online misconduct (Kowalski, Giumetti, Schroeder, & Lattanner, 2014; Pearson, Andersson, & Porath, 2005). Youth can easily copy all of their friends on a message or forward gossip to their entire address book, making it easier to harm others and to repeat the harm over and over again with a single click.

- In a study of middle and high school cyberbullying, Mishna, Cook, Gadalla, Daciuk, and Solomon (2010) found that those engaging in cyberbullying admitted to the following (in descending order): name calling, pretending to be someone else, spreading rumors, threatening, sending one person's private photos to someone else, or sending someone unwelcome sexual texts or photos. The majority of this behavior occurred through instant messaging, followed by social networking sites, e-mail, Internet games, and other websites.

Most of the cyberbullies targeted friends, while others targeted students at school, strangers, and students at another school, and most indicated they did not feel anything in response, while others reported feeling guilty, powerful, popular, or better than the other students. Interestingly, only 16% reported feeling guilty.

B. Assessment

a. Risk factors: Potential risk factors for cyberaggression are substance abuse, other forms of aggression, property damage, and poor mental health, including low self-esteem and depression. Modecki, Barber, and Vernon (2013) found that developmental increases in problem behavior across grades 8 to 10 predict both cyberaggression and victimization in grade 11, developmental decreases in self-esteem predicted both aggression and victimization in grade 11, and early depressed mood predicted both aggression and victimization later on.

b. Sexting: Döring (2014) reviewed all 50 sexting papers in the PubMed and PsychInfo databases, published between 2009 and 2013. They found that most papers (79%) address what they term "deviance discourse," viewing adolescent sexting as a risk behavior, link to sexual objectification, violence, risky sexual behavior, and negative consequences such as bullying by peers and criminal prosecution under child pornography laws. The other papers address the "normalcy discourse," where sexting is seen as normal intimate communication within romantic and sexual relationships. Viewing this as two schools of thought, there are no underlying specific cues for which to assess.

c. Cyberbullies: There are no definitive traits to look for; however, there are potential traits noted in the literature. Unlike traditional bullying, bully–victims are common in cyberbullying. Perpetrators of cyberbullying tend to engage in rule breaking and aggression. Both males and females engage in cyberbullying. Cyberbullying occurs in middle school and continues through the college years, but the younger bullies are less likely to use texts, picture bullying, and instant messaging. Motives include having a history of bullying or cyberbullying victimization, desire to demonstrate technical skills, seeing it as fun, and a desire to feel powerful. Children with low affective empathy (experience emotions of others) have been found to participate in more cyberbullying behaviors than those with low cognitive empathy (understand emotions of others; Ang & Goh, 2010). Cyberbullies are also more likely than those who do not bully to report perpetration of violence toward peers, use computers for several hours a day, use tech-devices, have perceived technological expertise, and give their password to friends. Traditional bullies are more likely to engage in moral disengagement, seeing their actions as benign, less harmful, or the fault of the victim; this may also pertain to cyberbullies. Cyberbullies may also have weaker emotional bonds with their parents, less frequent discipline from their parents, and less frequent parental monitoring (Kowalski et al., 2014).

C. Diagnosis

Cyberaggression is often comorbid with adverse developmental outcomes. Cyberaggression has been linked to anxiety, depression, and somatic symptoms.

D. Levels of Prevention/Intervention

a. Primary

- Encourage schools to address with students the potential consequences of sexting and other electronic forms of sexual communication. Peer education and dramatization may be helpful. Health care providers should include questions about cyberdelinquent behaviors on their growing list of assessment questions, and clinicians should provide teens and parents with information designed to discourage this practice.

- The National Crime Prevention Council recommends teaching teens about the ethical and legal rules of the Internet. Discuss how their actions on the Internet are not really anonymous and that real people are affected by cybercrimes.

- Discuss netiquette: Think before you post; choose words wisely; do not use the Internet as a weapon; remember that cyberspace is forever; and ask WWMT or WWDT—what would mom think or what would dad think—before engaging in risky Internet behavior (Whitson, 2012).

b. Secondary

Identify at-risk youth to allow for early intervention. For example, cyber- and face-to-face victimization have been demonstrated to predict cyberaggression, and addressing this victimization may decrease the risk for future aggression.

c. Tertiary

When you encounter a teen who is already engaging in cyberdelinquent behaviors, the goals should be to halt the activity, prevent or minimize psychological trauma, and assist with legal consequences. To prevent future cyberdelinquency, reinforce the primary prevention strategies. Assess the teen's psychological state, especially the teen who is already compromised by psychiatric disorders. Ask whether he or she is being teased because of the photos, and determine suicidality status. Refer the teen for counseling when indicated. To assist with legal consequences, encourage the parents to meet with an attorney.

E. Parenting Tips

a.   The National Crime Prevention Council provides signs that a teen may be cyber-bullying. However, these can be signs of other cyberdelinquent behaviors, too:

- Stops using the computer or turns off the screen when someone approaches
- Becomes anxious when using the computer or cell phone
- Is secretive about their computer activity
- Spends excessive time on the computer
- Becomes angry or upset when technology privileges are limited or taken away

b.   Here is a list of helpful tips for parents and teenagers to prevent/avoid sexting.

Tips for teens:

- Think twice before you click the send button. Once you send or post your photos, you cannot change your mind, and things never truly disappear in cyberspace.
- The receiver may not react the way in which you expect.
- If your boyfriend/girlfriend asks you to send a suggestive photo, say, "No." Do not do it on a dare, either. No one is worth compromising your reputation.
- Your photos may be shared with other classmates and posted on social media sites where they can go viral and everyone can see them, including your parents, friends, and teachers as well as police, potential employers, college admissions personnel, scholarship committee members, and sex offenders.
- Think about how classmates will react to you or what they will say behind your back. One photo can severely damage your reputation.
- Nothing is really anonymous; your photos can be traced back to you.
- You can be arrested, charged, and convicted for possessing and distributing child pornography, even when sending a photo of yourself. You may even be labeled a sex offender.
- If someone sends you a suggestive photo of himself or herself, tell a responsible adult (parent, teacher, and counselor). Do not forward it because it is a crime, and you will be held as responsible as the person who originally sent it.
- If you are sharing your photos with someone you only know online, you may be sharing them with a sex offender, and that sex offender may use your photos to blackmail you into doing things that you do not want to do.

Tips for parents:

- If you are not tech savvy, start learning. Get instructional materials, take a course, or, better yet, have your child teach you.

- Know what your children are doing in cyberspace.
- Talk with them about relationships and the importance of their reputations. Make sure that they understand that their cell and online activities are not truly private or anonymous.
- Set rules for technology use, and make sure to include consequences for breaking the rules. Consider limiting the number of texts or other messages that they can send.
- Know whom your children are spending time with, online and on the phone.
- Monitor and limit their device use. The simplest way to do this is to keep tech toys out of their bedrooms. Keep computers, tablets, and other devices in an area where they can be monitored, and have cell phones and other interactive devices turned in before bedtime to prevent nightly text fests and potential sexting.
- If you are concerned that something is wrong, talk with your child. Monitor his or her computer and phone use. It is your right and obligation as a parent when your child's health and safety are compromised.

Resources

Connect Safely: www.connectsafely.org/tips-to-help-stop-cyberbullying/

Cyberbullying Research Center: http://cyberbullying.org/

National Crime Prevention Council: Cyberbullying: www.ncpc.org/topics/cyberbullying

Safe Teens: Teen Sexting Tips: www.safeteens.com/teen-sexting-tips/

School Superintendents Association: Sexting: http://aasa.org/content.aspx?id=3390

Stop Cyberbullying: www.stopcyberbullying.org/

References

Ang, R. P., & Goh, D. H. (2010). Cyberbullying among adolescents: The role of affective and cognitive empathy, and gender. *Child Psychiatry and Human Development, 41*, 387–397. doi:10.1007/s10578-010-0176-3

Bowker, A. (1999). Juveniles and computers: Should we be concerned? *Federal Probation, 63*(2), 40–43.

Bowker, A. (2000). The advent of the cyberdelinquent. *FBI Law Enforcement Bulletin, 69*(12), 7–11.

Döring, N. (2014). Consensual sexting among adolescents: Risk prevention through abstinence education or safer sexting? *Cyberpsychology: Journal of Psychosocial Research on Cyberspace, 8*(1), article 9. doi:10.5817/CP2014-1-9

Hinduja, S., & Patchin, J. W. (2014). *Cyberbullying fact sheet: Identification, prevention, and response.* Cyberbullying Research Center. Retrieved from http://cyberbullying.org/Cyberbullying-Identification-Prevention-Response.pdf

Kowalski, R., Giumetti, G., Schroeder, A., & Lattanner, M. (2014). Bullying in the digital age: A critical review and meta-analysis of cyberbullying research among youth. *Psychological Bulletin, 140*(4), 1073–1137. doi:10.1037/a0035618.

Marcum, C., Higgins, G., & Ricketts, M. (2014). Juveniles and cyber stalking in the United States: An analysis of theoretical predictors of patterns of online perpetration. *International Journal of Cyber Criminology, 8*(1), 47–56.

Martinez-Rather, K., & Vandiver, D. (2014). Sexting among teenagers in the United States: A retrospective analysis of identifying motivating factors, potential targets, and the role of a capable guardian. *International Journal of Cyber Criminology, 8*(1), 21–35.

Mishna, F., Cook, C., Gadalla, T., Daciuk, J., & Solomon, S. (2010). Cyber bullying behaviors among middle and high school students. *American Journal of Orthopsychiatry, 80*(3), 362–374. doi:10.1111/j.1939-0025.2010.01040.x

Mishna, F., Khoury-Kassabri, M., Gadalla, T., & Daciuk, J. (2012). Risk factors for involvement in cyber bullying: Victims, bullies and bully–victims. *Children and Youth Services Review, 34*, 63–70.

Modecki, K., Barber, B., & Vernon, L. (2013). Mapping developmental precursors of cyber-aggression: Trajectories of risk predict perpetration and victimization. *Journal of Youth and Adolescence, 42*, 651–661. doi:10.1007/s10964-012-9887-z

Molesworth, M., & Denegri-Knott, J. (2007). Cyberdelinquency. In G. Ritzer (Ed.), *Blackwell encyclopedia of sociology.* Retrieved from www.blackwellreference.com/public/tocnode?id=g978 1405124331_chunk_g97814051243319_ss1-204

National Institute of Justice. (2007). Stalking. Retrieved from www.nij.gov/topics/crime/stalking/pages/welcome.aspx

NYS Division of Criminal Justice Services. (n.d.). Cyber bullying: General information. Retrieved from www.criminaljustice.ny.gov/missing/i_safety/cyberbullying.htm

Patton, D., Eschmann, R., & Butler, D. (2013). Internet banging: New trends in social media, gang violence, masculinity and hip hop. *Computers in Human Behavior, 29*, A54–A59.

Pearson, C.M., Andersson, L., & Porath, C.L. (2000). Assessing and attacking workplace incivility. *Organizational Dynamics, 29*, 123-137.

Rice, E., Gibbs, J., Winetrobe, H., Rhoades, H., Plant, A., Montoya, J., & Kordic, T. (2014). Sexting and sexual behavior among middle school students. *Pediatrics, 134*(1), 2013–2991.

Rice, E., Rhoades, H., Winetrob, H., Sanchez, M., Montoya, J., Plant, A., & Kordic, T. (2012). Sexually explicit cell phone messaging associated with sexual risk among adolescents. *Pediatrics, 130*(4), 667–673.

Strassberg, D., McKinnon, R., Sustaíta, M., & Rullo, J. (2013). Sexting by high school students: An exploratory and descriptive study. *Archives of Sexual Behavior, 42*(1),15–21.

Temple, J., & Choi, H. (2014). Longitudinal association between sexting and sexual behavior. *Pediatrics, 134*(5), e1287–e1292.

U.S. Department of Justice Attorney's Office. (2015). Task Forces. Pittsburgh High Tech Crimes Task Force. Retrieved from www.justice.gov/usao-wdpa/task-forces#pitt_tech

Whitson, S. (2012). Teaching netiquette to kids. *Psychology Today.* Retrieved from https://www.psychologytoday.com/blog/passive-aggressive-diaries/201210/teaching-netiquette-kids

CHAPTER 9

Cybervictimization

A. Description

Cybervictims are those persons who are the targets of the perpetrators of cybercrimes, such as the sexual solicitation of minors on the Internet, and other negative behaviors conducted via communications technology. Other behaviors include cyberbullying, cyberstalking, and sexting harassment. Online victimization from harassment and sexual solicitation affects a relatively small part of the population when compared with victimizations such as assaults, child maltreatment, and property crimes, and it often occurs with offline victimization; however, cybervictimization can independently cause psychological distress (Mitchell, Finkelhor, Wolak, & Ybarra, 2011).

   a.   Online sexual solicitation of youth decreased in 2010, likely because of several factors. Youth have moved from chat rooms to social networking sites and may be limiting their contact to people they know, which can reduce unwanted sexual solicitations. Youth may also be more cautious because of Internet education, as well as the publicity surrounding the arrests and prosecutions of persons who commit Internet crimes against children (Jones, Mitchell, & Finkelhor, 2012). However, there are still children being victimized, and victimization can occur on social networking sites. These victimizations include solicitations to engage in sexual talk or activities (e.g., masturbating via webcam); aggressive solicitations that include offline contact or attempts for offline contact; and exposure to sexual materials online (Mitchell, Jones, Finkelhor, & Wolak, 2014).

   b.   While some youth may not be affected by cyberbullying, others can be devastated. Cyberbullying can be more harmful than traditional bullying because the victim may feel that there is no escape. Cyberbullying can take place any time of day or night and anywhere the child has a communication device, even the child's bedroom, which should be a place of safety. Hurtful material may be posted globally and become irretrievable. Unlike victims of traditional bullying, victims of cyberbullying may not know the identity of the bully, creating frustration, fear, and feelings of helplessness.

c.   Cyberstalking: Victims may be stalked via e-mail, instant messages, chat rooms, and social networking sites. Pereira and Matos (2015) stress the importance of adopting fear as a key criterion to the cyberstalking definition.

d.   Sexting harassment: Youth may discover that the sexual images they sent to a paramour have been forwarded to others and possibly posted on social media. This can lead to persistent sexual harassment from peers, which can lead to significant emotional harm to the youth whose images have been shared.

B. Assessment

a.   Risk factors: Children usually experience multiple and recurring risks, instead of a single risk factor. With sexual solicitation, girls are more likely to be targeted than boys, and adolescents are at greater risk than younger children. Personal risks include low self-esteem, susceptibility to persuasion, immaturity, mental health issues, and increased time spent online. Children with disabilities may still be marginalized online, and thus more susceptible. Dysfunctional family dynamics, lack of family cohesion, and social vulnerability can also increase risk (Whittle, Hamilton-Giachritsis, Beech, & Collings, 2013). Cyberbullying victims are more likely than nonvictims to spend multiple hours online each day. Youth at greater risk for sexual solicitation include those with sexual orientation concerns, those who have been sexually or physically abused, and those who take risks online (e.g., providing personal information in association with other risk behaviors, discussing sex online).

b.   Sexual solicitation focuses chiefly on older youth, ages 16 or 17, with youth ages 13 to 15 reporting being distressed by the solicitations. Few children were 11 to 12, and girls are targeted more often than boys. Few solicitations are reported to the authorities, chiefly because the youth did not view the solicitation as serious enough (Mitchell et al., 2014). Assessing for sexual solicitation via the Internet should be part of the routine assessment for sexual abuse, especially those youth in the target age group.

c.   Cyberbullying: Victims of cyberbullying suffer the same effects as those who are victimized by traditional bullying. Victims may exhibit signs of depression (such as lack of interest in school or pleasurable activities, changes in sleep and eating patterns, depressed mood, and withdrawal), develop school phobias, complain about somatic symptoms such as headaches and abdominal pain, or demonstrate aggressive behaviors. Victims of cyberbullying may not tell their parents about the problem for fear of losing their technical devices, which means they may simply suffer in silence.

d.   Cyberstalking: Not much is known about adolescent cyberstalking. However, in adults, the impact of cyberstalking seems to be similar to that of offline stalking.

Victims may feel anger, aggression, and hopelessness. They can experience sleep disturbance, distrust toward others, and inner unrest (DreBing, Bailer, Anders, Wagner, & Gallas, 2014).

e.   Sexting harassment: Youth at risk for victimization may experience mood disorder, suicide, adjustment reactions, somatic symptoms, or some form of psychiatric sequelae (Korenis & Billick, 2014). Health care providers should assess all youth regarding their use of technology, including whether or not they are sexting. Since most youth sext within the context of beginning or maintaining a romantic relationship, this discussion may be weaved into the assessment of their dating and sexual behaviors.

f.   Cybervictims may be reluctant to discuss their victimization because they are fearful of losing their technology privileges. They may also feel that cyberspace is "their world" and are not psychologically ready to discuss it with adults, regardless of the danger. Thus, the health care provider needs to gain the youth's trust to detect victimization (Carter & Wilson, 2015). Given the media exposure of youth who have committed suicide after sexting harassment and cyberbullying, it is prudent to assess cybervictims for suicidal ideation.

C. Diagnosis

Cybervictimization is associated with aggression, and cases of suicide have occurred in vulnerable youth. A victim of cyberbullying may also exhibit somatic symptoms (headaches, stomachaches, nausea) and sleep problems; college victims may exhibit problematic alcohol abuse.

D. Levels of Prevention/Intervention

a.   Primary

Teach youth how to minimize their risk of cybervictimization (modified from New York State Division of Criminal Justice Services [n.d.]):

- Know the risks; when you send something via e-mail or text, or post something on a website, there is no expectation of privacy.
- Be careful about the information you post online or send via text or e-mail.
- Friends today may be enemies tomorrow, and they may forward or post your sensitive information to someone else.
- If you break up with an intimate partner, change all your passwords.

- Keep intimate things private; do not post intimate photos anywhere, and do not e-mail them.
- Do not get too comfortable when in cyberspace, as you may do something you would not do face-to-face.

b. Secondary

Focus on at-risk youth. High levels of Internet use (e.g., at least 3 hours/day) is associated with multiple forms of cybervictimization. Stress Internet safety and the potential consequences. Talk with adolescents about the dangers of engaging in an online relationship with an adult. Acknowledge their interest in romantic relationships, but discuss the risks and criminal nature, as well as avoidance skills. Especially focus on youth at risk, including children who had been sexually abused, youth with sexual orientation concerns, and those youth who engage in high-risk-taking behavior online (Wolak, Finkelhor, Ybarra, & Mitchell, 2010).

c. Tertiary

School health care providers may be required to report cybervictimization and may be held criminally or monetarily liable if they fail to do so. All health care providers are mandated to report child abuse, as in the cases of online sexual exploitation.

E. Parenting Tips

a. Know the signs that your child may be a cybervictim: suddenly stops using his or her device(s), appears anxious when using device(s); appears anxious about being at school or outside; appears angry, depressed, or frustrated after using phone or media; becomes abnormally withdrawn; or avoids talking about online activities (Hinduja & Patchin, 2014). Other signs include: child spending large amounts of time online, especially at night; pornography on your child's computer; child receives phone calls from an adult you do not know; child receives gifts from someone you do not know; and child uses someone else's account (Federal Bureau of Investigation [FBI], n.d.).

b. Discuss the danger of sexual exploitation.

c. Not all children are honest about their online behavior. Learn the secretive language that children use, such as PAW (parents are watching), POS (parent over shoulder), PIR (parent in room), P911 (parent emergency), and LMIRL (let's meet in real life).

d. Should you suspect your child is communicating with a sexual predator: talk to your child about your suspicions; review your child's computer for any signs of sexual communication or pornography; use caller ID to determine who is calling your child; obtain a device to see what numbers are called from your home; monitor your child's live Internet communications, especially social networking sites. Contact your local police immediately for the following: your child or anyone at home receives child pornography; your child is sexually solicited; or your child receives sexually explicit images (FBI, n.d.).

e. Use apps that can prevent bullying (Apple and Android):

APP	URL	FEATURES
Substance Abuse and Mental Health Services Administration (SAMHSA)	http://store.samhsa.gov/apps/knowbullying/index.html	Conversation starters Tips for ages 7–13 and teens Warning signs Reminders Social media Section for educators
Cyberbully Hotline	www.cyberbullyhotline.com/mobile-app.html	Provides rapid response to cyberbullying
Professor Garfield Cyberbullying	https://learninglab.org/	Helps identify cyberbullying behavior Provides antibullying strategies
STOPit	http://stopitcyberbully.com/	Helps report and deter inappropriate behaviors Apps for K-12 and higher education

Resources

Center for Cyber Victim Counseling: www.cybervictims.org

Cyberbullying: http://kidshealth.org/teen/homework/problems/cyberbullying.html

CyberTipline: www.missingkids.org/cybertipline

Stop Cyberbullying: www.stopcyberbullying.org

References

Carter, J., & Wilson, F. (2015). Cyberbullying: A 21st century health care phenomenon. *Pediatric Nursing, 41*(3), 115–125.

DreBing, H., Bailer, J., Anders, A., Wagner, H., & Gallas, C. (2014). Cyberstalking in a large sample of social network users: Prevalence, characteristics, and impact upon victims. *Cyberpsychology, Behavior, and Social Networking, 17*(2), 61–67.

Federal Bureau of Investigation. (n.d.). *A parent's guide to internet safety.* Retrieved from www.fbi.gov/stats-services/publications/parent-guide/parentsguide.pdf

Hinduja, S., & Patchin, J. W. (2014). *Cyberbullying fact sheet: Identification, prevention, and response.* Cyberbullying Research Center. Retrieved from http://cyberbullying.org/Cyberbullying-Identification-Prevention-Response.pdf

Jones, L., Mitchell, K., & Finkelhor, D. (2012). Trends in youth Internet victimization: Findings from three youth Internet safety surveys 2000–2010. *Journal of Adolescent Health, 50*(20), 179–186.

Korenis, P., & Billick, S. (2014). Forensic implications: Adolescent sexting and cyberbullying. *Psychiatric Quarterly, 85*, 97–10. doi:10.1007/s11126-013-9277-z

Mitchell, K., Finkelhor, D., Wolak, J., & Ybarra, M. (2011). Youth internet victimization in a broader victimization context. *Journal of Adolescent Health, 48*(2), 128–134.

Mitchell, K., Jones, L., Finkelhor, D., & Wolak, J. (2014). *Trends in unwanted online experiences and sexting* (Final report). Durham, NH: Crimes Against Children Research Center, University of New Hampshire. Retrieved from www.unh.edu/ccrc/pdf/Full%20Trends%20Report%20Feb%202014%20with%20tables.pdf

New York State Division of Criminal Justice Services. (n.d.). "Sexting." Retrieved from www.criminaljustice.ny.gov/missing/i_safety/sexting-dangers-teens.htm

Pereira, F., & Matos, M. (2015, August). Cyber-stalking victimization: What predicts fear among Portuguese adolescents? *European Journal on Criminal Policy and Research*, 1–18. Advance online publication.

Whittle, H., Hamilton-Giachritsis, C., Beech, A., & Collings, G. (2013). A review of young people's vulnerabilities to online grooming. *Aggression and Violent Behavior, 18*, 135–146.

Wolak, J., Finkelhor, D., Ybarra, M., & Mitchell, K. (2010). Online "predators" and their victims: Myths, realities, and implications for prevention and treatment. *Psychology of Violence, 3*(8), 13–35. doi:10.1037/2152-0828.1.S.13

CHAPTER 10

Dangerous Driving

A. Description

From a public health perspective, motor vehicle accidents (MVAs) are one of the most serious health issues facing adolescents (National Research Council, Institute of Medicine, & Transportation Research Board Program Committee for a Workshop on Contributions from the Behavioral and Social Sciences in Reducing and Preventing Teen Motor Crashes, 2007).

a.   The Centers for Disease Control and Prevention (CDC, 2015) reported that the number of passenger vehicle drivers ages 16 to 19 involved in fatal crashes decreased by 55% (from 5,724 to 2,568) from 2004 to 2013. They also noted that possible contributors to the decline are graduated driver licensing (GDL), safer vehicles, less driving, and adolescents waiting longer to get their licenses. The percentage of students who drive varies substantially according to where they live, and driving prevalence was higher in the midwestern and mountain states; however, the number of teen drivers declined. This was attributed to a number of factors, including alternate transportation and graduated licensing, but it also represented the concern that other youths are obtaining their licenses after age 18. These youths may not be getting the amount of supervised driving practice they would have received at younger ages (CDC, 2015). Jacobsohn and colleagues (2012) found that most parents reported 50 to 75 hours of practice driving for their novice adolescent driver.

b.   Texting/e-mailing while driving remains a considerable problem, with more than 40% of youths surveyed in the 2013 Youth Risk Behavior Survey (YRBS) admitting to texting/e-mailing during the 30 days before the survey (Kann et al., 2014). Text messaging while driving can result in injuries and fatalities. Caird, Johnston, Willness, Asbridge, and Steel (2014) conducted a meta-analysis of 28 studies that included dependent variables such as eye movements, stimulus detection, reaction time, collisions, lane positioning, speed, and headway. They found that texting affects drivers' ability to effectively direct attention to the roadway, respond to vital traffic events, control a vehicle within a lane, and maintain speed and headway. Thus, texting compromises the safety of the driver, passengers, and other road users.

B. Assessment

a.   Risk factors: Several factors influence adolescent risk-taking, including ego-centrism. Adolescents devote tremendous attention to their own cognitive abilities, magnifying the importance of their own ideas and displaying a form of cognitive arrogance. As a result, they may refuse to listen to another person's view or advice. They focus so much on themselves that they develop their own personal fable, complete with feelings of infallibility (Elkind, 1967). Yet they also conform and take risks because "everyone else does it." These cognitions can result in careless attitudes about driving, when they think "nothing bad will ever happen to me."

b.   Risk-taking behavior and age form a lethal combination behind the wheel. The American Academy of Pediatrics Committee on Injury, Violence and Poison Prevention and its Committee on Adolescence (2006) and the National Research Council et al. (2007) identified reasons why adolescents are at greater risk for MVAs:

- Inexperience: Adolescents' overall judgment and decision-making processes are not fully developed. As novice drivers, they lack the experience and ability to perform several complex driving tasks, such as detecting and responding to hazards, controlling the vehicle, and integrating speed. Teens experience their highest rate of crashes during the first month after they get their licenses. These deficits disappear with years of experience, and the crash rate actually decreases quickly over their first 5 months of driving. Thus, experience, not age, is critical, and traditional drivers education programs tend to provide only 6 hours of actual driving training.

- Risk taking: The prefrontal cortex, which is responsible for executive decision making and impulse control, does not fully mature until the early- to mid-20s. Adolescents' driving habits may be highly influenced by emotions, peer pressures, and other stressors, predisposing them to take more risks. Males tend to be more prone to risk taking, particularly with speeding, for which the 15- to 20-year-old age group ranks highest in fatal crashes.

- Adolescent passengers: Adolescents have a greater chance of crashing when they have a friend in the car; the risk doubles with two passengers and nearly quadruples with three or more passengers. This passenger effect is not seen with adult drivers and is less pronounced with 18- and 19-year-old drivers. The presence of a male passenger results in the driver traveling at a higher speed and engaging in other risky behaviors regardless of whether the adolescent driver is male or female.

- Night driving is more difficult for new drivers, and teen drivers have a higher rate of nighttime crashes than other age groups. While nighttime driving curfews for younger drivers restrict adolescents from driving after midnight, the majority of fatal crashes happen within the 3 hours before midnight. These crashes are probably also associated with speeding, having teen passengers, and alcohol use, but fatigue and lack of experience also play possible roles.

- Substance use: Fatal teen alcohol-related crashes have decreased considerably, but adolescents drink and drive less than adults and still have higher crash rates when they drink, especially at low and moderate blood alcohol levels. The combination of even moderate combined alcohol and marijuana use can result in a substantial deterioration in driving performance, including slowed reaction time. Many prescription medications can have a damaging effect on driving ability, especially when mixed with alcohol.

- Seat belts: The risk of injury is higher in adolescents because of their lower rate of seat belt use; airbags alone are not adequate protection against injury.

- Vehicles: The seat belt usage problem can be intensified in rural areas, where pickup trucks can be prone to rollover on impact, roads are not as well maintained, and where medical assistance may be a great distance away. Adolescents are also more likely to drive older cars, which have fewer safety features than newer ones. Teens are also drawn to sports cars, which may enhance their urge to speed.

- Distractions contribute to crashes for all ages. Cell phone use (for phone calls), including hands-free models, increases crash risk, but is actually less risky than eating, drinking, and adjusting the climate control or radio. However, as noted earlier, texting or e-mailing while driving can prove to be fatal.

- Unlicensed drivers (regardless of whether the license has been revoked, suspended, or not yet earned) are usually male and young, and tend to have a fatal nighttime crash, recent conviction for driving while intoxicated, or multiple license suspensions.

- Attention deficit hyperactivity disorder (ADHD): Adolescent drivers with ADHD are more likely to be involved in a car crash than youths who do not have the disorder. They are also more likely to have repeat traffic citations and license suspensions or revocations. Driving performance seems to improve with psychostimulant medication, particularly longer acting controlled-release dosing, which can decrease errors related to inattentiveness. Teens with ADHD, as well as autistic spectrum disorder, experience more difficulties related to executive functions, visual–motor integration, and motor skills (Monahan, Classen, & Helsel, 2013).

- Sleep deprivation: Inadequate sleep increases the chance of crashing, especially if it interacts with other factors, such as speed, alcohol, texting, night driving, and inexperience.

c. Assess for readiness to drive. The National Research Council et al. (2007) described five critical elements that adolescents need to drive safely:

- Skills: The ability to operate the vehicle and to recognize hazards, as well as the capability to react appropriately to unexpected events.
- Knowledge: Traffic rules, operating procedures, and an understanding of risks and their potential consequences.
- Experience: Sufficient practice and familiarity with the consequences of bad judgment that fosters good judgment.
- Maturity: Capacity for reasoning, judgment, and decision making.
- Environment: Safe surroundings in which to learn to drive.

d. Assess general health status, since it can affect driving. Medication use, attention deficit, and substance abuse may interfere with driving ability and warrant intervention. A driver's license may be prohibited for a teen who has a newly diagnosed seizure disorder. Other problems are more subtle; for example, a youth with anorexia nervosa can have lowered blood pressure that may result in fainting, a serious hazard when driving.

e. Assessment questions can focus on judgment and decision-making skills, level of accountability, and safety knowledge. Ask what the youth would do if he or she received a text from a friend that warranted only a yes-or-no reply. Ask whether the youth rides with someone who has been drinking, and about his or her own use of drugs and alcohol, especially when driving. Ask how the youth would get home if he or she and friends used alcohol and the youth was driving. What would the youth do if he or she were driving a new girlfriend or boyfriend who offered a joint at a red light? Who is at fault if the youth crashes the car after his or her best friend gives the youth a couple of beers? Ask about the frequency of seat belt usage, and verify this with the parent or guardian if possible. Does the youth use seat belts every time or only on trips with parents? Does the youth insist that passengers wear seat belts? What would he or she do if a passenger refused? How would he or she respond in emergency situations, such as a tire blowout or skidding? Whom would the youth contact in an emergency, and how would he or she contact that person (Muscari, 1999)?

C. Diagnosis, Including Differential Diagnoses, When Appropriate

a. Rule out health problems that may cause driving difficulties, such as medications, attention difficulties, autistic spectrum disorder, and substance abuse (including binge drinking).

D. Levels of Prevention/Intervention

a. Primary

Talk to parents of young children about positive role modeling when driving. Riding in a vehicle with an impaired driver may increase a teen's chance of future driving while intoxicated (DWI) after licensure (Li, Simons-Morton, Vaca, & Hingson, 2014). Young drivers who held a higher perception of parents as not committed to safety and who experienced lower perceived parental monitoring had a higher rate of risky driving events (Taubman-Ben-Ari, Musicant, Lotan, & Farah, 2014).

b. Secondary

- Routine physical exams, such as those required when a teenager applies for a driver's permit, are golden opportunities for clinical interventions that can reduce teen driver crashes. Remind teens of the National Highway Traffic Safety Administration's "5 to Drive":
  - No cell phones while driving
  - No extra passengers
  - No speeding
  - No alcohol
  - No driving or riding without a seat belt
- For teens with attention deficit or autistic spectrum disorder, recommend referral to an occupational therapy (OT) driver rehabilitation program, in lieu of traditional driver's education. An OT program will provide a therapeutic approach to cognitive and executive functions, visual–motor integration.

c. Tertiary

Consider reducing driving risks by withholding your signature from the forms of teens who do not use seat belts or who have other unsafe driving-related behaviors and refusal to change. Always discuss the rationale for your decision, and develop a plan for constructive behavior changes with input from the adolescent and parents.

E. Parenting Tips

The Centers for Disease Control and Prevention (CDC; www.cdc.gov/parentsarethekey/danger/index.html) provides tips for parents to minimize teen crash risk by focusing on the eight danger zones:

a. Danger Zone #1: Driver Inexperience

- Provide at least 30 to 50 hours of supervised driving practice over at least 6 months.

- Practice on a variety of roads, at different times of day, and in varied weather and traffic conditions.
- Stress the importance of continually scanning for potential hazards including other vehicles, bicyclists, and pedestrians.

b.   Danger Zone #2: Driving With Teen Passengers

- Follow your state's GDL system for passenger restrictions. If your state does not have such a rule, limit the number of teen passengers your teen can have to zero or one.
- Keep this rule for at least the first 6 months that your teen is driving.

c.   Danger Zone #3: Nighttime Driving

- Make sure your teen is off the road by 9 or 10 p.m. for at least the first 6 months of licensed driving.
- Practice nighttime driving with your teen when you think your teen is ready.

d.   Danger Zone #4: Not Using Seat Belts

- Require your teen to wear a seat belt on every trip. This simple step can reduce your teen's risk of dying or being badly injured in a crash by about half.

e.   Danger Zone #5: Distracted Driving

- Do not allow activities that may take your teen's attention away from driving, such as talking on a cell phone, texting, eating, or playing with the radio.
- Learn more about distracted driving.

f.   Danger Zone #6: Drowsy Driving

- Young drivers are at high risk for drowsy driving, which causes thousands of crashes every year. Teens are most tired and at risk when driving in the early morning or late at night.
- Know your teen's schedule so you can be sure he or she is well rested before getting behind the wheel.

g.   Danger Zone #7: Reckless Driving

- Make sure your teen knows to follow the speed limit and adjusts his or her speed to match road conditions.
- Remind your teen to maintain enough space behind the vehicle ahead to avoid a crash in case of a sudden stop.

h.   Danger Zone #8: Impaired Driving

- Be a good role model: Never drink and drive.
- Reinforce this message with a Parent–Teen Driving Agreement.

- Learn more about impaired driving.
- Get the stats on teen drinking and driving.

Resources

American Academy of Pediatrics Parent-Teen Driving Agreement: www.cdc.gov/parentsarethekey/agreement/index.html

American Automobile Association (AAA) Teen Driver Safety: http://exchange.aaa.com/safety/teen-driver-safety/#.VkJqE7erRD8

American Occupational Therapy Association: www.aota.org/

Children's Hospital of Philadelphia Teen Driver Source: www.teendriversource.org/for_parents#pages

Contract to Drive: http://driveithome.org/get-involved-stay-involved/new-driver-deal/

Digital Driving Coach: http://driveithome.org/digital-driving-coach/

What Works: Motor Vehicle-Related Injury Prevention: www.thecommunityguide.org/about/What-Works-Motor-Vehicle-factsheet-and-insert.pdf

References

American Academy of Pediatrics Committee on Injury, Violence and Poison Prevention and Its Committee on Adolescence. (2006). The teen driver. *Pediatrics, 118*(6), 2570–2581. doi:10.1542/peds.2006-2830

Caird, J., Johnston, K., Willness, C., Asbridge, M., & Steel, P. (2014). A meta-analysis of the effects of texting on driving. *Accident Analysis & Prevention, 71*, 311–318.

Centers for Disease Control and Prevention. (2015). Driving among high school students—United States, 2013. *MMWR. Morbidity and Mortality Weekly Report, 64*(12), 313–317.

Elkind, D. (1967). Egocentrism in adolescents. *Child Development, 38*, 1025–1034.

Jacobsohn, L., García-España, J., Durbin, D., Erkoboni, D., & Winston, F. (2012). Adult-supervised practice driving for adolescent learners: The current state and directions for interventions. *Journal of Safety Research, 43*(1), 21–28.

Kann, L., Kinchen, S., Shanklin, S. L., Flint, K. H., Kawkins, J., Harris, W. A., . . . Centers for Disease Control and Prevention. (2014). Youth risk behavior surveillance—United States, 2013. *MMWR. Surveillance Summaries, 63*(Suppl. 4), 1–168.

Li, K., Simons-Morton, B., Vaca, F., & Hingson, R. (2014). Association between riding with an impaired driver and driving while impaired. *Pediatrics, 133*(4), 620–626.

Monahan, M., Classen, S., & Helsel, P. (2013). Pre-driving evaluation of a teen with attention deficit hyperactivity disorder and autism spectrum disorder. *Canadian Journal of Occupational Therapy, 80*(1) 35–41. doi:10.1177/0008417412474221

Muscari, M. (1999). Maximum mileage: Preventing teen auto deaths. *Advance for Nurse Practitioners, 7*(2), 61–62.

National Research Council, Institute of Medicine, and Transportation Research Board Program Committee for a Workshop on Contributions from the Behavioral and Social Sciences in Reducing and Preventing Teen Motor Crashes. (2007). *Preventing teen motor crashes: Contributions from the behavioral and social sciences, workshop report.* Washington, DC: The National Academies Press.

Taubman-Ben-Ari, O., Musicant, O., Lotan, T., & Farah, H. (2014). The contribution of parents' driving behavior, family climate for road safety, and parent-targeted intervention to young male driving behavior. *Accident Analysis and Prevention, 72*, 296–301.

CHAPTER 11

Depression and Suicidal Ideation

A. Description

Transient depression is common, especially among adolescents, but clinical depression is pervasive. Clinical depression is a common and debilitating problem during childhood, adolescence, and young adulthood, and most adult depression has roots in adolescence. It is a mood disorder manifested by overwhelming feelings of sadness, guilt, hopelessness, helplessness, loss of pleasure, fatigue and low energy, appetite and sleep changes, and thoughts of suicide.

a. The onset of puberty is associated with an increase in depression among adolescents, particularly among adolescent girls (Center for Behavior Health Statistics and Quality, 2012).

b. Development influences the expression of depressive symptoms. Young children may manifest irritability, as opposed to typical depressive features.

c. Primary care providers can have a huge impact on suicide prevention. Approximately 45% of suicide victims contacted their primary care physician within a month of their death (Luoma, Martin, & Pearson, 2002; Reed, n.d.), and up to 67% of persons who attempt suicide receive medical care as a result of their attempt (SAMHSA, 2012).

d. Suicide is a leading cause of death in people ages 15 to 24, and rates for younger teens are rising. Females attempt suicide more often than males, but males are more successful in actually committing suicide because they use more lethal weapons. Most victims of suicide have a psychiatric illness, particularly major depression or bipolar disorder. Other victims frequently had severe anxiety, exhibited violent and impulsive behavior, had no plans for the future, or were deficient in social skills. Most attempted suicides, and completed suicides are preceded by a precipitant, such as a relationship breakup, family or school violence, rejection, sexual abuse, pregnancy, or a sexually transmitted disease. Drugs and alcohol play a key role in suicide, as do exposure to suicide in family or friends, and availability of weapons. "Copycat" suicides remain common among teenagers, especially vulnerable ones.

B. Assessment

a. Risk factors for depression include a low socioeconomic status, family history of depression, low birth weight, maternal age under 18 years, parental conflict, emotional dependence, decreased physical activity, overeating, poor sleep patterns, ineffective coping skills, low self-esteem, negative body image, negative thinking styles, experiencing or witnessing abuse or violence (traumatic events in general), having a chronic medical illness or other psychiatric illness, poor peer relationships, antisocial peers, bullying victimization, poor school performance, loss of a relationship, and substance abuse. Stressful life events can potentially predict later depression in youth, including exposure to peer stress and the loss of a relationship. The risk of depression is higher in females and youth who are gay, lesbian, bisexual, or transgender (Clarke, Jansen, & Cloy, 2012; Cohen et al., 2015; Giardino, 2014).

b. The American Academy of Pediatrics and the U.S. Preventive Services Task Force (USPSTF) recommend routine annual screening for depression in adolescents (ages 12 through 18), provided that there are adequate systems in place for diagnosis, treatment, and monitoring; the USPSTF notes there is insufficient evidence to assess the balance between benefits and harms for screening children ages 7 to 11 (Corona, McCarty, & Richardson, 2013). Evidence was insufficient for routine screening of younger children in primary care; using screening tools for children with at least one risk factor may be more helpful than universal screening (B-level recommendation for ages 12 to 18; I-level for ages 11 and under; Clarke et al., 2012; USPSTF, 2015).

c. Depressed children become sad, losing interest in the activities that please them most. They criticize themselves and believe that others criticize them. They feel pessimistic, helpless, and unloved. They experience difficulty making decisions, have trouble concentrating, and may neglect their appearance and hygiene. Feelings of hopelessness can arise and evolve into thoughts or actions of suicide. Depressed children and teens often act irritable and sometimes become aggressive. Some teens feel a surge of energy, occupying every minute of their day with activity to avoid their depression. Depressed youths may become anxious and have separation fears, and they may have somatic complaints, such as headaches, stomachaches, and other aches and pains. But detecting depression in children can be difficult. Young children with depression may also have separation anxiety, which masks the symptoms of depression; adolescents may show temporary improvement when with peers. Youth of all ages may present with physical complaints and have difficulty identifying their mood states (Garland & Solomons, 2002).

d. Screening tests include:

- Child Depression Inventory 2 (CDI-2; www.mhs.com/product.aspx?gr=edu& id=overview&prod=cdi2) to evaluate depressive symptoms in youth ages 7 to 17.
- Beck Depression Inventory for Primary Care for adolescents ages 12 to 18 (copy with scoring available in: www.aafp.org/afp/2012/0901/p442.pdf).
- Reynolds Child Depression Scale (RCDS-2) for children ages 7 to 13 (needs to be purchased).
- Reynolds Adolescent Depression Scale, Second Edition (RADS-2) for youths age 11 to 20 years (needs to be purchased).

e. There are no specific laboratory tests for pediatric depression; however, other etiologies should be ruled out. Suggested testing includes: complete blood count with differential to look for anemia and infection; blood urea nitrogen, electrolytes, creatinine clearance, creatinine, and urine osmolality to rule out renal disorders; and triiodothyronine (T3), thyroxine (T4), and thyroid-stimulating hormone (TSH) to rule out thyroid disease.

f. Risk factors for suicide include: suicidal history (history of prior suicide attempts, aborted suicide attempts, or self-injurious behavior); current/past psychiatric disorders (mood disorders, anxiety disorders, psychotic disorders, alcohol/substance abuse, chronic pain, attention deficit hyperactivity disorder, traumatic brain injury, posttraumatic stress disorder, conduct disorder, borderline and antisocial personality disorders—comorbidity and recent onset of illness increase risk); key symptoms (anhedonia, impulsivity, hopelessness, anxiety/panic, insomnia, command hallucinations); family history (suicide attempts or psychiatric disorders requiring hospitalization); precipitants/stressors/interpersonal (triggering events leading to humiliation, shame, or despair [e.g., loss of relationship, work, financial or health status—real or anticipated], ongoing medical illness, intoxication, family turmoil/chaos, history of physical or sexual abuse, social isolation, bullying); change in treatment (discharge from psychiatric hospital, provider or treatment change); access to firearms or other lethal methods; local epidemics of suicide ("contagion factor"); and unwillingness to seek help (American Foundation for Suicide Prevention, 2015; Centers for Disease Control and Prevention [CDC], 2015; SAMHSA, n.d.). The risk of suicide is higher in youth who are gay, lesbian, bisexual, or transgender; military and veterans, youth in justice or welfare settings, youth who engage in nonsuicidal self-injury; and American Indians and Alaska Natives (SAMHSA, 2014).

g. Protective factors for suicide include: internal (problem-solving and conflict resolution skills; ability to cope with stress; cultural and religious beliefs; frustration tolerance) and external (responsibility to children or beloved pets; positive therapeutic relationships; social supports; effective treatment for mental, physical, and substance abuse disorders; SAMHSA, 2014).

h.   Warning signs of suicide include: talking about killing themselves, having no reason to live, being a burden, feeling trapped, or unbearable pain; increased substance use; searching online for ways to kill themselves; reckless behavior; aggression; rage; withdrawal; isolation; too much or too little sleep; visiting, calling, and texting people to say goodbye; giving away favorite possessions (American Foundation for Suicide Prevention, 2015).

i.   Health care providers should routinely screen for suicidal ideation and conduct a lethality assessment (thoughts, intent, and plan) to determine whether a youth is at risk and whether that risk is urgent or emergent. Assessment should include risk and protective factors, and a lethality assessment, ascertaining ideation (frequency, intensity, and duration), plan (timing, location, means, availability of means, preparation), behaviors (past attempts, aborted attempts, rehearsals, nonsuicidal injuries), and intent (extent to which youth expects to carry out plan and belief that plan will be lethal). Also explore reasons to die versus reasons to live (SAMHSA, n.d.).

The following chart is representative of risk and interventions, not actual determinations. This is to assist with assessment as there is no substitute for clinical judgment, best practice, and collateral professional collaboration.

	HIGH	MEDIUM	LOW
Risk factors	Psychiatric disorders	Multiple risks	Modifiable risk factors
	Acute precipitating event		
Protective factors	Not relevant	Few protective factors	Strong protective factors
Social supports	No resources	Limited	Adequate
	Unwilling to use	Limited willingness	Willing to access
	Isolated, withdrawn	Some social contacts	Regular social contacts
PLAN			
Time frame	Today	Within 7 days	Maybe sometime
Method	Thought out	Has an idea	Unclear
Availability	Has means	Can get means	Not readily available
Location	Chose location	Knows some places	Not planned

(continued)

	HIGH	MEDIUM	LOW
Chance of intervention	No one near; isolated	Others available if called	Others present most of time
Mood	Upset	Unsettled	Calm*
	Crying/agitated	Irritable/distracted	In control*
	Severely depressed	Moderately depressed	Situational sadness
BEHAVIORS			
Eating	Too much/too little	Has appetite	Normal
Health	Aches	No energy	Listless
Isolation	Wants to be alone	Alone at times	No
Recklessness	Risk taking	Considers risks	Safe behaviors
Sleep	Too much/too little	Tired/restless	Sleep problems rare
Talks of death	States desire for death	Has made comments	No comments made
Possessions	Gives them away	Plans to give away	No plans for possessions
EMOTIONS			
Depression	Overwhelming	Moderate	Mild
Helpless	Always	Sometimes	No
Worthless	Constantly	Sometimes	No
Restless	Yes; cannot focus	Easily distracted	No
Substance use	Daily	Regularly	Experimental
PRIOR ATTEMPTS			
Self	High lethality attempt or multiple moderate attempts	Previous low lethality attempt; threats	No prior suicidal behavior
Significant others	Recently committed suicide	Recently attempted suicide	No prior suicidal behavior

(continued)

	HIGH	MEDIUM	LOW
Possible interventions	Admission with suicide precautions, unless significant change in risk	Admission may be necessary, depending on risk	Outpatient referral
		Develop a crisis prevention plan	Symptom reduction
		Give emergency numbers	Give emergency numbers

*Can also mean the youth are calm and in control about their decision to commit suicide.
Developed from: California State University (n.d.); National Association of Secondary School Principals (2015); SAMHSA (n.d.); Syracuse University School of Education (n.d.).

j. Screening tools for suicide include the Suicide Assessment Five-step Evaluation and Triage (SAFE-T) by SAMHSA (www.integration.samhsa.gov/images/res/SAFE_T.pdf), the Columbia Suicide Severity Rating Scale (C-SSRS; http://cssrs.columbia.edu), and the Suicide Ideation Questionnaire (SIQ; www4.parinc.com/Products/Product.aspx?ProductID=SIQ).

C. Diagnosis

The most common mood disorders found in children and adolescents are major depressive disorder, reactive depression, dysthymic disorder, and bipolar disorder. Mood disorders such as depression increase the risk for suicide, which reaches its peak during the adolescent years. About two thirds of children and adolescents with depression also have another mental health disorder, such as an anxiety disorder, a disruptive or antisocial disorder, an eating disorder, or a substance abuse disorder. Sex differences for major depression emerge at ages 12 to 17 years with females being three times more likely than males to have had a major depressive episode in the past 12 months (Center for Behavior Health Statistics and Quality, 2012).

a. Diagnosing childhood depression is challenging at best, even for seasoned mental health care professionals, owing to both its heterogeneous presentation and its comorbidity with other disorders, including anxiety disorders, attention deficit hyperactivity disorder (ADHD), and conduct disorder (Allgaier et al., 2014). Major depressive disorder (MDD) is a serious condition that causes significant impairment in important life functions. The *Diagnostic and Statistical Manual of Mental*

Disorders, 5th Edition (*DSM-5*), published by the American Psychiatric Association (APA, 2013), identifies several behaviors as indicative of MDD. These include depressed mood, decreased interest in formerly pleasurable activities (anhedonia), significant appetite and weight change that can translate into failure to meet expected weight gain in growing children, persistent sleep disturbance, agitation or loss of energy, decreased inability to concentrate, and suicidal ideation. Childhood onset MDD may be a precursor of bipolar disorder, and thus health care providers should assess for symptoms that may indicate the development of a manic state (Giardino, 2014).

b. Persistent depressive disorder, formally called dysthymia, is similar to major depression, with fewer symptoms and a more chronic course. Because of its persistent nature, persistent depressive disorder tends to interfere with normal development. The child feels depressed for most of the day, on most days, and for several years, with an average duration of 4 years. Some are depressed for so long they do not recognize their state as abnormal and thus do not complain of being depressed. Characteristics of persistent depressive disorder include low energy or fatigue, changes in eating and/or sleeping patterns (too much or too little of either), poor concentration and hopelessness, and like MDD, the child may present with symptoms such as irritability, social withdrawal, and somatic complaints (Forrest, 2014). Most affected children eventually experience an episode of major depression.

c. Premenstrual dysphoric disorder (PMDD) indicates serious premenstrual suffering that interferes with social or occupational/academic functioning to the point where it causes significant distress requiring treatment. The *DSM-5* (APA, 2013) identifies several behaviors as indicative of PMDD. These include menstrual mood swings, irritability, fatigue, major appetite or sleep disturbances, and a feeling of being overwhelmed or out of control. The female may also experience headache, breast swelling or tenderness, joint or muscle pain, and bloating. It should be noted that not everyone is in agreement over terming this a disorder. For example, Browne (2015) considers it a socially constructed diagnosis, and notes that more research is needed and that women should not be labeled as mentally ill to have their distress taken seriously.

d. As per the *DSM-5* (APA, 2013), differentiate normal sadness and grief from depression. Bereavement can cause suffering, but it does not usually induce MDD. The two may coexist, but the symptoms and functional impairment are more severe, and the prognosis is worse compared with bereavement alone. MDD is most likely to be induced by bereavement in youth with other risks for depression (Halverson, 2015).

e. Medical differential diagnoses include: anemia, infection (e.g., mononucleosis, HIV), sleep disorders, chronic fatigue, hypoglycemia, thyroid disease, inflammatory bowel disease, collagen vascular disease, central nervous system disorder, and malignancy. Psychiatric differential diagnoses include ADHD, substance abuse, bipolar disorder, eating disorders, anxiety disorders, somatic disorders, conduct disorder, and psychotic disorders (Clarke et al., 2012; Giardino, 2014; Halverson, 2015).

D. Levels of Prevention/Intervention

a. Primary

Merry et al. (2011) examined randomized controlled trials of psychological and educational prevention programs for youths ages 5 to 19 and found that, compared with no intervention, depression prevention programs were effective, showing a decrease in episodes of depressive illness over a year; data supported both targeted and universal programs. They did recommend further research to identify the most effective programs.

b. Secondary

Effective treatment of depressive disorders warrants identification of at-risk youth, especially those who have a first-degree relative with depression, and early detection (Garland & Solomons, 2002). Prevention of suicide warrants identification of at-risk youth, monitoring for warning signs, and early intervention.

c. Tertiary

Initial treatment depends upon age, severity, number of previous episodes, chronicity, contextual issues (e.g., exposure to adverse childhood experiences [ACEs], family conflict, academic problems), previous response and adherence to treatment, and motivation. Current evidence-based interventions include cognitive behavioral therapy (CBT), pharmacotherapy, or a combination of both for children and adolescents with MDD. Safety is a priority, and risk assessment should be ongoing (Giardino, 2014). Children and adolescents with mild depression can be managed with symptom monitoring and active support. Those with moderate-to-severe depression can be treated with psychotherapy and/or antidepressants, which may involve referral to a mental health professional. Little is known about treating children under age 12, who may be candidates for earlier referral to mental health specialty care (Cheung, Kozloff, & Sacks, 2013).

- Active monitoring is preferred over watchful waiting to discourage passivity and encourage what primary care providers can do before formal treatment. Primary care providers can: work with the teen to develop self-management goals and to review his or her progress on these goals regularly; schedule frequent visits; promote healthy lifestyle and stress management techniques; recommend a peer support group; follow up via telephone or electronically; and provide educational materials. Psychoeducation is critical and can include understanding the disorder and its treatments, warning signs of suicide, addressing modifiable risk factors, availability of services, removal or securing of weapons, and how to access care after hours (crisis hotlines, emergency departments). Parents should also be informed of behaviors that require immediate provider contact, such as suicidal ideation, impulsivity, irritability, restlessness, pressured speech, or psychomotor agitation (Clarke et al., 2012; Zuckerbrot et al., 2007).

- CBT, one of the best supported therapies for depression and a therapy found effective in the treatment of childhood depression, rests on the belief that one's thoughts, feelings, and behaviors affect one another. Negative thoughts induce negative feelings that predispose to and/or are exacerbated in depression. The goal of CBT is to modify the negative thoughts and behaviors to break the depressive cycle. Important elements of CBT include increasing pleasurable activities (behavioral activation), building coping skills, improving communication skills, reducing negative thoughts (cognitive restructuring), and improving problem-solving skills and assertiveness to reduce hopelessness (Clarke et al., 2012; Zuckerbrot et al., 2007).

- Interpersonal therapy for adolescents (IPT-A), which shows good support, is founded on the principle that depression occurs in an interpersonal context. The goal of IPT-A is to identify and manage the interpersonal problems that contribute to or result from the patient's depression. Critical elements of IPT-A include identifying interpersonal problem areas, improving interpersonal problem-solving skills, and modifying communication patterns (Clarke et al., 2012; Zuckerbrot et al., 2007).

- Psychopharmacology is used when the youth have: moderate and severe depression, a prior episode of depression, previous medication treatment for depression, family history of depression, family history of depression with substantial response to medication, modification of environmental stressors without improvements in mood, or evidence-based psychotherapy (such as CBT, IPT-A) that has been unsuccessful. The selective serotonin reuptake inhibitors (SSRIs) fluoxetine and escitalopram are the only FDA-approved medications for MDD in youths, and there is superior efficacy when combined with CBT. Given the reports of suicide with SSRIs and depression, clients should be carefully monitored (Clarke et al., 2012; Zuckerbrot et al., 2007).

- Depression treatment should continue for 6 months after remission.

- If there is limited improvement with first-line medications, chronic depression, or comorbid substance abuse, psychiatric consultation is strongly recommended (Clarke et al., 2012). Indications for hospitalization are major depression with psychotic features and people with significant suicidal risk, including those for whom an outpatient safety plan is not feasible (Giardino, 2014).

- Intervention for suicidal youth: low risk (crisis intervention, safety planning, outpatient referral, symptom reduction, give emergency numbers); moderate risk (admission may be necessary; depending on risk, develop a crisis prevention plan and give emergency numbers); and high risk (admission with suicide precautions, unless significant change in risk; California State University, n.d.; National Association of Secondary School Principals, 2015; SAMHSA, n.d.; Syracuse University School of Education, n.d.).

E. Parenting Tips

Teach parents how to prevent suicide (American Academy of Pediatrics, 2015; Nevada Division of Public and Behavioral Health Office of Suicide Prevention, n.d.):

a.   Trust your instincts. If you think your child is in trouble, you are probably right.

b.   Talk with your teen, making plenty of time to listen to him or her—both what is and what is not said.

c.   Share your feelings, and let your teen know he or she is not alone.

d.   Encourage healthy stress management—proper eating, exercise, activity, and rest.

e.   Spend quality (and quantity) time with your child.

f.   Develop a good relationship with your child.

g.   Provide a safe and stable emotional and physical home environment.

h.   Be supportive, not intrusive.

i.   Encourage healthy expression of emotions.

j.   Take all threats of self-harm and suicide seriously.

k.   Watch for warning signs, and call your health care provider if you notice that your child:

- Appears sad, depressed, irritable, or hostile
- Neglects appearance
- Alters eating or sleeping habits
- Engages in risky behaviors
- Focuses on songs, literature, movies, or art about death, separation, and loss
- Gives away prized possessions to siblings or friends
- Hints that he or she might not be around anymore
- Loses interest in favorite things or activities

- Shows trouble concentrating or thinking clearly
- Talks about feeling hopeless or guilty
- Talks about suicide or death
- Uses drugs or alcohol
- Withdraws from friends or family
- Hurts himself or herself (cutting, severe dieting)
- Exhibits any suicidal behavior

1. Make sure firearms are stored safely, or move them elsewhere until the crisis is over.

Resources

Depression

American Academy of Child and Adolescent Psychiatry, Depression Resource Center: www.aacap.org/AACAP/Families_and_Youth/Resource_Centers/Depression_Resource_Center/Home.aspx

Guidelines for Adolescent Depression in Primary Care (GLAD-PC) toolkit: www.gladpc.org

National Institutes of Health, Depression: www.nimh.nih.gov/health/topics/depression/index.shtml

Suicide

American Association of Suicidology: www.suicidology.org

American Psychiatric Nurses Association Psychiatric-Mental Health Nurse Essential Competencies for Assessment and Management of Individuals at Risk for Suicide: www.apna.org/i4a/pages/index.cfm?pageID=5684

Emergency Nurses Association Clinical Practice Guideline: www.ena.org/practice-research/research/CPG/Documents/SuicideRiskAssessmentCPG.pdf

Mental Health America: www.nmha.org

National Hopeline Network (http://hopeline.com): 1-800-SUICIDE (1-800-784-2433)

National Suicide Prevention Lifeline (www.suicidepreventionlifeline.org): 1-800-273-TALK (1-800-273-8255)

Nineline (www.covenanthouse.org/homeless-youth-programs/nineline): (1-800) 999-9999 (specializes in homeless youth)

SAMHSA-HRSA Center for Integrated Health Solutions Suicide Prevention in Primary Care: www.integration.samhsa.gov/about-us/esolutions-newsletter/suicide-prevention-in-primary-care

Suicide Prevention Education Association: www.helppreventsuicide.org

Suicide Prevention Resource Center: www.sprc.org

Suicide Prevention Resource Center, Suicide Prevention Toolkit for Rural Primary Care: www.sprc .org/for-providers/primary-care-tool-kit?sid=508

Trevor Helpline (www.thetrevorproject.org): 1-800-850-8078 (specializes in LGBTQ youth suicide prevention)

U.S. Surgeon General and the National Action Alliance for Suicide Prevention 2012 National Strategy for Suicide Prevention, Goals and Objectives for Action: www.surgeongeneral.gov/library/reports/ national-strategy-suicide-prevention/full_report-rev.pdf

References

Allgaier, A., Krick, K., Opitz, A., Saravo, B., Romanos, M., & Schulte-Kome, G. (2014). Improving early detection of childhood depression in mental health care: The Children's Depression Screener (ChilD-S). *Psychiatric Research, 217*(3), 248–252. doi:10.1016/j.psychres.2014.03.037

American Academy of Pediatrics. (2015). *10 things parents can do to prevent suicide.* Retrieved from www.healthychildren.org/English/health-issues/conditions/emotional-problems/Pages/Ten-Things-Parents-Can-Do-to-Prevent-Suicide.aspx

American Foundation for Suicide Prevention. (2015). *Suicide risk factors.* Retrieved from www.afsp. org/understanding-suicide/suicide-risk-factors

American Psychiatric Association. (2013). *Diagnostic and statistical manual of mental disorders* (5th ed.). Washington, DC: Author.

Browne, T. (2015). Is premenstrual dysphoric disorder really a disorder? *Bioethical Inquiry, 12,* 313–330. doi:10.1007/s11673-014-9567-7

California State University. (n.d.). *Suicide risk assessment summary sheet.* Retrieved from www.csus .edu/indiv/b/brocks/Workshops/District/2.Suicide%20Risk%20Assessment%20Summary.pdf

Center for Behavior Health Statistics and Quality. (2012). Depression triples between the ages of 12 and 15 among adolescent girls. In: *Data Spotlight.* Rockville, MD: Substance Abuse and Mental Health Services Administration. Retrieved from www.samhsa.gov/data/sites/default/files/NSDUH-SP77-AdolescentGirlsDepression-2012/CBHSQ-NSDUH-Spotlight-077-AdolescentGirlsDepression-2012.pdf

Centers for Disease Control and Prevention. (2015). *Suicide: Risks for suicide.* Retrieved from www.cdc.gov/ViolencePrevention/suicide/riskprotectivefactors.html

Clarke, M., Jansen, K., & Cloy, A. (2012). Treatment of childhood and adolescent depression. *American Family Physician, 86*(5), 442–448.

Cohen, J., Spiro, C., Young, J., Gibb, B., Hankin, B., & Abela, J. (2015). Interpersonal risk profiles for youth depression: A person-centered, multi-wave, longitudinal study. *Journal of Abnormal Child Psychology, 43*, 1415–1426. doi:10.1007/s10802-015-0023-x

Corona, M., McCarty, C., & Richardson, L. (2013, July 1). Screening adolescents for depression. In: *Contemporary Pediatrics.* Retrieved from http://contemporarypediatrics.modernmedicine.com/contemporary-pediatrics/content/tags/depression/screening-adolescents-depression

Cheung, A.H., Kozloff, N., & Sacks, D. (2015). Pediatric depression: An evidence-based update on treatment interventions. *Current Psychiatry Reports, 15*, 381–388. doi 10.1007/s11920-013-0381-4

Forrest, J. (2014). Pediatric dysthymic disorder. *Medscape Emedicine.* Retrieved from http://emedicine.medscape.com/article/913941-overview

Garland, E., & Solomons, K. (2002). Early detection of depression in young and elderly people. *BCMJ, 44*(9), 469–472.

Giardino, A. (2014). Pediatric depression. In: *Medscape Emedicine.* Retrieved from http://emedicine.medscape.com/article/914192-overview

Halverson, J. (2015). Depression. In: *Medscape Emedicine.* Retrieved from http://emedicine.medscape.com/article/286759-overview

Luoma, J., Martin, C., & Pearson, J. (2002). Contact with mental health and primary care providers before suicide: a review of the evidence. *American Journal of Psychiatry, 159*(6), 909–916.

Merry, S., Hetrick, S., Cox, G., Brudevold-Iversen, T., Bir, J., & McDowell, H. (2011). Psychological and educational interventions for preventing depression in children and adolescents. *Cochrane Database of Systematic Reviews, 2011*(12). doi:10.1002/14651858.CD003380.pub3

National Association of Secondary School Principals. (2015). *A school suicide lethality assessment.* Retrieved from www.principals.org/Content.aspx?topic=A_School_Suicide_Lethality_Assessment

Nevada Division of Public and Behavioral Health Office of Suicide Prevention. (n.d.). *What can parents do to prevent youth suicide?* Retrieved from http://suicideprevention.nv.gov/Youth/WhatYouCanDo/

Reed, J. (n.d.). *Primary care: A crucial setting for suicide prevention.* Washington, DC: SAMHSA-HRSA Center for Integrated Health Solutions. Retrieved from www.integration.samhsa.gov/about-us/esolutions-newsletter/suicide-prevention-in-primary-care

SAMHSA. (n.d.). *SAFE-T: Suicide assessment five-step evaluation and triage.* Retrieved from www .integration.samhsa.gov/images/res/SAFE_T.pdf

SAMHSA. (2012). Results from the 2010 National Survey on Drug Use and Health: Mental Health Findings. Center for Behavioral Health Statistics and Quality, Substance Abuse and Mental Health Services Administration, U.S. Department of Health and Human Services. http://archive.samhsa.gov/ data/NSDUH/2k10MH_Findings/2k10MHResults.htm#2.3

SAMHSA. (2014). *Populations at risk for suicide.* Retrieved from www.samhsa.gov/suicide-prevention/ at-risk-populations

Syracuse University School of Education. (n.d.). *Determination of risk and intervention.* Retrieved from http://soe.syr.edu/academic/counseling_and_human_services/modules/Suicide_Risk/determi nation_of_risk_and_intervention.aspx

U.S. Preventive Services Task Force. (2015). *Draft evidence review for depression in children and adolescents: Screening.* Retrieved from www.uspreventiveservicestaskforce.org/Page/Document/ draft-evidence-review110/depression-in-children-and-adolescents-screening1

Zuckerbrot, R. A., Cheung, A.H., Jensen, P.S., Stein, R.E., & Laraque, D. (2007). GLAD-PC Steering Group. Guidelines for adolescent depression in primary care (GLAD-PC): I. Identification, assessment, and initial management. *Pediatrics,* 120(5), e1299-e1312.

CHAPTER 12

Disordered Eating and Body Image

A. Description

Healthy body image is critical to adolescent development, and teens often diet and worry about their weight and appearance. However, for some youth these concerns become fixed and distorted, resulting in psychopathology. Eating disorders, particularly binge-eating disorder, anorexia nervosa, and bulimia nervosa, are serious, complex chronic disorders, which can be life-threatening. Body dysmorphic disorder results in a persistent fixation on one's appearance to the point of functional impairment. These disorders usually begin during adolescence, but can begin during mid to late childhood.

    a. Anorexia nervosa is a potentially life-threatening disorder that has been called the relentless pursuit of thinness. Affected youth refuse to maintain a body weight at or above a minimally normal weight for their height and age. They weigh less than one-fifth their normal weight for their height, build, and age, yet they firmly believe that they are overweight. Anorectics have intense fear of gaining weight or becoming fat, even when underweight, as well as a disturbance in the way in which their body weight or shape is experienced; females may have missed at least three consecutive menstrual cycles. This body image disturbance can range from a mild distortion to a severe delusion and is not related to the degree of weight loss. These teens may be preoccupied with their entire body or a specific body area, such as the abdomen, thighs, and buttocks.

    b. Bulimia nervosa signifies the chaotic eating patterns that characterize this disorder. Bulimic individuals have recurrent binge-eating episodes during which they eat a relatively large amount of food in a short period of time, feeling out of control during the binge. These episodes are accompanied by repeated compensatory mechanisms to prevent weight gain, including self-induced vomiting, laxative and/or diuretic abuse, ipecac (medication to induce vomiting) abuse, fasting, and excessive exercise. Like anorectics, bulimics are constantly concerned with their body shape and weight. Bulimic individuals develop an intense preoccupation with food that progressively interferes with their educational, vocational, and/or social activities. Shame follows their binging, and they are usually quite distressed by their symptoms. Bulimic individuals are also at risk for impulsive behaviors such as substance abuse, shoplifting, and promiscuity, increasing their chances for chemical dependency and sexually transmitted diseases.

c.   Binge-eating disorder (BED), which became a formal diagnosis in the *Diagnostic and Statistical Manual of Mental Disorders, 5th Edition* (*DSM-5;* American Psychiatric Association [APA], 2013) and is the most common eating disorder, results in a person frequently consuming large amounts of food and feeling unable to stop eating. The affected adolescent feels shame about the behavior, wants to stop, but is unable to do so.

d.   The main characteristic of body dysmorphic disorder (BDD) is persistent and intrusive preoccupations with a real but minor or imagined defect in one's appearance. These youths see themselves as ugly and tend to avoid social interactions with others from fear that others will notice their flaws, significantly interfering with normal adolescent development with high levels of distress and suicidal ideation and attempts (Phillips et al., 2006).

e.   Eating disorders are serious problems that are associated with a high mortality rate. Eating disorders can create numerous physical complications: anemia, constipation, bloating, heart damage, and sudden death. Hypotension can result in dizziness and fainting. Amenorrhea, along with low calcium intake, can lead to osteoporosis well before they reach middle age. These adolescents may not be able to concentrate and may be moody and withdrawn. Binging can lead to stomach rupture and obesity with its associated problems. Enlarged saliva glands result from overuse because of binging and irritation from the stomach acid bath of vomiting. At the least, self-induced vomiting can cause dental decay, but it can also lead to erosion of the esophagus and serious electrolyte imbalance, particularly potassium depletion, which can produce fatal heart arrhythmias. Some teens with bulimia resort to using syrup of ipecac to induce vomiting. They may take excessive dosages, which can prove fatal because ipecac is cardiotoxic. Some resort to other purgative measures to lose weight, including laxative or diuretic abuse, diet pills, and even enemas. All of these can lead to various problems, including dehydration and electrolyte imbalance. Psychiatric complications/comorbidities of eating disorders include mood disorders, anxiety, substance abuse, and suicide.

f.   Males also suffer from these disorders and may go undetected since they have been seen as "female disorders" (an issue addressed when the diagnostic criteria were revised for the *DSM-5*). Although the literature is sparse regarding adolescent males and BDD, adult males also obsess about their hair, but tend to focus on their genitals and body build, may excessively lift weights, and have substance abuse disorders (Phillips, Menard, & Fay, 2006). Surprisingly, there is still minimal research on male eating disorders.

B. Assessment

a. Risk factors include: family history of eating or mood disorders or substance abuse, poor self-esteem, restrictive dieting, weight changes, transitional or situational stressors. More research is needed to ascertain differences, if any, in risk between males and females with eating disorders; however, there is some evidence that males reported less somatization, obsessive-compulsivity, interpersonal sensitivity, and anxiety, but no differences in binging, vomiting, laxative and diet pill use, or substance abuse (Mazzeo & Bulik, 2009; Raevuori, Keski-Rahkonen, & Hoek, 2014; Welch, Ghaderi, & Swenne, 2015). Post-traumatic stress disorder (PTSD) and depression were associated with BED in male veterans (Raevuori et al., 2014).

b. Further attention is required for evidence of excessive weight concern, inappropriate dieting, patterned weight loss, amenorrhea, or failure to achieve appropriate height and weight increases (Rosen & The Committee on Adolescence, 2010).

c. Manifestations (Ahmed, 2014; Bernstein, 2014, 2015; Rosen & The Committee on Adolescence, 2010; Yager, 2014):

- Signs common to anorexia and bulimia nervosa: distorted body image, preoccupation with body shape and weight.
- Signs of anorexia nervosa include: extreme weight loss (take into account weight that should have been gained with growth), history of amenorrhea, difficulty concentrating and making decisions, fainting or dizziness, lethargy, food obsessions, constipation, flat or anxious affect, irritability, resting bradycardia, hypotension, orthostatic lowered pulse and blood pressure, hypothermia, acrocyanosis, cold extremities, dry skin, hypercarotenemia, lanugo, peripheral edema, thinning hair, facial atrophy, breast atrophy, click or murmur (mitral valve prolapse), and delayed or interrupted puberty. Clients with anorexia nervosa also may display perfectionism, lack of age-appropriate sexual activity, denial of hunger even when starving, dependency, immaturity, social isolation, and obsessive-compulsive behavior.
- Signs of bulimia include: feelings of being out of control with eating behavior; binge eating; using dietary supplements, herbal products or enemas to lose weight; self-induced vomiting; history of amenorrhea, lightheadedness, dizziness, palpitations (related to dehydration, possible hypokalemia), abdominal pain, blood in vomitus, trouble swallowing, constipation/obstipation, bloating,

Russell sign (calluses on knuckles from self-induced emesis), sialoadenitis (parotitis most frequently reported), angular stomatitis, palatal scratches, oral ulcerations, dental enamel erosions, pharyngeal irritation, arrhythmia.

- Signs of BED include: overweight or obesity (but may be normal weight); binging in response to emotional triggers; eating large amounts of food in a discrete time period; eating rapidly during binges; eating until uncomfortably full; and feeling guilty, ashamed, or depressed about eating. The youth do not regularly compensate for extra calories through purging or excessive exercise.

- Signs of BDD include preoccupation with one or more body areas (usually face, hair, skin, nose, chest, and abdomen) with the perception that the body part(s) is/are abnormal without evidence of physiological illness. They firmly believe that they are deformed, despite their "flaws" not being visible to others. Youths with BDD may perform compulsive behaviors to try to hide their perceived flaws, including camouflage (make-up, clothing), avoiding mirrors, and seeking plastic surgery. Some also engage in skin picking. They experience a high level of distress, including suicidal ideation. BDD can remit and exacerbate, with the focus shifting from one body part to another over time.

d. Screening test: The SCOFF questionnaire (Morgan, Reid, & Lacey, 1999) screens for anorexia and bulimia, awarding 1 point for each positive response. A score of 2 or more is likely indicative of anorexia or bulimia:

- Do you make yourself Sick because you feel uncomfortably full?
- Do you worry you have lost Control over how much you eat?
- Have you lost more than One stone (approximately 15 pounds) in a 3-month period?
- Do you believe yourself to be Fat when others say you are too thin?
- Would you say that Food dominates your life?

e. Diagnostic testing: While there are no definitive diagnostic tests, testing is warranted because of the physiological effects of some of these disorders. Initial testing should include complete blood count, complete chemistry panel, and urinalysis. Usually, results are normal; other findings/suggestions are as follows (Ahmed, 2014; Bernstein, 2014, 2015; Rosen & The Committee on Adolescence, 2010; Yager, 2014):

- If the physical examination for a client with BED suggests medical conditions, conduct appropriate testing for disorders such as hypothyroidism and Prader–Willi syndrome.

- There are no specific diagnostic tests for BDD; however, clients considering cosmetic surgery should be first evaluated for BDD by a psychiatric professional since they are usually unsatisfied with the results and present with new complaints after the procedure.

DIAGNOSTIC TESTING	ANOREXIA	BULIMIA
Complete blood count	Low WBC Thrombocytopenia	Normal; exclude anemia or occult hematological problems
Comprehensive blood chemistry panel	Hyponatremia: excess water intake or the inappropriate secretion of antidiuretic hormone Hypokalemia: diuretic or laxative use Hypoglycemia: lack of glucose precursors in the diet or low glycogen stores; may also be because of impaired insulin clearance Elevated blood urea nitrogen (BUN): dehydration Liver functions may be mildly elevated High cholesterol noted in starvation	Hyperamylasemia: significant vomiting because of hypersecretion of the salivary glands Hypokalemic metabolic alkalosis: severe vomiting Normokalemic metabolic acidosis: laxative abuse rule out hyponatremia, hypocalcemia, hypophosphatemia, and hypomagnesemia
Serum vitamin D	Obtain if osteoporosis suspected	
Pregnancy test	Always rule out pregnancy in amenorrhea	
Urinalysis	Specific gravity elevated in dehydration	
Urine toxicology	Assess for comorbid substance abuse	
Electrocardiogram (for any cardiovascular symptoms, electrolyte abnormalities, or significant weight loss or purging)	QT-interval prolongation may indicate risk for cardiac arrhythmias and sudden death Sinus bradycardia, ST-segment elevation, T-wave flattening, low voltage, and rightward QRS axis may be noted, but are considered clinically insignificant	
Bone densitometry	Consider for females who have amenorrhea for more than 6 to 12 months	

C. Diagnosis

a.   Body image is dynamic and shaped by perceptions, emotions, physical sensations, and external influences, including family, peers, and the media. Puberty intensifies body image concerns, especially when it occurs earlier or later than expected norms. Nonpathological body image concerns are not obsessive, and they do not interfere with the youth's activities of daily living. Males can be just as concerned with body image as females, usually focusing on society's image of a perfect muscular male.

b.   Referred to as the "relentless pursuit of thinness," anorexia nervosa is a potentially life-threatening disorder. The *DSM-5* (APA, 2013) identifies several behaviors as indicative of anorexia nervosa. These include disturbance in how one's body weight or shape is perceived (e.g., believing one is fat even when emaciated), fear of gaining weight, and restriction of energy intake. Youth may solely restrict intake or may binge/purge. Anorexia nervosa is staged as mild (mild body image distortion, weight loss 90% or less of weight for height, no signs of excessive weight loss, and use of potentially harmful weight control measures), and moderate/established (definite body image distortion, weight loss 85% of weight for height with weight gain refusal, signs of excessive weight loss with denial of the same, uses unhealthy means to lose weight; Bernstein, 2014).

c.   The term "bulimia" is derived from the Greek *boulimia* for ox or extreme hunger. Bulimia nervosa is characterized in the *DSM-5* by binge eating; feeling out of control during the binging; and compensatory measures to counteract weight gain, including self-induced vomiting, laxative and/or diuretic abuse, extreme dieting, and compulsive exercise. Persons with bulimia nervosa also have distorted views of their body weight (APA, 2013).

d.   Although first recognized in the 1950s, BED was only recently branded as a psychiatric disorder. According to the *DSM-5*, BED is characterized by binge-eating episodes and a feeling of lack of control and significant distress over the binging (APA, 2013). People with BED are usually ashamed of their behaviors and attempt to conceal them from others (Bernstein, 2015).

e.   BDD is a preoccupation with an imagined physical flaw or a disproportionate concern over a slight actual irregularity. The affected individual engages in repetitive thoughts or behaviors in response to the body image concern, and experiences considerable distress due to it. Consistent with the repetitive thoughts and behaviors, BDD is classified in the obsessive-compulsive and related disorders section of the *DSM-5* (Ahmed, 2014; APA, 2013).

f.   Differential diagnoses for eating disorders include: cardiac valvular disease, malabsorption syndromes; inflammatory bowel disease; chronic infections; thyroid disease; hypopituitarism, Addison disease; central nervous system lesions; cancer; and other psychiatric disorders including depression, obsessive-compulsive disorder, anxiety, and substance abuse (Bernstein, 2014, 2015; Yager, 2014). Differential diagnoses for BDD are social phobia, panic disorder, obsessive-compulsive disorder, premenstrual dysphoric disorder, avoidant and narcissistic personality disorders, PTSD, dysthymia, major depression, and chronic depression (Ahmed, 2014; Phillips et al., 2006).

g. Comorbidity is very common in eating disorders, including: mood disorders, obsessive-compulsive disorder, somatization disorder, substance abuse, and personality disorders (typically cluster B disorders [dramatic/erratic] with bulimia, and cluster C disorders [avoidant/anxious] with anorexia). Eating disorders have been found in youth with type 1 diabetes. They engage in typical eating disordered behaviors and may also underdose or omit insulin to induce hyperglycemia; these behaviors increase both short- and long-term diabetic-related complications, including diabetic ketoacidosis, retinopathy, neuropathy, and nephropathy, creating a higher mortality (Colton et al., 2015). BDD has a strong association with obsessive-compulsive disorder (OCD).

D. Levels of Prevention/Intervention

a. Primary

Health care providers can promote healthy development, encourage healthy eating habits, reinforce healthy body image, foster open communications between parents and child, and promote healthy self-esteem. Use caution when counseling regarding obesity prevention, and avoid statements such as "You may want to lose a little weight." There are a variety of successful prevention programs developed for various settings. Programs that target high-risk populations and that are interactive, multisession, and aimed at older adolescents appear to be most effective (Rosen & The Committee on Adolescence, 2010).

b. Secondary

- Secondary prevention focuses on early detection and intervention. Health care providers should observe and screen for the risks and subtle signs of these disorders and begin initial counseling and education regarding healthy nutrition.

c. Tertiary

- Eating disorders are difficult to treat, especially when presenting with comorbid diagnoses, and treatment depends on the severity of the illness. Primary health care providers play a critical role in assessment, monitoring of treatment progress, screening for and managing medical complications, and coordinating care with psychiatric and nutritional professionals. Target goal weight is individualized on the basis of age, height, pubertal stage, previous growth trajectories, and premorbid weight, and goal weight should be reevaluated regularly for growing youth. Return to menses is an objective measure in post-menarcheal females (Rosen & The Committee on Adolescence, 2010).

- Youths who are psychiatrically or medically unstable require inpatient treatment, as recommended by the American Academy of Pediatrics (Rosen & The Committee on Adolescence, 2010). These criteria are as follows:

  - Psychiatric criteria:
    - Suicide risk
    - Refusal to eat
    - Failure to respond to outpatient treatment

  - Medical criteria:
    - Less than 75% of ideal body weight or continuous weight loss despite intensive treatment
    - Body fat less than 10%
    - Systolic blood pressure less than 90 mmHg
    - Arrhythmia
    - Heart rate less than 50 beats in daytime; less than 45 beats in nighttime
    - Orthostatic changes in pulse greater than 20 beats per minute or blood pressure greater than 10 mmHg
    - Hypothermia less than 96°F
    - Intractable vomiting
    - Hematemesis

  - The APA recommends that hospitalization occur before the onset of medical instability as manifested by abnormal vital signs, physical findings, or laboratory tests. It further notes that hospitalizing pediatric clients even when declining weight loss is not as severe as the level recommended for adult hospitalization can avert irreversible effects of physical growth and development (Yager et al., 2010).

- Most youth can be treated on an outpatient basis utilizing a multidisciplinary approach.

  - Nutrition: Refeeding should be managed by a nutrition specialist versed in eating disorder management, as anorexia nervosa can result in starvation-related hypophosphatemia and dangerous variations in potassium, sodium, and magnesium levels. Refeeding should be a slow process, with assessment of vitamins A and D, calcium, linolenic acid, retinol, and pantothenic acid levels. Proper management minimizes the risk of refeeding syndrome, which can be fatal. Refeeding syndrome is a metabolic complication that can occur when nutritional support is given to severely malnourished patients: Metabolism shifts from catabolic to anabolic; insulin is released on carbohydrate consumption, which activates cellular uptake of potassium, phosphate, and magnesium, thus reducing the serum concentrations of these electrolytes, resulting in serious complications, such as arrhythmias (Crook, Hally, & Panteli, 2001). Youth with bulimia nervosa require a structured meal plan to help reduce episodes of dietary restriction that results in the urge to binge/purge. Nutritional counseling can also help clients increase the variety of foods eaten (Yager, 2014).

- Psychotherapies include insight-oriented, cognitive behavioral therapy (CBT), interpersonal, motivational, family and group, among others. CBT has been shown to be very effective for both anorexia and bulimia nervosa, and is the treatment of choice for BED. Family therapy may be helpful when family dynamics figure prominently in the triggers for the youth's disorder. Dialectical behavior therapy (DBT) may help reduce binge eating because it is useful in reducing sudden intense surges of emotion (Greenberg et al., 2010).

- Psychopharmacological treatment in anorexia nervosa is generally ineffective, although selective serotonin-reuptake inhibitors (SSRIs) may help with relapse prevention. SSRIs are typically used in the treatment of bulimia, with fluoxetine (Prozac) the only one approved by the Food and Drug Administration (FDA) for bulimia. Bupropion (Wellbutrin) is relatively contraindicated because of the risk for seizures in clients with eating disorders. Topiramate (Topamax) significantly decreases binge eating in bulimia and BED, and may be an option for patients who do not respond to SSRIs. However, side effects can be considerable, including weight loss, so it may be problematic in those who are normal or underweight (Bernstein, 2014, 2015; Yager, 2014).

- Treatment for BDD includes CBT and SSRIs. BDD clients with delusional symptoms may benefit from the antipsychotic agent pimozide in addition to an SSRI. Since more than 90% of BDD clients report symptoms that are unchanged or exacerbated after surgical procedures, plastic or cosmetic surgery to correct the perceived defect in BDD is contraindicated (Ahmed, 2014).

E. Parenting Tips

a. The following are signs that your child may have an eating disorder. Should you suspect that he or she has a problem, contact your health care provider.

- Recent weight loss or weight fluctuations of more than 5 lb (bulimia)
- A fear of gaining weight or of being fat
- Preoccupation with being fat or with a specific body part

- Signs of purging behaviors: going into the bathroom right after meals (to vomit); scrape or scar on her knuckles (sticking her fingers down her throat to induce vomiting); laxatives or diuretics found in room
- Having a distorted image of body's size or shape
- A preoccupation with thoughts of food, calories, and weight
- Restrictive eating patterns, such as skipping meals, fasting, or eliminating entire food groups
- Preference for eating alone
- Preoccupied with food-related items, like cookbooks
- Telling family what to eat and commenting on calorie content of family members' food
- Loss of periods or delayed onset of puberty and menarche (first period)
- Being underweight
- Exercising compulsively (gets stressed if exercise ritual is broken)
- Shows extreme denial about weight loss and eating disorder
- Withdraws from friends and family, or has very superficial friendships
- Wearing bulky clothing to hide weight loss
- Shoplifting
- Large quantities of household food missing frequently; stealing money or items to buy food
- Recent or past event in life that was very stressful

b.   Tips for coping with mealtimes when your child has an eating disorder (National Health Service, United Kingdom, 2015):

- Ask your child's treatment team for suggestions.
- Shop and plan meals together.
- Create agreement about meals with the entire family to help set everyone's expectations.
- Avoid talking about calories, fat content, and portion sizes of food.
- Keep meal time lighthearted.
- If your child attempts to take over the cooking as a means of control, have him or her set the table instead.
- Avoid focusing on the affected child.
- Plan an activity after the meal to distract the child from purging.
- If things go wrong, just move on.

Resources

BDD Alliance: www.bddalliance.org

Binge Eating Disorder Association: http://bedaonline.com

Healthy Body Image: http://chhs.unh.edu/sites/chhs.unh.edu/files/docs/fs/adolescent_resources/ Health_Body_Image.pdf

Kids and Eating Disorders: http://kidshealth.org/kid/health_problems/learning_problem/eatdisorder.html

National Eating Disorder Association: www.nationaleatingdisorders.org

National Institute of Mental Health Eating Disorders: www.nimh.nih.gov/health/publications/eating-disorders-new-trifold/index.shtml

References

Ahmed, I. (2014). Body dysmorphic disorder. In: *Medscape Emedicine*. Retrieved from http://emedicine.medscape.com/article/291182-overview

American Psychiatric Association. (2013). *Diagnostic and statistical manual of mental disorders* (5th ed.). Washington, DC: Author.

Bernstein, B. (2014). Anorexia nervosa. In: *Medscape Emedicine*. Retrieved from http://emedicine.medscape.com/article/912187-overview#a2

Bernstein, B. (2015). Binge-eating disorder (BED). In: *Medscape Emedicine*. Retrieved from http://emedicine.medscape.com/article/2221362-overview

Colton, P., Olmsted, M. P., Daneman, D., Farquhar, J. C., Wong, H., Muskat, S., & Rodin, G. M. (2015). Eating disorders in girls and women with type 1 diabetes: A longitudinal study of prevalence, onset, remission, and recurrence. *Diabetes Care, 38*(7), 1212–1217.

Crook, M., Hally, V., & Panteli, J. (2001). The importance of refeeding syndrome. *Nutrition, 17*, 632–637.

Greenberg, J., Markowitz, S., Petronko, M., Taylor, C., Wilhelm, S., & Wilson, G. (2010). Cognitive-behavioral therapy for adolescent body dysmorphic disorder. *Cognitive and Behavioral Practice, 17*, 248–258.

Mazzeo, S., & Bulik, C. (2009). Environmental and genetic risk factors for eating disorders: What the clinician needs to know. *Child and Adolescent Psychiatric Clinics of North America, 18*(1), 67–82. doi:10.1016/j.chc.2008.07.003

Morgan, J., Reid, F., & Lacey, J. (1999). The SCOFF questionnaire: Assessment of a new screening tool for eating disorders. *British Medical Journal, 319*(7223), 1467–1468.

National Health Service, United Kingdom. (2015). Eating disorders: Advice for parents. Retrieved from http://www.nhs.uk/Livewell/eatingdisorders/Pages/eating-disorders-advice-parents.aspx

Phillips, K., Didie, E., Menard, M., Pagano, M., Fay, C., & Weisberg, R. (2006). Clinical features of body dysmorphic disorder in adolescents and adults. *Psychiatry Research, 141*(3), 305–314. doi:10.1016/j.psychres.2005.09.014

Phillips, K., Menard, M., & Fay, C. (2006). Gender similarities and differences in 200 individuals with body dysmorphic disorder. *Comprehensive Psychiatry, 47*, 77–87. doi:10.1016/j.comppsych.2005.07.002

Raevuori, A., Keski-Rahkonen, A., & Hoek, H. (2014). A review of eating disorders in males. *Current Opinions in Psychiatry, 27*(6), 426–430.

Rosen, D., & The Committee on Adolescence. (2010). Clinical Report—Identification and management of eating disorders in children and adolescents. *Pediatrics, 126*(6), 1240–1253. doi:10.1542/peds.2010-2821

Welch, E., Ghaderi, A., & Swenne, I. (2015). A comparison of clinical characteristics between adolescent males and females with eating disorders. *BMC Psychiatry, 15*, 45, 1–7. doi:10.1186/s12888-015-0419-8

Yager, J. (2014). Bulimia nervosa. In: *Medscape Emedicine*. Retrieved from http://emedicine.medscape.com/article/286485-overview

Yager, J., Devlin, M. J., Halmi, K. A., Herzog, D. B., Mitchell, J. E., Powers, P., & Zerbe, K. J. (2010). *Practice guideline for the treatment of patients with eating disorders* (3rd ed.). Retrieved from http://psychiatryonline.org/pb/assets/raw/sitewide/practice_guidelines/guidelines/eatingdisorders.pdf

CHAPTER 13

Firesetting

A. Description

Juvenile firesetting, which accounts for approximately half of all arson arrests, results in considerable morbidity, mortality, and financial loss. Many juvenile fires go undetected or unsolved, and thus the true extent of this problem is unknown, and adult fire behavior is the result of supervised childhood fire activities (Dolan, McEawan, Doley, & Fritzon, 2011). Not all juvenile firesetting is pathological; juvenile firesetting elevates to this level when it is recurrent (more than three times), unsupervised, and associated with psychosocial dysfunction and significant life stressors (Gaynor, 2002).

   a.   Most children understand the basic safety factors and risks of fire by age 10 years. Fire behavior follows a development sequence in children and presents on at least three different levels: fire interest, firestarting, and firesetting. These categories represent increasing levels of involvement with fire. Preventive measures allow most children to learn age-appropriate, fire-safe behaviors. However, some children become involved in fire risk behaviors owing to a number of factors that include emotional disorders, family dysfunction, and chronic stress. These factors can lead to such behaviors as unsupervised firestarting, and repeated, intentional, and malicious firesetting (Gaynor, 2002; Putnam & Kirkpatrick, 2005).

   - Fire interest: Most children begin to demonstrate fire interest between 3 and 5 years of age. This interest may be expressed through questioning, usually about the physical properties of fire, and dramatic play such as dressing up as firemen or playing with fire trucks. This level and interest is healthy and provides children with a way to explore and learn about the productive values of fire. It is also the time when parents should begin to teach children about fire.

   - Firestarting: Firestarting begins when children experiment with ignition sources, particularly matches and lighters. Most boys between ages 3 and 9 experiment with firestarting materials at least once. This best occurs with the older ones (if developmentally capable) in an adult-supervised, controlled environment, such as lighting candles on a birthday cake, so that children learn how to handle themselves. Unfortunately, many firestarts take place in unsupervised settings. Most unsupervised firestarts are single episodes primarily motivated by curiosity, and fires resulting from these incidents are accidental or unintentional, and the children will make an attempt either to put the fire out or get help. Single-episode, unsupervised firestarts usually do not result in a significant fire. However, if children continue to participate in unsupervised firestarts, the probability of starting a significant fire increases dramatically. (The term "fireplay" is often used to convey a low level of intent to inflict harm and an absence of malice.)

- Firesetting: Most children have learned many of the rules of fire safety by age 10 and are capable of engaging in age-appropriate firestarting behaviors such as helping to light the family barbecue or building a campfire. With proper guidance, most children achieve a sense of competency and mastery over this powerful yet controllable aspect of their physical environment. However, for some children, fire interest leads to unsupervised firestarts and repeated firesetting. Children ages 7 to 10 may be involved in repeated firesetting. Although intentional, it may not be motivated by psychological or social problems, but can lead to devastating consequences. Other children are motivated by psychological or social problems, and their firesetting consists of a series of planned firestarts that take place over weeks, months, or years, with fire severity varying from small burns to fires that require fire department suppression. These children search for ignition sources and conceal them until needed, and they often gather flammable materials and/or accelerants to hasten the pace of their fires. Their targets often hold specific meaning for them, and once the fire burns, they rarely attempt to extinguish it. Instead, many watch it burn, often from a place where they are safe and undetectable. Some children run away and come back later to view the devastation; others call the fire department and act as the first on the scene. Some volunteer to suppress the fire.

- Arson: Both unsupervised firestarting and pathological firesettting may be classified as arson if the fire causes damage and the juvenile acted intentionally or recklessly. Intent may be difficult to establish if the juvenile lacks emotional maturity or has mental illness.

b.   Firesetting can serve as a gateway to future delinquent and violent acts, indicating a poor prognosis for these troubled youth. Juvenile firesetting behavior is a frightening yet reliable predictor of adult criminality, and its consequences can be tragic and costly. Fires set by youths destroy more than $300 million worth of property and claim the lives of approximately 300 people, with children being the predominant victims of these fires, accounting for 85 of every 100 lives lost (Putnam & Kirkpatrick, 2005).

c.   Young children typically set fires out of curiosity and close to home; they tend to respond with fear and try to put them out. Adolescents usually set fires away from home and in groups; they typically get excited by the fire and often stay to watch the emergency response (Dolan et al., 2011).

d.   Juvenile firesetting may indicate that fire can be an instrument of power or a weapon, as opposed to merely being a product of curiosity. Children typically have less power than adults in society, and many rights and privileges are determined by age, such as voting and drinking alcohol. Access to firearms and other weapons is restricted, but matches and lighters are relatively accessible to youth inclined to act in harmful ways, and a pack of matches can be a formidable weapon used to act out negative behaviors. The most substantial and pervasive problem for these juveniles seems to be difficulty processing emotions. They tend to feel overwhelmed by negative feelings and do not know how to properly deal with them. Consequently, feelings related to problems such as insecurity and perceived rejection progress into frustration and anger, and they are still unable to face or adequately address these disturbing sensations. This inability to properly express feelings is usually what drives them to set fires, allowing them to ultimately achieve a sense of relief or domination, or to accomplish an indirect form of revenge, cleansing themselves of their persistent and disabling emotions. The underlying reason for setting fires lies among a broad spectrum of emotions that range from basic boredom to intense suicidal ideation, but some general tendencies typically align with the sex of the individual. Boys seem to set fires more for the purposes of destruction or rebellion, while girls typically obtain a sense of excitement from fire or use it as a means of self-injury. Regardless of the gender or purpose of firesetting, the act is often reinforced instantaneously, increasing the likelihood of the behavior being repeated in the future. There is an association between firesetting and abuse. One study showed that, when compared with nonabused children, children with histories of maltreatment demonstrated more frequent fire involvement, more versatility regarding ignition sources and targets, and a greater likelihood of an immediate family stressor as a motive for firesetting. They were more likely to become involved with fire out of anger and demonstrated a trend toward higher rates of recidivism. Overall, juvenile firesetting most likely has multiple causes, and firesetters may be of many different types.

B. Assessment

a.   Risk factors: There is still little research on risk factors; however, possible factors include child maltreatment, fire interest with antisocial behavior, binge drinking, frequent cannabis use, and sensation-seeking. Firesetting is more common in males, during the afternoon hours, and in the month of July, when outside fires are more common. The most common heat sources are lighters and matches, the most common location is a bedroom, and the most common ignited object is a mattress or bedding (Burnett & Omar, 2014; Campbell, 2014; MacKay, Paglia-Boak, Henderson, Marton, & Adlaf, 2009).

b. Health care providers can screen children and adolescents to identify those who are at risk and ensure that these children obtain appropriate interventions. Juveniles and their families can be described according to three risk levels that represent the likelihood that the child will become involved in future firesetting. Each level of risk represents a successively more severe form of firesetting behavior (Gaynor, 2002).

- Little risk: About 60% to 70% of juveniles involved in unsupervised firestarting are motivated by curiosity and experimentation. Most of these children are at little risk for becoming involved in future firesetting if they receive the proper supervision and education. The majority of these children are young boys between the ages of 3 and 7 who come from all types of social and economic backgrounds. Young girls participate in unsupervised firestarts, but do so less frequently than young boys. Low-risk children do not exhibit significant psychological problems. Their family and peer relationships are intact and stable, and their school performance and behavior meet expectations. This risk group includes the curious and mild cognitively impaired firesetters.

- Definite risk: Of children and adolescents identified with firesetting histories, 30% to 40% fall into the definite risk category. These juveniles are very likely to engage in future firesetting incidents. The earlier they are identified, evaluated, and provided appropriate interventions, the better their chances of avoiding involvement in future firesetting. There are two major classes of definite risk juveniles: troubled/crisis and delinquent.

- Definite risk-troubled juveniles: These juveniles can be described as the cry-for-help type that start fires to bring attention to their psychological distress. In most cases, it is their emotional conflict that motivates their firesetting. The source of this emotional conflict can vary greatly, and can include such things as family turmoil, abuse, neglect, unresolved difficulties in school, and other recent or chronic stressful life events. Fire safety and prevention education may be helpful, but it will not address their primary psychological problems. Therefore, they should be referred to the appropriate mental health agencies. If these youth and their families receive the help they need in a timely fashion, the chances are reasonably good that their firesetting behavior will not recur.

- Definite risk-delinquent juveniles: Delinquent juveniles exhibit a certain pattern of aggressive, deviant, and criminal behavior. These behaviors emerge at a young age, and occur with greater frequency and intensity as the juvenile matures. What begins as stubborn and disobedient behavior as a preschooler can lead to lying and stealing as a young child, and to firesetting, petty theft, and vandalism as a teenager. Serious emotional or family dysfunction also may contribute to this pattern of antisocial behavior. The longer this delinquent behavior pattern continues, the harder it is to reverse. Therefore, early identification is critical. They can be referred to mental health, social service, and other community agencies, and, if their firesetting is classified as an arson crime, they can be referred to the juvenile justice system. These juveniles present one of the biggest and costliest challenges to their families and their communities.

- Extreme risk: This group represents less than 1% of firesetting youth. These juveniles suffer from significant mental dysfunction, such as the psychotic disturbances of schizophrenia and affective disorders, as well as organically impaired disturbances of mental retardation and fetal alcohol syndrome. These children are beyond most fire safety and prevention programs currently available and are a significant danger to themselves or others.

c.   Several types of juvenile firesetters have been described by various sources (American Psychological Association, 2004; Gaynor, 2000; Kolko, 2002):

- Curiosity/experimental/accidental firesetters are typically young boys or girls who lack the understanding of fire's destructiveness. They act without malice, and are usually opportunistic, impulsive, and unsupervised. They have ready access to ignition sources, such as matches and lighters, and are frightened by their acts, which contributes to their low risk of setting further fires.

- Cry for help/troubled/crisis firesetters are typically boys who use fire to express their emotions. They usually have underlying disorders, such as attention deficit hyperactivity disorder (ADHD) or depression, and family stressors, and may not understand the consequences of their actions. They usually have set two or more fires when identified, and will continue to set fires until their needs are met or identified and channeled appropriately.

- Cognitively impaired firesetters are developmentally disabled or impaired children who lack good judgment, but avoid intentional harm. However, they may cause significant property damage.

- Sociocultural firesetters set fires because of support from their peer or community group, including those who set fires during riots or in religious fervor.

- Pathological/emotionally disturbed/extreme firesetters include boys and girls of all ages. They have psychiatric diagnoses and chronic histories of school, behavioral, and social emotional problems. This group includes those who are thought-disordered firesetters (set fires in direct response to disordered thinking; a misperception of reality; and thinking errors that may revolve around religious, political, personal, or even counterintuitive agendas and result in related targets for firesetting); compulsive firesetters (who are commonly known as pyromaniacs and fall under the diagnostic category of impulse control disorders; they are remorseful, but have a need to set fires); and disordered coping firesetters (behavior is a learned and deliberate response to a sense of disequilibrium; there is poor interpersonal empathy, but they do not understand the impact of their behavior.

- Delinquent/criminal firesetters tend to be teens with a history of firesetting, gangs, truancy, antisocial behavior, or drug/alcohol abuse. They typically target schools, open fields, dumpsters, or abandoned buildings, and are characterized by group-influenced behavior often occurring under the influence of drugs and/or alcohol. Fire often serves as a cover-up for another crime such as vandalism or property destruction, and is only one of a number of negative and/or delinquent behaviors.

- Thrill seeker firesetters begin setting fires in early to midadolescence and appear to have an attraction toward danger for its own sake. They do it for excitement and to experience the rush brought on by the peril and possibility of discovery and apprehension, often entering into a "game" with fire investigators and police in which each fire is regarded as a triumph of the arsonist over authority.

- Revenge-based firesetters usually begin experimenting with incendiaries and explosives during the school-age years, and often "grow into" firebombing activity in addition to acts of arson. Fueled by rage, they identify their targets in a methodical and purposeful manner and determine the type of havoc they wish to create.

d.   DelBove and McKay (2011) stated that existing juvenile firesetting typologies have been relatively arbitrary and univariate. They examined 240 juvenile firesetters, ages 4 to 17, who were referred to an arson prevention program. Although their typologies are empirically based, it should be noted that a population of children in need of a specialized program is less likely to be one-time curious or accidental firesetters, and may already be representative of a more troubled population:

- Conventional-limited (CL) cluster: This group has the least severe firesetting behavior with the fewest risk factors, oldest age of onset, lowest level of fire interest, least number of firesetting events, and fewest targets and ignition sources. These youth also had the lowest levels of attention and skills deficits, low externalizing behavior, and the most contact with biological parents.

- Home-instability moderate (HM) cluster: These children had younger age firesetting onset, more fire interest, and more targets and ignition sources. They also exhibited antisocial motivation related to their firesetting, had the lowest involvement with parents and the highest abuse rate, and showed poor academic performance.

- Multi-risk persistent (MP) cluster: This group had the youngest age of firesetting onset, high levels of fire interest, and the highest number of firesetting incidents and ignition sources. They were also antisocial motivated, with less than half expressing remorse for their actions. Most had been in contact with the child welfare system, but had experienced less abuse than the HM cluster. They also experienced poor academic performance, and high social skill deficit, attention difficulties, and externalizing behaviors.

What these typologies do show is that juvenile firesetters are a very diverse group with different levels of severity and varying underlying factors for their firesetting behaviors. It is of key importance to health care providers to understand each individual child's needs to better implement an intervention plan.

C. Diagnosis, Including Differential Diagnoses, When Appropriate

The most common associated disorder is conduct disorder, as well as ADHD and oppositional defiant disorder (all common disorders in delinquency). When the Minnesota Multiphasic Personality Inventory-Adolescent (MMPI-A) was administered, adolescent male firesetters were found to be more pathological, demonstrating higher scores on clinical scales of mania, psychasthenia (irrational fear, fascination, and obligation), and schizophrenia. The high mania scores are indicative of the juvenile being impulsive and challenging as well as hyperactive, while heightened psychasthenia suggests increased levels of anxiety and a tendency toward being compulsive and unsure of one's self. The schizophrenia scale includes psychotic tendencies; however, it also measures difficulties socializing and controlling behaviors, academic problems, and "intense, acute situational distress," which may be more relevant to characteristics of firesetters. Firesetters also had noticeably greater scores on several content scales, including depression, alienation, anger, conduct problems, family problems, school problems, and negative treatment indicators. Thus, adolescent male firesetters display a particular range of psychological difficulties as compared with nonfiresetters.

D. Levels of Prevention/Intervention

a. Primary

Health care providers should include age-appropriate fire-safety anticipatory guidance in their wellness visits and other forms of child injury prevention teachings, such as health fairs and other community programs.

b. Secondary

Health care providers can work with their community or regionally based juvenile firesetting prevention program to:

- Organize and coordinate community-based screening, assessment, and intervention programs.

- Identify and provide for the child's and family's needs (fire safety education, counseling, social services, etc.) using community resources.
- Assist parents/caregivers and all who work with children to better understand children's involvement with fire, along with when and where to go for help.

At-risk children should also be referred for psychiatric evaluation and treatment.

c.   Tertiary

Juvenile firesetting is a multifaceted phenomenon that warrants a diversified approach to prevention relying on structural, situational, and social interventions (Uhnoo, Perrson, Ekbrand, & Lindgren, 2015). Tertiary prevention should aim at recidivism prevention for those children who are at risk for repeated firesetting. This is part of the continuum of a juvenile firesetting prevention program. Intervention depends on the child's typology.

- Curious firesetters respond well to fire safety education, whereas cognitively impaired firesetters may need special education, intensive fire education, and behavior management.
- Thought-disordered firesetters require appropriate and aggressive treatment of their thinking errors while under therapeutic supervision to reduce the possibility of additional acts of firesetting. Resolution of their thought disorder generally causes the disappearance of firesetting as a high-risk behavior.
- Delinquent firesetters require interventions that include restitution and criminal punishment.

d.   Health care providers should be aware of, and can become involved with, their community juvenile firesetting intervention program. According to the Pennsylvania Office of the State Fire Commissioner (n.d.), a juvenile firesetting intervention program should be part of a community- or regionally based network that offers a continuum of care. The program should be designed to provide a range of intervention services including prevention, education, immediate treatment, and graduated sanctions to juveniles and their families. Community and regional intervention programs should be diverse in composition and include multiple disciplines that continually have contact with juveniles. These services include: public and private school systems, fire service professionals, mental health professionals, school social workers and counselors, children and youth social service workers, juvenile justice probation officers, law enforcement, and other like team members. All of these professionals should be part of the planned and coordinated effort to reduce child-set fires. Treatment for firesetting usually occurs in the least restrictive environment; however, juveniles may need to be confined to a secure facility, residential treatment center, or hospital, depending on the seriousness of the offense and based on the needs of the juvenile. Although many juvenile firesetters can be maintained in the community with appropriate supervision, careful assessment is critical to provide the appropriate level of care. The assessment must consider the child, family, environment, facts about the fire, and other fire history, as well as the child's reaction to the fire and sense of accountability. Consideration should also be given to ensure that the child does not pose a risk to others and that the public safety is protected. The teaming up of mental health and fire department professionals to treat juvenile firesetters is becoming an increasingly popular occurrence. Treatment programs that incorporate a collaborative and comprehensive approach to the treatment of juvenile firesetting are gaining popularity, and the outcomes of these programs show impressive potential to decrease the prevalence of juvenile firesetting behavior.

E. Parenting Tips (Adapted from the National Fire Protection Association Parent Safety Tips About Young Firesetters, n.d.)

a. Once your children ask about fire or show an interest in fire by playing with fire trucks or cooking on a play stove, it is time to begin educating them about fire. They especially need to understand that fire is hard to control, fast, and very harmful.

b. Have clear rules and consequences about fire misuse.

c. Discourage unsupervised fire starts.

d. Keep matches and lighters out of children's reach and sight, preferably in a locked cabinet or container, and do not leave them any place where children may be unsupervised.

e. Use child-resistant lighters, but realize that child-resistant does not mean child-proof.

f. Do not ask your child to get you your lighter or matches.

g. A child who has an interest in fire may develop firestarting behaviors that can lead to firesetting. Do not wait for it to get to that point; speak to your health care provider.

Resources

Counseling Children Who Play With Fire: www.communityhealthstrategies.com/counseling-children-whoplay-with-fire/

Hartford Insurance Fire Safety Tips and Fun Games for Children: www.thehartford.com/our-company/fire-safety-for-kids

KidsHealth Fire Safety: http://kidshealth.org/parent/firstaid_safe/home/fire.html

National Fire Protection Association Sparky the Fire Dog: www.nfpa.org/safety-information/sparky-the-fire-dog

Safe Kids Fire Safety: www.safekids.org/fire

U.S. Fire Administration Sesame Street Fire Safety Program: www.usfa.fema.gov/

References

American Psychological Association. (2004). *Types of fire-setters.* Retrieved from www.apa.org/monitor/julaug04/types.aspx

Burnett, A., & Omar, H. (2014). *Firesetting and maltreatment.* Pediatrics Faculty Publications (Paper 105). Retrieved from http://uknowledge.uky.edu/cgi/viewcontent.cgi?article=1104& context= pediatrics_facpub

Campbell, R. (2014). *Playing with fire* (NFPA No. USS17). Quincy, MA: National Fire Protection Association.

DelBove, G., & McKay, H. (2011). An empirically derived classification system for juvenile firesetters. *Criminal Justice and Behavior, 38*(8), 796–817. doi:10.1177/0093854811406224

Dolan, M., McEawan, T., Doley, R., & Fritzon, K. (2011). Risk factors and risk assessment in juvenile fire-setting. *Psychiatry, Psychology and Law, 18*(3), 378–394.

Gaynor, J. (2002). *Juvenile firesetters intervention handbook* (Under Contract EME-97-RP-0015 from the Federal Emergency Management Agency, U.S. Fire Administration). Washington, DC: Socio Technical Research Applications, Inc. Retrieved from http://poage.com/JFSDocs/USFA%20FA210% 20Juvenile%20Firesetter%20Intervention%20Handbook.pdf

Kolko, D. (Ed.). (2002). *Handbook on firesetting in children and youth.* Boston, MA: Academic Press.

MacKay, S., Paglia-Boak, A., Henderson, J., Marton, P., & Adlaf, E., (2009). Epidemiology of firesetting in adolescents: Mental health and substance use correlates. *Journal of Child Psychology and Psychiatry, 50*(10), 1282–1129. doi:10.1111/j.1469-7610.2009.02103.x

National Fire Protection Association. (n.d.). Children and fire safety tips. Retrieved from www.nfpa .org/safety-information/for-consumers/causes/young-firesetters/children-and-fire-safety-tips

Pennsylvania Office of the State Fire Commissioner. (n.d.). Pennsylvania's juvenile firesetting inter vention protocol. Retrieved from www.osfc.pa.gov/Prevention%20and%20education%20Programs/ JUVENILE%20FIRE-SETTER%20INTERVENTION/Pages/Juvenile-Firesetter-Intervention-Protocal.aspx

Putnam, C., & Kirkpatrick, J. (2005). *Juvenile firesetting: A research overview* (Juvenile Justice Bulletin, NCJ 207606). Washington, DC: Office of Juvenile Justice and Delinquency Prevention. Retrieved from www.ncjrs.gov/pdffiles1/ojjdp/207606.pdf

Uhnoo, S., Perrson, S., Ekbrand, H., & Lindgren, S. (2015). Juvenile school firesetting in Sweden: Causes and countermeasures. *Journal of Scandinavian Studies in Criminology and Crime Prevention, 16*(1), 25–40. doi:/10.1080/14043858.2014.989668

CHAPTER 14

Gambling

A. Description

Gambling is defined as the playing of games to win (or lose) money or possessions, or the betting of money or other valuables ("Gambling," 2016). Some games are chiefly about chance (lotteries), some involve skill (darts), and others involve both (cards). It is a popular recreation activity for fun, excitement, and the "high" of winning, and most people do not develop problems with it. Adolescent gambling may not sound like a primary care topic, yet it is prevalent. A meta-analysis by Blinn-Pike, Worthy & Jonkman (2010) suggested that 77% to 83% of adolescents were involved in some type of gambling.

a. Although illegal, and thus attractive to them, adolescents engage in many types of gambling, including self-organized (cards, dice, sports betting) and legalized (lotteries and casino games), both live and virtual.

b. The expansion of legalized gambling and increased advertising has resulted in youth being exposed to gambling at a much younger age. Today's youth are the first generation to grow up in a time when gambling is legal, actively promoted, and glamorized. This has resulted in increased rates of youth gambling, with *DSM* prevalence estimates rivalling those of alcohol.

c. The *Diagnostic and Statistical Manual of Mental Disorders, 5th Edition (DSM-5),* published by the American Psychiatric Association (APA, 2013), replaced *DSM-IV-TR's* Pathological Gambling with Gambling Disorder, which now requires four instead of five criteria for diagnosis and excludes the "illegal acts" criterion. Gambling Disorder is also now listed under the Substance-Related and Other Addictive Disorders section, instead of being categorized as an impulse control disorder as done in the previous edition (Leeman & Potenza, 2012; Rennert et al., 2014). The onset of gambling disorder can occur during adolescence or young adulthood with a course that develops over the years with a pattern of gambling that increases in both intensity and frequency. Most persons report one or two types of gambling that are particularly problematic, even though they may participate in many forms.

Patterns may be regular or episodic, and the disorder may go into remission or be persistent, and persons may alternate among abstinence, nonproblematic gambling, and problematic gambling (APA, 2013).

d.   Adolescents usually begin gambling with family members or friends. Development of an early-life gambling disorder seems to be associated with impulsivity and substance abuse, but many youth do grow out of the gambling disorder over time.

B. Assessment

a.   Risk factors for problem/pathological gambling vary per study and include non-peer involvement gambling, heavy alcohol use, poor academic functioning, internalizing psychopathology such as depression, elevated probability among children who live at home without siblings, learning disorders, sensation seeking, and superstitious thinking. Male and female adolescents seem to follow different paths in gambling with probabilistic reasoning ability and the perception of economic profitability in males, and parental gambling behavior in females (Donati, Chiesi, & Primi, 2013; Parker, Summerfeldt, Kloosterman, Keefer, & Taylor, 2013; Portenza et al., 2012).

b.   Playing video games is not likely to be a risk factor for pathological gambling in adolescents (Delfabbro, King, Lambos, & Puglies, 2009).

c.   Various descriptions and typologies have been proposed. In a study of 154 patients ages 17 to 25, Jimenez-Murcia and colleagues (2013) found three typologies of adolescent pathological gambling: less psychopathology and more functional personality traits (Type I); major emotional distress, shame, immaturity, hostility, and negative feelings (Type II); and the most severe psychopathological profile with the most psychopathological disturbances and schizotypal traits (Type III). Floros and colleagues (2013) examined adolescent online gambling, associated school performance, and psychopathology and found two profiles: those who had higher psychopathology, less prosocial behavior, higher Internet addiction scores with higher frequencies of online activities, moderate levels of truancy, and lower expectations of school achievement; and those who had less psychopathology, more prosocial behavior, less Internet involvement, but skipped school more frequently and whose prospects of high school completion were slimmer than those of the first group.

d.   The South Oaks Gambling Screen: Revised for Adolescents (SOGR-RA) is a 12-item screen for youth ages 12 to 17 that rates gambling on four levels. It has been shown to be suitable for use as a screening tool in adolescents (Chiesi, Donati, Galli, & Primi, 2013) and can be found at www.ncpgambling.org/files/NPGAW/SOGS_RA.pdf.

C. Diagnosis

a. Differentiate experimental from problem gambling. Experimental gambling is just that— experimental—with youths gambling to try out the experience or to participate in activities with friends or family. It does not cause them any significant distress. Transition age youth may be social or even professional gamblers. Social gambling occurs in a social context, and professional gamblers have discipline and limit their risk. Consider the following to screen for a gambling problem: at least once per week threshold, gambling more than planned, and behaviors that suggest they are hiding their gambling behaviors from others (Gupta, Pinzon, & Canadian Paediatric Society Adolescent Health Committee, 2012).

b. Gambling disorder, also known as gambling addiction or compulsive gambling, is an impulse-control disorder whereby a person has the need to gamble regardless of the consequences. The *DSM-5* (APA, 2013) identifies several behaviors as indicative of gambling disorder. These include persistent gambling that results in impairment or distress. The person is preoccupied with gambling, needs to gamble with more and more money to achieve a level of excitement, is unsuccessful at stopping his or her gambling, and becomes irritable when attempting to stop. The youth may lie to cover up the gambling behavior, use gambling to relieve negative moods, rely on bailouts from others, and may also jeopardize his or her schooling or relationships because of gambling.

c. The gambling is not due to a manic episode. Specifiers relate to severity, frequency, and remission. Severity levels are mild (meets 4–5 criteria), moderate (meets 6–7 criteria), and severe (meets 8–9 criteria). The disorder is episodic if the youth met the criteria at one point in time but symptoms have subsided between gambling periods for the last several months; the disorder is persistent if the youth met the criteria and experienced continuous gambling symptoms for multiple years. Youths would be in early remission if they had once met full criteria and have not met them for at least 3 months but less than 12 months; they are in sustained remission if none of the criteria are met for 12 or more months, after once meeting criteria.

d. The following have been found as comorbidities of gambling-related problems: low grades, risk-taking, personality disorders, substance abuse (including tobacco), and mood disorders. Problem gambling has also been associated with attention deficit hyperactivity disorder (ADHD), anxiety, conduct disorders/delinquent behaviors, illicit activities, and significant psychosocial problems (Gupta et al., 2012; Petry & Tawfik, 2012).

e. Differential diagnoses should be considered. Excessive gambling with loss of judgment can occur during a manic episode; in these cases, the youth does not exhibit problematic gambling when not manic. Gambling can be part of conduct disorder and antisocial personality disorder (youths 18 and older).

D. Levels of Prevention/Intervention

a. Primary

The literature on prevention is limited. The general approach is to reduce risk levels by enhancing protective factors, including family cohesion and school connectedness, as well as strengthening youth coping abilities and the surrounding environment. This focuses on increasing resiliency, so that if they do gamble, they know what to do if they experience difficulty. No one prevention strategy should be used to the exclusion of others, and prevention program content should fit the developmental level of the targeted population. Abstinence programs may work for younger children to delay the onset of gambling behavior, but can have a negative effect on adolescents (Problem Gambling Institute of Ontario, n.d.). The Stacked Deck Program is an effective, school-based program for adolescents (grades 9 through 12) that teaches facts about gambling and related risks, encourages responsible decisions about gambling, and aims to prevent problem gambling. The program includes resources, handouts, parent information, and six interactive lessons for youth: gambling history including the "house edge"; signs and symptoms of problem gambling; gambling misconceptions and inappropriate thinking styles; essential life skills including good decision making and problem solving (determining the odds and weighing the pros and cons of one's actions); barriers to good decision making; and skills retention (optional lesson; Williams, Wood, & Currie, 2010).

b. Secondary

Screen for those at higher risk for gambling problems, which include those adolescents whose parents gamble, provide low levels of parental monitoring, and have higher levels of inadequate disciplinary practices (Gupta et al., 2012). The general approach is to reduce risk levels by enhancing protective factors, including family cohesion and school connectedness, as well as strengthening youth coping abilities and the surrounding environment. This focuses on increasing resiliency, so that if they do gamble, they know what to do if they experience difficulty.

c. Tertiary

Problem gambling falls into the category of developmental addictions with links to substance abuse and other impulse control behaviors. There is no gold standard of treatment, and it is generally believed that gambling problems should be treated in the same manner as other behavioral addictions (Gupta et al., 2012).

E. Parenting Tips

Your child may have a gambling problem if he or she (American Academy of Pediatrics, 2015):

a. Has gambling items, such as lottery scratch cards, betting sheets, and casino chips

b. Watches an excessive amount of televised sports and has an intensive interest in the outcome of sporting events

c. Visits a casino, despite being underage

d. Spends excessive time online and/or checks the Internet frequently

e. Accumulates unexplained debts

f. Flashes large amounts of money or buys expensive items

g. Cuts school or work

h. Is anxious or nervous

i. Steals

Resources

Family First Aid Help for Troubled Teens: Teen Gambling: www.familyfirstaid.org/issues/teen-gambling/

Gambling Addiction: http://kidshealth.org/teen/your_mind/problems/gambling.html

Problem Gambling: Early Intervention Makes a Difference (90-minute online course for primary care providers): www.problemgambling.ca/EN/ResourcesForProfessionals/Pages/CoursesandTraining.aspx

Self-Help Gambling Tools: www.problemgambling.ca/gambling-help/HomePage.aspx

Teen Gambling: It's a Bad Bet: http://gamingcontrolboard.pa.gov/files/compulsive/compulsive_gaming_week/Teen_Gambling.pdf

The YMCA Youth Gambling Project: www.ymcagta.org/en/who-we-work-with/educators/gambling/index.html

References

American Academy of Pediatrics. (2015). Teen gambling: How can I tell if my son or daughter is having a problem with gambling? Retrieved from www.healthychildren.org/English/ages-stages/teen/substance-abuse/Pages/Teen-Gambling.aspx

American Psychiatric Association. (2013). *Diagnostic and statistical manual of mental disorders* (5th ed.). Washington, DC: Author.

Blinn-Pike, L., Worthy, S.L., & Jonkman, J.N. (2010). Adolescent gambling: A review of an emerging field of research. *Journal of Adolescent Health, 47*(3), 223-236. doi: 10.1016/j.jadohealth.2010.05.003.

Chiesi, F., Donati, M., Galli, S., & Primi, C. (2013). The suitability of the South Oaks Gambling Screen-Revised for Adolescents (SOGS-RA) as a screening tool: IRT-based evidence. *Psychology of Addictive Behavior, 27*(1), 287-293. doi:10.1037/a0029987

Delfabbro, P., King, D., Lambos, C., & Puglies, S. (2009). Is video-game playing a risk factor for patho-logical gambling in Australian adolescents? *Journal of Gambling Studies, 25*(3), 391–405. doi:10.1007/s10899-009-9138-8

Donati, M., Chiesi, F., & Primi, C. (2013). A model to explain at-risk/problem gambling among male and female adolescents: Gender similarities and differences. *Journal of Adolescence, 36,* 129–137.

Floros, G., Paradisioti, A., Hadjimarcou, M., Mappouras, D. G., Karkanioti, O., & Siomos, K. (2013). Adolescent online gambling in Cyprus: Associated school performance and psychopathology. *Journal of Gambling Studies, 31,* 367–384. doi:10.1007/s10899-013-9424-3

Gambling. (2016). *Merriam-Webster's dictionary online.* Retrieved from www.merriam-webster.com/dictionary/gamble

Gupta, R., Pinzon, J., & Canadian Paediatric Society Adolescent Health Committee. (2012). Gambling in children and adolescents. *Paediatric Child Health, 17*(5), 263–264.

Jimenez-Murcia, S., Granero, R., Stinchfield, R., Fernández-Aranda, F., Penelo, E., Savvidou, L. G., ... Menchón, J. M. (2013). Typologies of young pathological gamblers based on sociodemographic and clinical characteristics. *Comprehensive Psychiatry, 54*(8), 1153–1160.

Leeman, R., & Potenza, M. (2012). Similarities and differences between pathological gambling and substance use disorders: A focus on impulsivity and compulsivity. *Psychopharmacology, 219,* 469–490. doi:10.1007/s00213-011-2550-7

Parker, J., Summerfeldt, L. J., Kloosterman, P. H., Keefer, K. V., & Taylor, R. N. (2013). Gambling behaviour in adolescents with learning disorders. *Journal of Gambling Studies, 29,* 231–239. doi:10.1007/s10899-012-9312-2

Petry, N., & Tawfik, Z. (2012). Comparison of problem-gambling and non–problem gambling youths seeking treatment for marijuana abuse. *Journal of the American Academy of Child and Adolescent Psychiatry, 40*(11), 1324–1331.

Portenza, M., Wareham, J. D., Steinberg, M. A., Rugle, L., Cavallo, D. A., Krishnan-Sarin, S., & Desai, R. A. (2011). Correlates of at-risk/problem internet gambling in adolescents. *Journal of the American Academy of Child and Adolescent Psychiatry, 50*(2), 150–159.e3. doi:10.1016/j.jaac.2010.11.006

Problem Gambling Institute of Ontario. (n.d.). *Youth and gambling: Prevention.* Retrieved from www.problemgambling.ca/EN/ResourcesForProfessionals/Pages/YouthAndGamblingPrevention.aspx

Rennert, L., Denis, C., Peer, K., Lynch, K., Gelernter, J., & Kranzler, H. (2014). *DSM-5* gambling dis-order: Prevalence and characteristics in a substance use disorder sample. *Experimental and Clinical Psychopharmacology, 22*(1), 50–6. doi:10.1037/a0034518.

Williams, R., Wood, R., & Currie, S. (2010). Stacked deck: An effective, school-based program for the prevention of problem gambling. *Journal of Primary Prevention, 31*(3), 109–125. doi:10.1007/s10935-010-0212-x

CHAPTER **15**

Gang Membership

A. Description

There is no one accepted definition of a gang; however, the National Youth Gang Survey (NYGS, n.d.) requests that their recipients define youth gangs as "a group of youths or young adults in your jurisdiction that you or other responsible persons in your agency or community are willing to identify as a 'gang.'" Youth gangs, which can be formal or informal, typically consist of at least three members and have a distinguishable name, hand sign, or symbol. One of their primary objectives is criminal activity, which differentiates them from other youth social groups such as fraternities, sororities, or social clubs.

    a.   Members range from "wannabes" (young children who want to be gang members) to hard-core members (original/old gangsters, or OGs). Active members self-admit to membership and have gang-related tattoos and a history of street crime; associate gang members tend to come and go from the gang as they please. Wannabes may be very dangerous because they are motivated to be part of a gang and are willing to do anything to prove it; they may also be instructed by OGs to prove they "have the heart" for gang activity by committing a violent crime, including killing a rival gang member. OGs are the leaders who are usually well-versed in the criminal justice system because of "being busted" (arrested), which helps them earn respect. OGs are involved in major crimes, including narcotics sales, robberies, shootings, and murder (Akiyama, 2012).

    b.   Most children who join gangs do so at a very early age, between 11 and 15. Pyrooz and Sweeten (2014) found gang membership as early as age 5, with the bulk joining after age 10. The majority of children who join gangs face a number of negative consequences, including: substance abuse; high-risk sexual behaviors; teen pregnancy; school dropout; family problems; unstable employment; and violence and serious offenses that can lead to arrest, conviction, incarceration, and the increased risk of experiencing violent victimization. Societal costs are also high, such as weakened informal social-control mechanisms and decreased property values (Simon, Ritter, & Mahendra, 2013).

c.   Although some children are forced to join gangs, this is an unusual occurrence. More common reasons include the individual child's need for acceptance, for excitement, to follow the family tradition, for glamour, identity or profit, response to peer pressure, or the need for protection or socialization.

- Acceptance: When children feel that they are not getting the attention they feel they deserve at home, they start looking for love in other places, and often find what they are looking for in a gang. The gang becomes their substitute family.

- Excitement: Some children enjoy the high of committing crime and getting away with it. Many commit their crimes just to be chased by the police. These children are thrill seekers who live for the adrenaline rush of being in a gang.

- Family tradition: Some join because another family member, usually a sibling, joined.

- Glamour: Movies and music have glamorized gangs, making them attractive to children who are feeling chronically bored.

- Identity: Being a gang member is better than being nothing.

- Profit: It is becoming more common for gang members to turn toward using the gang to make a profit through illegal activities, such as selling narcotics, robberies, burglaries, auto thefts, and other property crimes. Many gangs specialize in a specific criminal activity.

- Peer pressure: If children hang around gangs and gang members, it is almost guaranteed that they are being pressured to join the gang.

- Protection: In bad neighborhoods, kids often have to join a gang just to survive because it is often easier to join the gang than to be victimized on a daily basis.

- Socialization: The best parties are gang parties. Easy access to liquor, narcotics, and girls is attractive to potential young recruits, and young males who have a hard time socializing find that girls often like gang members.

d.   The "three Rs" of gang life are:

- Reputation/rep is a critical concern to gang members. The rep extends to each individual and the gang as a whole. Gang members gain status by having the most "juice" (power), based largely on one's rep. The manner in which one gains juice is important, so many members embellish their past gang activities to impress the listener, freely admitting to crimes. To even so much as gain membership, a person must be "jumped in" by being "beaten down" until the leader calls for it to end. Afterward, they all hug each other to further the "G thing," an action that bonds members together. Young members frequently talk of this fellowship as the reason they joined the gang.

- Respect is something that they carry to the extreme, for each member, the gang, their territory, and various other things, real or perceived. Some gangs require that members always show disrespect ("dis") for rival gangs through hand signals, graffiti, or a simple "mad dog" or stare down. If a member fails to dis a rival, causing a violation to his fellow posse (gang members), he will be "beaten down" by his own gang as punishment.

- Revenge/retaliation shows that no challenge goes unanswered in gang culture. Many drive-by shootings follow an event perceived as a dis. Typically, a confrontation takes place between a gang set and a single rival gangbanger. The gang member leaves, only to return with his "home boys" to complete the confrontation and keep his rep intact.

e. Gang members engage in Internet "banging," trading insults or threats that can lead to physical violence; they also brag about fights and murders, all to promote gang affiliation or interest in joining, gaining notoriety and reputation, sharing information on rival gangs, and network (Patton, Eschmann, & Bulter, 2013).

B. Assessment (History, Physical, Diagnostic Screening/Testing, Where Appropriate)

a. Risk factors, as well as protective factors, are similar to those for the development of aggressive and delinquent behaviors (see Chapter 3). For children ages 0 to 5, key risks include hypervigilance to threat, cognitive impairment, insecure attachment to caretaker, and early aggressive behavior. For children ages 6 to 12, critical risks include poor parental monitoring, social information-processing skill deficits, antisocial beliefs, poor school performance, and negative relationships with peers that include being rejected and victimized by peers. Protective factors for children at risk include secure attachment and effective parenting, higher levels of social–emotional competence, and academic success (Guerra, Dierkhising, & Payne, 2013).

b. Identifying a gang member is not an easy task. The best place to identify and refer is in primary care or school health. However, at-risk youth and gang-involved youth may not attend school or have primary care providers. Thus, most realistic locations may be the emergency department when gang members come in for treatment of trauma wounds, or through creative collaboration with law enforcement.

c. Akiyama (2012) suggests that youth have some level of gang involvement if they do any of the following: openly admit to being in a gang; are obsessed with a particular color of clothing (e.g., blue = Crips; black/gold = Latin Kings; gray = Tiny Rascal Gang; and red = Bloods); wear jewelry with distinct designs; wear a colored handkerchief on one side of the body (left = Crip side; right = Blood side); prefer a specific brand of clothing (British Knights = BK = Blood Killer; K-SWISS = Killing Slobs When I See Slobs; and Calvin Klein = CK = Crip Killer); use hand signals when engaging other youth; have paint or permanent marker stains on hands or clothing or are in possession of graffiti paraphernalia (markers, spray paint, bug spray, or starch cans); or display unusual drawings or graffiti on textbooks, bedsheets, mirrors, or bathroom walls.

d.   Health care providers may be able to assess where a juvenile is with regard to gang membership by assessing for the following levels of involvement (Winston-Salem Police Department et al., n.d.):

- Fantasy—Gang knowledge minimal, possibly from media
- Fringe—Casually associates with gang members and may admire them
- Associate—Regularly associates with gang members, considers them normal or admirable, and considers joining them
- Member—Participates in gang crimes and related activities, and sees them as the only authority
- Hard-core—Totally committed to the gang and is considered hard-core by self and other members

e.   Do not forget the girls, who join gangs in large numbers. Young girls join gangs for similar reasons as boys. Factors include deprivation, disengagement, and poor self-esteem. Many of these girls have mental health problems, including self-harming behaviors and suicidal risk (Allen, 2013).

C. Diagnosis, Including Differential Diagnoses, When Appropriate

Possible diagnoses may include conduct disorder, antisocial personality disorder (18 years old and older), and substance abuse.

D. Levels of Prevention/Intervention

a.   Primary

Gangs create a significant burden on public health systems, and preventing youth from joining gangs is crucial to the lasting reduction of youth gang activity (Simon et al., 2013). Provide access to needed services such as prenatal and infant care, after school activities, truancy and dropout prevention, and job programs. Given the young age at which children may join gangs, prevention efforts should begin early, before age 12, with the implementation of evidence-based, effective prevention programs, such as Gang Resistance Education and Training (G.R.E.A.T.), which is a law-enforcement instructed, school-based curriculum to prevent delinquency, youth violence, and gang membership. Preventing youth from joining gangs is far more effective in warding off consequences than persuading active gang members to leave (Simon et al., 2013).

b. Secondary

Identify families and at-risk youth, ages 7 through 14, and strengthen their engagement with school and meaningful school-related activities. Encourage supportive teacher–student relationships (Ang, Hua, Chan, Cheong, & Leaw, 2015). Community partnerships can reinforce and enhance existing strengths of communities and families with activities such as effective parenting classes, mentoring, life-skills training, case management, and supervised recreation. Additional prevention for females includes preventing sexual abuse and intimate partner violence (Simon et al., 2013).

c. Tertiary

Increase access to health care, but take precautions so that youth are not attacked in retaliation by rival gangs or other gang members (a good approach is to treat rival gang members at different locations), and promote a healthy lifestyle. Health care providers can also: act as liaison between the youth, their families, and other agencies; teach about major causes of morbidity and mortality among youth, such as motor vehicle accidents, homicide, and suicide; teach about major health issues common to the participants' age group, such as drug use, obesity, mental health, and sexual health; and refer for appropriate mental illness and substance abuse treatment, as well as social services. It is also important for health care providers to understand their regional gangs, which can be accomplished with the assistance of law enforcement, to both better assist these youth in reentering into healthy lifestyles, and to keep themselves and their staff safe (Akiyama, 2012).

E. Parenting Tips

Teach parents to:

    a. Spend quality time with your child and convey a strong sense of family.

    b. Supervise your child's activities, and know his or her whereabouts at all times.

    c. Know your child's friends and their families.

    d. Be a positive role model.

    e. Teach values, and let your child know why you think gangs are dangerous.

    f. Get involved in your child's activities.

    g. Stress the importance of schooling, and encourage good study habits.

    h. Create rules; set limits; and be consistent, firm, and fair.

    i. Respect your child's feelings and attitudes.

    j. Foster healthy self-esteem.

k.   Help your child develop self-control and deal effectively with problems.

l.   Tell your child not to:

- Associate with gang members or wannabe members
- Communicate with gang members
- Hang out near or where gangs hang out
- Approach strangers in cars
- Wear gang-related clothing
- Wear gang-initialed clothing (BK [British Knights] also stands for Blood Killer)
- Use words like "slob" where gang members may be, like malls
- Attend parties sponsored by gangs
- Hang out near graffiti or take part in graffiti activity
- Use any type of hand signal in public

m.   Teach your child what to do if approached by a gang member. The best response is to walk away. Tell your child not to respond with the same gesture as a gang member could be "false flagging," using a sign of a rival gang, which could result in violence.

n.   Contact your school if any gang activity takes place there. If they are not helpful, contact the police.

o.   Look for signs of gang activity in your community, especially graffiti and young people hanging out on corners or near school property.

Resources

COPS Gang Tool Kit: www.cops.usdoj.gov/Default.asp?Item=1309

Facts for Teens: Youth Gangs: www.safeyouth.org

Female Gangs: A Focus on Research: www.ncjrs.gov/pdffiles1/ojjdp/186159.pdf

Gang Ink (Gang tattoos): www.gangink.com

Gang Resistance Education and Training (G.R.E.A.T.). www.great-online.org/

Offices of Juvenile Justice and Delinquency Prevention Comprehensive Gang Model: A Guide to Your Community's Youth Gang Problem: www.nationalgangcenter.gov/Content/Documents/Assessment-Guide/Assessment-Guide.pdf

Parent's Quick Reference Card Recognizing and Preventing Gang Involvement: www.cops.usdoj.gov/html/cd_rom/school_safety/pubs/COPS07.pdf

References

Akiyama, C. (2012). Understanding youth street gangs. *Journal of Emergency Nursing, 38*(6), 568–570.

Allen, D. (2013). Why girls fall into gang culture. *Nursing of Children and Young People, 25*(8), 8–9.

Ang, R., Hua,V., Chan, W., Cheong, S., & Leaw, J. (2015). The role of delinquency, proactive aggression, psychopathy and behavioral school engagement in reported youth gang membership. *Journal of Adolescence, 41,* 148–156.

Guerra, N., Dierkhising, C., & Payne, P. (2013). How should we identify and intervene with youth at risk of joining gangs? A developmental approach for children ages 0–12. In T. Simon, N. Ritter, & R. Mahendra (Eds.), *Changing course: Preventing gang membership* (pp. 63–74). Washington, DC: U.S. Department of Justice.

National Gang Center. (n.d.). *National Youth Gang Survey Analysis.* Retrieved from www.national-gangcenter.gov/Survey-Analysis

Patton, D., Eschmann, R., & Butler, D. (2013). Internet banging: New trends in social media, gang violence, masculinity and hip hop. *Computers in Human Behavior, 29,* A54–A59.

Pyrooz, D., & Sweeten, G. (2014). Gang membership between ages 5 and 17 years in the United States. *Journal of Adolescent Health, 56*(4), 414–419. doi:10.1016/j.jadohealth.2014.11.018

Simon, T., Ritter, N., & Mahendra, R., (Eds.). (2013). *Changing course: Preventing gang membership.* Washington, DC: U.S. Department of Justice.

Winston-Salem Police Department, Winston-Salem/Forsyth County Schools, Forsyth County Sheriff's Office, City of Winston-Salem and the Winston-Salem State University Center for Community Safety. (n.d.). Gangs: A guide for parents, teachers and other concerned citizens. Retrieved from http://toknc.com/documents/files/GangGuide2.pdf

CHAPTER 16

Hoarding

A. Description

Hoarding is the excessive acquisition of objects and the unwillingness to part with them. Previously considered only as a symptom of obsessive compulsive disorder (OCD), hoarding is now recognized in the *Diagnostic and Statistical Manual of Mental Disorders, 5th Edition (DSM-5)*, published by the American Psychiatric Association (APA, 2013) as a discrete disorder with distinct treatment needs. It is also now known that many persons with hoarding disorder (HD) report having first experienced symptoms as children or adolescents (Ivanov et al., 2013).

a. The key feature of HD is the person's long-standing, persistent, irrational difficulty in parting with possessions, regardless of their value.

b. Frost (2013) notes that hoarding is a complex disorder believed to be associated with four underlying characteristics. The first includes core vulnerabilities, such as emotional dysregulation and a family history of hoarding and perfectionism. Second, those who hoard seem to have difficulty processing information, which can manifest in problems with attention, memory, categorization, and decision making. Third, people who hoard develop powerful emotional attachments to a greater variety of objects than those who do not hoard, and they feel safe when surrounded by their possessions and anguished at the thought of losing them. Finally, those who hoard believe in the necessity of not wasting objects or losing the opportunities that the objects represent; they believe they need to save objects to remember events or people or because the objects' aesthetic beauty contributes to the problem.

c. Children who hoard develop an overwhelming attachment to their possessions, resulting in cluttered rooms and family tension.

d. One study found a prevalence of 2% in 15-year-old twins ($n = 3,974$), with a significantly higher prevalence in girls than boys (Ivanov et al., 2013).

B. Assessment

    a.   Identify risk: Risk factors for hoarding include traumatic events and having a relative who hoards.

    b.   Hoarding symptoms generally begin in early adolescence (ages 12–13), but have been noted in children as young as 3 years (Frost, 2013; Munroff, Bratiotis, & Steketee, 2011).

    c.   Hoarding ranges from mild (minimal impact on life) to severe (serious dysfunction in day-to-day living).

    d.   HD was recently recognized as a distinct disorder, both in adults and in children. The *DSM-5* (APA, 2013) identifies the following behaviors as indicative of HD: difficulty parting with possessions, even when of no value, because of a perceived need to save them; the accumulation of these possessions to the point where living space is cluttered; and significant distress resulting from the hoarding behavior. Possession accumulation in children may be limited because of their inability to attain excessive items, and clutter may be limited to areas of their rooms, such as under the bed; however, they would still need to feel the need to possess their hoard, be unable to part with the possessions, and have significant distress to meet the criteria for HD.

    e.   Children's hoarding may be contained (under the bed or in the closet), and not readily visible. Hoarded objects may also be limited because of children's limited resources, and these items may include old clothes, books, fast-food containers, broken items, and old food. Children may also steal their hoarded items.

    f.   A key symptom is children's attachment to their possessions. They worry about them to the point of impairment, creating a major source of friction with their parents, and become distressed when the objects are taken away from them or even if the parent rearranges their hoarded items. The hoarding may also interfere with the child's normal activities, as the child may not want to go to school or play with friends because of the child's difficulty in leaving the hoarded items behind. Storch and colleagues (2011) noted clinically that children who hoard tend to collect items that have emotional value for them (an item that belonged to a deceased relative, even though it no longer has use), fear not having the item, and/or feel the need to save it.

    g.   Hoarded items result in actual or potential injury, health hazard, fire hazard, or legal issues (child stealing objects).

    h.   The Structured Interview for Hoarding Disorder (SIHD; Nordsletten et al., 2013) was designed to assist clinicians with the diagnosis of HD in persons ages 16 years and older. The instrument is available via the International OCD Foundation's website (www.iocdf.org) and may be beneficial in the primary care setting to help develop assessment interview questions.

i.   The Hoarding Rating Scale is a Likert-style self-report instrument that is useful as a screening tool. It is also available via the International OCD Foundation's website.

C. Diagnosis, Including Differential Diagnoses, When Appropriate

a.   HD is often a disorder of exclusion after careful evaluation of the motivations underlying the hoarding activity. Collateral information should be collected from the child's family. Photographs of the hoarded items may also be beneficial.

b.   For HD in children, assess for the three key characteristics: cluttered space from having too many possessions, difficulty parting with possessions regardless of value, and significant distress or functional impairment.

c.   Differential diagnoses

- Collecting behavior: Essentially, children collect because they want to, whereas other children hoard because they have to. Collectors deliberately seek out specific items, such as comic books, rocks, insects, feathers, toy cars, dolls, stamps, and movie/licensed character memorabilia. Collectors take pride in their collections. They categorize, carefully display, and enjoy talking about them. Collections may be large, but they do not cause distress or uncontrolled clutter. Children tend to begin to cultivate an interest in collections around age 8 years, when they develop problem-solving and organizational skills.

- Food insecurity: Children who are fostered or adopted and who have come from neglectful situations may hoard food because of food insecurity. They may steal food from the pantry/cupboards and hide it in their furniture or clothing. Although this behavior diminishes with time, it may recur during times of stress.

- Hoarding as part of OCD: In children with OCD, the thoughts about hoarding are distressing (ego-dystonic) within the context of OCD. These thoughts are not distressing (ego-syntonic) or repetitive in HD, nor do they result in rituals developed to control the thoughts. Instead, in HD, the acquisition and reviewing of hoarded items is associated with positive feelings. Distress comes from the consequences of hoarding (Frank et al., 2014; Frost, Stektee, & Tolin, 2012).

- Other conditions that may lead to hoarding behaviors: autistic spectrum disorder (restricted interests), brain injury, bulimia nervosa (usually food hoarding), psychotic delusions, and Prader–Willi syndrome (Storch et al., 2011).

d.   Comorbidities (which may also be differential diagnoses): Hoarding has high comorbid rates with attention deficit hyperactivity disorder, depression, generalized anxiety disorder, learning disorders, social anxiety, somatic complaints, and personality disorders (particularly obsessive compulsive personality disorder [OCPD]), as well as chronic medical conditions, and obesity (Frank et al., 2014).

D. Levels of Prevention/Intervention

a. Primary

Little is known about this disorder, and thus there is no known primary prevention at this time.

b. Secondary

Screen for risk factors by asking about hoarding behaviors in relatives and traumatic events in the child's lifetime. Be advised that, because of the ego-syntonic nature of HD, parents with this disorder may be oblivious to the fact that they have a disorder.

c. Tertiary

The main goal of treatment for older children is to assist them in recapturing the positive role of possessions in their lives, usually through a specific, empirically focused cognitive behavioral therapy (CBT) program. The behavioral plan includes stopping the acquisition of new items while providing incentives for the child to get rid of hoarded objects. Children learn how to decide which items to keep and which to discard, and they develop an understanding of why they need to hoard. The medications usually used as part of the treatment plan for hoarding are selective serotonin reuptake inhibitors (SSRIs); however, not all hoarders respond to medications. The treatment of children aged 8 years and younger typically involves a behavioral plan that begins with stopping the child from acquiring new possessions and then using incentives to gradually enable the child to get rid of hoarded objects. Compulsive hoarding can be difficult to treat, and it may be accompanied by comorbid disorders; therefore, this behavior warrants referral to a psychiatric provider experienced with this problem.

E. Parenting Tips

a. Do not allow the child to accumulate additional items.

b. Encourage donating old items to charities that are meaningful to the child. Create a special place or bin for this purpose.

c. Help the child to organize by making it a fun game. The child can also create a special place for treasured items.

d. Use plastic bins and open shelves to organize items, so that the child can still see his or her treasures while undergoing the decluttering process.

e. Be supportive; this process can be long and stressful.

Sometimes it is the parent, not the child, who has HD, and this can be very stressful, as well as dangerous, to the child who can suffer the consequences of cramped and unusable living space, dangerous conditions related to potential injury, fire and health hazards, and financial strain. The embarrassment of their living conditions can also take its toll, possibly even causing children to become isolated because of fear of their peers finding out about their home life. The International OCD Foundation's website has a pdf of agencies that should be involved when HD becomes disruptive to families; among those on the list is Child Protective Services. There is also an organization called Children of Hoarders that can provide supportive information: www.childrenofhoarders.com

Resources

The Compulsive Hoarding Center: http://anxietytreatmentexperts.com/compulsive-hoarding-center/

Hoarding Behaviors in Children: Social Workers' Perspectives (2012, Lap Lambert Academic Publishing) by Brianne Agan

International OCD Foundation: www.iocdf.org

The Oxford Handbook of Hoarding and Acquiring (2014, Oxford University Press) by Randy Frost, Ph.D. and Gail Stekette, Ph.D.

Stuff: Compulsive Hoarding and the Meaning of Things (2011, Mariner Books) by Randy Frost, Ph.D. and Gail Stekette, Ph.D.

References

American Psychiatric Association. (2013). Diagnostic and statistical manual of mental disorders (5th ed.). Washington, DC: Author.

Frank, H., Stewart, E., Walther, M., Benito, K., Freeman, J., Conelea, C., & Garcia, A. (2014). Hoarding behavior among young children with obsessive–compulsive disorder. Journal of Obsessive-Compulsive and Related Disorders, 3, 6–11.

Frost, R. (2013). Causes of hoarding. Retrieved from www.icarevillage.com/common-concerns-hoarding-frost-causes.aspx

Frost, R. O., Steketee, G., & Tolin, D. F. (2012). Diagnosis and assessment of hoarding disorder. *Annual Review of Clinical Psychology, 8*, 219–242.

Ivanov, V. Z., Mataix-Cols, D., Serlachius, E., Lichtenstein, P., Anckarsäter, H., Chang, Z., . . . Rück, C. (2013). Prevalence, comorbidity and heritability of hoarding symptoms in adolescence: A population based twin study in 15-year olds. *PLoS One, 8*(7), e69140. doi:10.1371/journal.pone

Muroff, J., Bratiotis, C., & Steketee, G. (2011). Treatment for compulsive hoarding: A review. *Clinical Social Work Journal, 39*, 406–423.

Nordsletten, A. E., Fernández de la Cruz, L., Pertusa, A., Reichenberg, A., Hatch, S. L., & Mataix-Cols, D. (2013). The Structured Interview for Hoarding Disorder (SIHD): Development, usage and further validation. *Journal of Obsessive Compulsive and Related Disorders, 2*(3), 346–350.

Storch, E. A., Rahman, O., Park, J. M., Reid, J., Murphy, T. K., & Lewin, A. B. (2011). Compulsive hoarding in children. *Journal of Clinical Psychology, 67*(5), 507–516. doi:10.1002/jclp.20794

CHAPTER 17

Hyperactivity

A. Description

Hyperactivity is a higher than developmentally normal level of activity; inattention is the lack of required focus to a task or event at hand; and impulsivity means doing things abruptly with little to no thought.

    a. Most children have times when they are inattentive, irritable, fidgety, disorganized, impulsive, distracted, or hyperactive. However, for most children, these behaviors occur sporadically, are developmentally appropriate, and do not cause distress or impairment. Attention deficit hyperactivity disorder (ADHD) is a psychiatric disorder where children have these types of behaviors most of the time both at home and at school, and these behaviors cause significant impairment or distress.

    b. In most cases, the disorder stabilizes in early adolescence and, in most children, symptoms subside between late adolescence and early adulthood. A few individuals experience the full range of ADHD symptoms into middle adulthood.

B. Assessment (History, Physical, Diagnostic Screening/Testing, Where Appropriate)

    a. Risk factors: The biggest risk for ADHD is having a genetic tendency for the disorder.

    b. The comprehensive history should include: prenatal, perinatal, and postnatal history; toddlerhood history; report of symptoms from parent/caretaker, school, and client; school/work performance; cardiac history and family history of sudden cardiac death.

    c. The comprehensive physical exam should include vision and hearing screen and a complete neurological evaluation.

d.   An electrocardiograph should be ordered prior to treatment; however, cardiology consultation and examination are warranted if there are any cardiac risk factors.

e.   Rating scales include:

- American Academy of Pediatrics, National Initiative for Children's Healthcare Quality Vanderbilt Assessment Scales for children 6 to 12 years of age. This is a free download for the 1st edition, available at www.nichq.org/childrens%20 health/adhd/resources/vanderbilt%20assessment%20scales. The 2nd edition is available for purchase, also via the website.

- The Child Behavior Checklist is available for ages 18 months to 18 years of age (parent/teacher or self-report) at store.aseba.org.

- The Conners 3rd edition (Conners 3), which is used for ages 2 years through adulthood, has been updated to provide a new scoring option for the *Diagnostic and Statistical Manual of Mental Disorders, 5th Edition* (*DSM-5*; American Psychiatric Association [APA], 2013), Symptom Scales, but also has an option for the *DSM, 4th Edition, Text Revision* (*DSM-IV-TR*): DSM Symptom Scales (www.mhs.com/product.aspx?gr=cli&id=overview&prod=conners3).

C. Diagnosis, Including Differential Diagnoses, When Appropriate

a.   ADHD should be considered in clients 4 years old and older who have a persistent pattern of inattention, hyperactivity, and/or impulsivity, or a combination of the two. The *DSM-5* (APA, 2013) identifies several behaviors as indicative of ADHD. Characteristics of inattention include lack of attention to detail, making careless mistakes, inability to stay on task or follow directions, forgetfulness, easily losing things, avoiding disliked tasks, and being easily prone to distraction. Characteristics of hyperactivity and impulsivity include fidgetiness; inability to stay seated or in line; excessive talking, running, or climbing; blurting out answers or interrupting others; difficulty playing quietly; and the appearance of being on the go all the time. To be diagnosed with ADHD, symptoms must be present before age 12 and must occur in two or more settings.

b.   Differential diagnoses and comorbidities are similar: anxiety disorders; autistic spectrum disorder; bipolar disorder; communication disorder; conduct disorder; depression; disruptive mood dysregulation disorder; dissociative disorders; eating disorder; fetal alcohol syndrome; fragile X syndrome; hearing loss; intellectual disability; intermittent explosive disorder; learning disability; neurofibromatosis; oppositional defiant disorder; personality disorder (particularly borderline or antisocial); post-traumatic stress disorder; psychotic disorders; seizure disorder; sleep disorder; speech and language disorder; substance-related disorders; thought disorder; Tourette syndrome or other tic disorders; somatic comorbidity; thyroid abnormalities; and vision disorder (Felt, Biebermann, Christner, Kochhar, & Harrison, 2014; Subcommittee on Attention-Deficit/Hyperactivity Disorder, Steering Committee on Quality Improvement and Management et al., 2013; Wilkes, 2015).

c.   Substances that can mimic ADHD include: steroids, antihistamines, anticonvulsants, caffeine, and nicotine (Post & Kurlansik, 2012).

D. Levels of Prevention/Intervention

a.   Primary

Initiatives that may lower the rates of ADHD include programs that promote maternal health during pregnancy, such as warnings against alcohol and cigarette use, and initiatives to reduce environmental toxins, such as lead and mercury (Halperin, Bedard, & Curchack-Litchtin, 2012).

b.   Secondary

Parent-focused interventions The Incredible Years and Triple P for preschoolers have demonstrated behavioral improvements that persist beyond the end of treatment (Halperin et al., 2012).

c.   Tertiary

- ADHD is a chronic condition; thus children and youth with ADHD have special care needs, and their care should follow the principles of chronic care and the medical home (AAP, 2011). Evidence-based (Quality A/strong recommendation) parent- and/or teacher-administered behavior therapy is the first line of treatment for children ages 4 to 5 years; methylphenidate is prescribed if behavior interventions do not provide significant improvement with continued moderate–severe disturbance in function. Medications reduce the main ADHD symptoms for most children. Psychostimulants (methylphenidate, dextroamphetamine, and mixed amphetamine salts such as dextroamphetamine/amphetamine [Adderall]) are the safest and most effective option, and are the first choice for ADHD treatment. Atomoxetine and alpha-2 receptor agonists (guanfacine, clonidine) are effective but are less effective than psychostimulants and have fewer supporting studies. Starting with a second-line drug may be an option because of strong family preference for a nonstimulant medication, concern about drug diversion (some long-acting stimulants reduce this risk), or comorbid conditions that might also be managed by a single medication (an anxiety or tic disorder). Other

medications used to treat ADHD include antidepressants, atypical antipsychotics, aripiprazole, and mood stabilizers. These are not Food and Drug
Administration (FDA) approved for treating ADHD and are used off-label for
treatment of comorbid conditions or when psychostimulants, atomoxetine,
or alpha-2 receptor agonists are ineffective (Felt et al., 2014).

- Pharmacotherapy is the primary treatment for ADHD in young adults. Medications used for children have been found to be safe and effective for adults,
with stimulants and antidepressants having similar effectiveness. Stimulants
and atomoxetine are first-line treatments, followed by antidepressants (Post &
Kurlansik, 2012).

- Monitor for the emergence and severity of medication side effects, many of
which are transient. These can be managed with dosage adjustment, drug
change, or adjunctive therapy. Measure weight and height twice each year
(Winthrow, Hash, & Holten, 2011).

- Evidence-based behavioral therapies, such as positive parent training, peer interventions, and classroom management, improve behavior, social skills, relationships, and academic functioning (Felt et al., 2014). Parental and classroom
interventions are considered to be more effective than cognitive behavioral
therapy (Winthrow et al., 2011).

E. Parenting Tips

To help your child manage ADHD (American Academy of Child and Adolescent
Psychiatrists, 2016; CHADD, n.d.; Tartakovsky, 2013):

a. Take control. Learn everything you can about ADHD and its treatment, including
medications and successful behavioral management; keep current, and know what to
expect as your child ages. You are the captain of your child's wellness team.

b. Find out if you or your partner has ADHD. It runs in families and can make
parenting difficult.

c. Do not blame yourself or your child for the ADHD. It is an illness, just like asthma
or diabetes.

d. Trust your instincts—if you think something is wrong, it probably is—talk to
your health care provider about it.

e. Know your child's rights—your child may be entitled to additional services or
accommodations in school, as per federal laws.

f. Talk to your child's high school guidance counselor and your health care provider when readying your child for college; you will want to choose a college that is

supportive and that has adequate resources for your child's emotional, academic, and social needs.

g. Communicate with your child, family, and health care team.

h. Follow the rules, both at home and at school, and make sure they are clear and consistent. But expect some rule breaking, and manage it appropriately when it happens.

i. Embrace challenges and wrestle with them one at a time.

j. Know when to compromise and when to adjust to change.

k. Help your child adjust to change and to make smart choices.

l. Foster your child's success in academics, activities, and friendships.

m. Boost your child's self-image, self-esteem, and self-confidence. Acknowledge successes, and help your child learn from mistakes. Give your child special time, and, most important, give unconditional love and show it.

n. Take care of yourself. Enjoy date nights with your partner, outings with friends, help from a support group, quiet alone time, or whatever helps you de-stress and refresh.

o. Celebrate being a family, and embrace your child's energy and enthusiasm.

Resources

American Academy of Child and Adolescent Psychiatry: www.aacap.org/AACAP/Families_and_ Youth/Resource_Centers/ADHD_Resource_Center/Home.aspx

Attention-Deficit Hyperactivity Disorder: http://familydoctor.org/familydoctor/en/diseases-conditions/attention-deficit-hyperactivity-disorder-adhd.html

American Academy of Pediatrics: www2.aap.org/pubserv/adhd2/1sted.html

Centers for Disease Control and Prevention: www.cdc.gov/ncbddd/adhd/materials.html

CHADD: www.chadd.org/

National Institute for Children's Health Quality: www.nichq.org/childrens-health/adhd/resources/ adhd-toolkit

National Institute of Mental Health: www.nimh.nih.gov/health/topics/attention-deficit-hyperactivity-disorder-adhd/index.shtml

References

American Academy of Child and Adolescent Psychiatrists. (2016, January). ADHD Resource Center. Retrieved from www.aacap.org/aacap/families_and_youth/Resource_Centers/ADHD_Resource_Center/Home.aspx

American Academy of Pediatrics Subcommittee on Attention-Deficit/Hyperactivity Disorder, Steering Committee on Quality Improvement and Management. (2011). ADHD: Clinical practice guideline for the diagnosis, evaluation, and treatment of attention-deficit/hyperactivity disorder in children and adolescents. *Pediatrics, 128*(5), 1007-1022; doi: 10.1542/peds.2011-2654

American Psychiatric Association. (2013). *Diagnostic and statistical manual of mental disorders* (5th ed.). Washington, DC: Author.

Children and Adults With Attention-Deficit/Hyperactivity Disorder. (n.d.). *Parenting a child with ADHD*. National Resource Center on ADHD. Retrieved from www.chadd.org/Portals/0/Content/CHADD/NRC/Factsheets/parenting2015.pdf

Felt, B. T., Biebermann, B., Christner, J. G., Kochhar, P., & Harrison, R. V. (2014). Diagnosis and management of ADHD in children. *American Family Physician, 90*(7), 456–464.

Halperin, J., Bedard, A., & Curchack-Litchtin, J. (2012). Preventive interventions for ADHD: A neurodevelopmental perspective. *Neurotherapeutics, 9*(3), 531–541.

Post, R., & Kurlansik, S. (2012). Diagnosis and management of attention-deficit/hyperactivity disorder in adults. *American Family Physician, 85*(9), 890–896.

Subcommittee on Attention-Deficit/Hyperactivity Disorder, Steering Committee on Quality Improvement and Management, Wolraich, M., Brown, L., Brown, R. T., DuPaul, G., Earls, M.,... Visser, S. (2011). ADHD: Clinical practice guideline for the diagnosis, evaluation, and treatment of attention-deficit/hyperactivity disorder in children and adolescents. *Pediatrics, 128*(5), 1007–1022.

Tartakovsky, M. (2013). Parenting kids with ADHD: 16 tips to tackle common challenges. *Psych Central*. Retrieved from http://psychcentral.com/lib/parenting-kids-with-adhd-16-tips-to-tackle-common-challenges

Wilkes, M. (2015). Pediatric attention deficit hyperactivity disorder. *Emedicine Medscape*. Retrieved from http://emedicine.medscape.com/article/912633-overview

Winthrow, L., Hash, P., & Holten, K. (2011). Managing ADHD in children: Are you doing enough? *Journal of Family Practice, 60*(4), E1–E3.

CHAPTER 18

LGBTQI2

A. Description

LGBTQI2 stands for lesbian (female attracted primarily to other females), gay (person attracted to members of the same sex, but often used for males), bisexual (person attracted to both males and females), transgender (usually used for persons who do not identify with their birth gender or the binary gender system), questioning (persons who are exploring their own sexual orientation, gender identity, or gender expression), intersex (person whose sexual anatomy or chromosomes do not match with traditional male or female markers; includes those born XXY) or two-spirit (no single definition; can be used for Native, Aboriginal, and First Nations persons who experience gender or sexual identity outside the binary gender system).

a. Sexual orientation, usually identified as heterosexual, homosexual, or bisexual, includes components of identity, attraction, and behavior in a person's emotional, sexual, and/or relational attraction to others. Gender identity is a person's sense of being male, female, or something else, whereas gender expression is how a person expresses his or her gender identity (body movement, dress, etc.). Gender nonconforming youth are those whose gender expression differs from how their family, culture, or society expects them to act, behave, and dress. Gender queer youth do not accept typical gender roles, are not exclusively masculine or feminine, have no gender or have two or more genders, or move between genders (Center of Excellence for Transgender Health, 2015; Substance Abuse and Mental Health Services Administration [SAMHSA], 2014).

b. Many families have strict cultural expectations about gender role behavior and have difficulty tolerating their child's nonconforming behavior. In general, family reactions vary, but there tends to be more acceptance and ambivalence than outright rejection, as previously assumed. Rejecting families become less rejecting with time, and most want to help their child and keep the family together, but do not know how. Those who reject their child's orientation and behaviors and try to change them often do so because they believe they are trying to help their child fit in and be accepted by others. Thus, accurate information from health care providers is critical.

c.   Two-spirit persons were traditionally respected as gifted and spiritual people who performed highly respected spiritual, medical, and economic roles as ceremonial leaders, shamans, medical doctors, caretakers, and teachers of children. Those who identify as two-spirit today view themselves as living in harmony with traditional Native values and beliefs; however, they often experience discrimination, encountering homophobia within their communities. Many modern constructs of Native masculinity and femininity today reject variations in the binary gender roles that have been adopted over time (Sheppard & Mayo, 2013).

B. Assessment (History, Physical, Diagnostic Screening/Testing, Where Appropriate)

a.   Risk factors: Family rejection during adolescence can lead to increased risk of suicide, depression, substance abuse, and engaging in unprotected intercourse (Ryan, Huebner, Diaz, & Sanchez, 2009). Factors that place sexual minority youths at greater risk for psychiatric disorders include homophobia (fear/hatred of homosexual persons), heterosexism (presumption that all people are or should be heterosexual), rejection by society, fear of harassment and violence, fear of rejection, moral or religious pressures, feelings of otherness, and poor social supports (Lambrese & Hunt, 2013).

b.   Protective factors: Family acceptance predicts better self-esteem, social support, and general health status, and is protective against depression, substance abuse, and suicidal ideation and behaviors (Ryan, Russell, Huebner, Diaz, & Sanchez, 2010). Other caring adults and school safety also act as protective factors.

c.   Health care professionals should be aware of their own biases and not assume heterosexuality. A comprehensive, developmentally appropriate, gender-neutral, and confidential adolescent history allows for the assessment of strengths, assets, and risks, allowing sexual minority youth to live productive and healthy lives as they transition through adolescence and young adulthood. Talk to all youth about sexual orientation, and ask about family and friends' reactions, feelings, and concerns.

d.   Stigmatization creates many issues for LGBTQI2 youth, including homelessness, altered body image, social anxiety, depression, suicidality, substance abuse, posttraumatic stress disorder, and other mental health issues. Many experience harassment and violence. Sexual minority youth are more likely to be kicked out of their homes or to have run away from their homes than heterosexual youth, and few shelters exist for this population. Homeless sexual minority youths are also more likely to engage in survival sex (selling themselves for sex to meet their needs for food, clothing, and shelter), and more likely to have more sexual partners, experience victimization, engage in substance abuse, and experience psychopathology than heterosexual homeless youths (Gamache & Lazear, 2009).

e.   Physical health risks are also a concern, and these include HIV/AIDS and other sexually transmitted diseases and pregnancy. Transgender youth who use street transgenic hormones can develop significant health problems, even if the hormones are pure (American Academy of Pediatrics Committee on Adolescence, 2013).

f.   Understand the youth's coming-out status. People choose to come out for many reasons, including: wanting to begin dating and wanting family to know; not wanting people to make assumptions about them; being tired of hearing stereotypes of negative labels; and feeling like they are living a lie and wanting to be accepted for who they are. However, there are also people who choose not to come out, and their reasons include: being unsure of who they are and how they feel; feeling the topic is private; fearing bullying, harassment, discrimination, or violence; and being concerned about how their family members will react (Nemours Foundation, 2015). Youth are coming out at earlier ages, with some children identifying as lesbian, gay, bisexual, or transgender in middle school (Shields et al., 2013), and families play a critical role in providing support. Thus, it is also important to assess the family's acceptance and cultural views of their child's gender and sexual preference orientations. Ask about family reactions to the youth's sexual orientation, gender identity, and gender expression.

g.   When assessing transgender youth, honor their preferred gender identity by using the pronouns and terminology that the youth prefer. Recognize that their bodies may have characteristics that do not conform to their gender identity. Their anatomy does not define them, even though that anatomy may require treatment. Transgender youth may also undergo hormonal or surgical treatment, and face fertility issues. Thus, health care providers should utilize evidence-based protocols when addressing prevention and screening.

C. Diagnosis

a.   Possible psychiatric problems/diagnoses are social anxiety, depression, posttraumatic stress disorder, eating disorders, and suicidality (Lambrese & Hunt, 2013).

b.   Children as young as 2 years may show features of gender dysphoria. The *Diagnostic and Statistical Manual of Mental Disorders, 5th Edition* (*DSM-5*), published by the American Psychiatric Association (APA, 2013), identifies several behaviors as indicative of gender dysphoria. The individuals experience significant difference between their birth gender and their experienced gender. This can be characterized by a strongly expressed desire to be their experienced gender, persistent preference for cross-dressing, rejection of clothes/games/toys typical of their birth gender, and a desire for those of their experienced gender. They may have a strong dislike for their sexual anatomy and a strong desire to have the anatomy of their experienced gender.

D. Levels of Prevention/Intervention

a.   Primary

Include LGBTQI2 books, brochures, flyers, and posters throughout the primary care agency. Many of these youths look for safe zone or rainbow stickers to indicate that a provider will be open and respectful in providing support and addressing needs (SAMHSA, 2012).

b.   Secondary

- To decrease risk and increase well-being through family engagement, SAM-HSA (2012) recommends the following measures:
    - Connect with families and caregivers by meeting them where they are, and view them as allies.
    - Let family members tell their story.
    - Enable family members to use respectful language to talk about sexual orientation and gender identity.
    - Educate families on the impact of family rejecting behaviors on their LGBT child.
    - Educate families on the impact of supportive and accepting behaviors on their LGBT child.
    - Even if families do not accept their children's sexual orientation and gender identity, they can still support their children and decrease rejecting behaviors to protect them from harm.
    - Little changes make a big difference in decreasing family rejecting behaviors and in increasing support for their LGBT children.
- Because many adolescents who identify as LGBTQI2 may have unpredictable sexual encounters, conversation about highly effective birth control methods and emergency contraception is important (American Academy of Pediatrics Committee on Adolescence, 2013). Suicide prevention is critical, warranting addressing depression and hopelessness (Mustanski & Liu, 2013).

c.   Tertiary

Provide education, support, and counseling to parents, families, foster parents, and caregivers who are engaging in rejecting behaviors. This includes using educational materials to help them understand the impact of their behaviors on their LGBT child (see Resources at the end of this chapter), and providing coaching, counseling, peer support, and family therapy. Refer children who meet the criteria for gender dysphoria. Retraditionalization (re-embracing traditional practices) can be an important tool in the healing process of two-spirits and their communities.

E. Parenting Tips

When your child comes out (i.e., telling people one is LGBTQI2):

a. "Coming out is a life-long journey of understanding and sharing one's gender identity and sexual orientation with others" (American Academy of Pediatrics, 2015).

b. Each child is unique, and coming out may be quick and easy for some, but long and difficult for others; however, most people come out gradually, usually first telling family, friends, or a counselor (American Academy of Pediatrics, 2015; Lazarus, 2013; Nemours Foundation, 2015):

- Coming out can be difficult because your child may be concerned about how you or other family members will react.
- Understand that human sexuality is complex and essentially genetic/epigenetic, not a conscious choice.
- Accept your child for who he or she is, and do not blame anyone for your child being who he or she is.
- Avoid criticism, disapproval, and rejection.
- Support your child, and provide unconditional love.
- Validate your child's sexual identity and preferences by telling your child that you want him or her to be happy in life.
- Do not demand or suggest that your child seek help to get straight.

Resources

Advocates for Youth: www.advocatesforyouth.org

American Academy of Child and Adolescent Psychiatrists. (2012). Practice parameter on gay, lesbian, or bisexual sexual orientation, gender nonconformity, and gender discordance in children and adolescents. *Journal of the American Academy of Child and Adolescent Psychiatry, 51*(9), 957–974.

American Academy of Pediatrics Committee on Adolescence. (2013). Office-based care for lesbian, gay, bisexual, transgender, and questioning youth. *Pediatrics, 132*(1), 198–203.

American Academy of Pediatrics Lesbian, Gay, Bisexual and Transgender Health and Wellness: www.aap.org/en-us/about-the-aap/Committees-Councils-Sections/solgbt/Pages/home.aspx

American Academy of Pediatrics Office-Based Care for Lesbian, Gay, Bisexual, Transgender, and Questioning Youth: http://pediatrics.aappublications.org/content/132/1/198.full?sid=baab3d90-dd2d-4618-8b7d-b3091d6eb732

American Psychological Association LGBT Youth Resources: www.apa.org/pi/lgbt/programs/safe-supportive/lgbt/default.aspx

Association for Lesbian, Gay, Bisexual & Transgender Issues in Counseling: www.algbtic.org/

Gender Spectrum: www.genderspectrum.org/

Makadon, K., Mayer, K., Potter, J., & Goldhammer, H. (2015). The Fenway *guide to lesbian, gay, bisexual and transgender health*, 2nd Edition. American College of Physicians. ISBN-13: 978-1938921001

National Coalition for LGBT Health: www.healthhiv.org/sites-causes/national-coalition-for-lgbt-health/

National Gay and Lesbian Task Force: www.thetaskforce.org

National LGBT Health Education Center: www.lgbthealtheducation.org/training/cme/

Parents, Families, and Friends of Lesbians and Gays: www.pflag.org. Substance Abuse and Mental Health Services Administration (SAMHSA). LGBT Training Curricula for Behavioral Health and Primary Care Practitioners: www.samhsa.gov/behavioral-health-equity/lgbt/curricula

Substance Abuse and Mental Health Services Administration (SAMHSA). LGBT Training Curricula for Behavioral Health and Primary Care Practitioners: www.samhsa.gov/behavioral-health-equity/lgbt/curricula

Transgender Health Information Program: http://transhealth.vch.ca/

Urban Native Youth Association Two-Spirit Youth Speak Out! www.unya.bc.ca/downloads/glbtq-twospirit-final-report.pdf

University of California San Francisco Center of Excellence for Transgender Health: www.transhealth.ucsf.edu/trans?page=home-00-00

World Professional Association for Transgender Health. (2013). Standards of care for the health of transsexual, transgender, and gender-nonconforming people. Retrieved from www.wpath.org/uploaded_files/140/files/IJT%20SOC,%20V7.pdf

References

American Academy of Pediatrics. (2015). *Coming out: Information for parents of LGBT teens.* Retrieved from www.healthychildren.org/English/ages-stages/teen/dating-sex/Pages/Four-Stages-of-Coming-Out.aspx

Center of Excellence for Transgender Health. (2015). *Transgender terminology.* Retrieved from www.transhealth.ucsf.edu/trans?page=protocol-terminology

Gamache, P., & Lazear, K. J. (2009). *Asset-based approaches for lesbian, gay, bisexual, transgender, questioning, intersex, two-spirit (LGBTQI2-S) youth and families in systems of care.* (FMHI pub. no. 252). Tampa, FL: University of South Florida, College of Behavioral and Community Sciences, The Louis de la Parte Florida Mental Health Institute, Research and Training Center for Children's Mental Health. Retrieved from http://rtckids.fmhi.usf.edu/rtcpubs/FamExp/lgbt-mono.pdf

Lambrese, J., & Hunt, J. (2013). Mental health needs of sexual minority youth: A student-developed novel curriculum for healthcare providers. *Journal of Gay & Lesbian Mental Health, 17,* 221–234.

Lazarus, C. (2013). What to do if your child comes out. *Psychology Today.* Retrieved from www.psychologytoday.com/blog/think-well/201312/what-do-if-your-child-comes-out

Mustanski, B., & Liu, R. (2013). A longitudinal study of predictors of suicide attempts among lesbian, gay, bisexual, and transgender youth. *Archives of Sexual Behavior, 42,* 437–448. doi:10.1007/s10508-012-0013-9

Nemours Foundation. (2015). Coming out. KidsHealth/TeensHealth. Retrieved from http://kidshealth.org/teen/your_mind/friends/coming-out.html

Ryan, C., Huebner, D., Diaz, R. M., & Sanchez, J. (2009). Family rejection as a predictor of negative health outcomes in White and Latino lesbian, gay and bisexual young adults. *Pediatrics, 123*(1), 346–352.

Ryan, C., Russell, S., Huebner, D., Diaz, D., & Sanchez, J. (2010). Family acceptance in adolescence and the health of LGBT young adults. *Journal of Child and Adolescent Psychiatric Nursing, 23*(4), 205–213.

Sheppard, M., & Mayo, J. (2013). The social construction of gender and sexuality: Learning from two spirit traditions. *The Social Studies, 104,* 259–270.

Shields, J. P., Cohen, R., Glassman, J. R., Whitaker, K., Franks, H., & Bertolini, I. (2013). Estimating population size and demographic characteristics of lesbian, gay, bisexual, and transgender youth in middle school. *Journal of Adolescent Health, 52*(2), 248–250.

Substance Abuse and Mental Health Services Administration. (2012). *Top health issues for LGBT populations information & resource kit.* HHS Publication No. (SMA) 12-4684. Rockville, MD: Author.

Substance Abuse and Mental Health Services Administration. (2014). *A practitioner's resource guide: Helping families to support their LGBT children* (HHS Publication No. PEP14-LGBTKIDS). Rockville, MD: Author.

CHAPTER 19

Missing Children

A. Description

Missing children are defined by Biehal and Wade (2002, p. 6) as "children and young people who spend time away from where they ought to usually live, without the consent of parents or carers, or because they have been forced to leave by parents and carers." The law of the United States defines "missing child" as "any individual less than 18 years of age whose whereabouts are unknown to such individual's legal custodian" (Cornell University Law School, n.d.).

    a. Children, especially children with autism, may wander, while others may run away, become lost in unfamiliar places or during disasters, or be abducted. Children who go missing, especially those who end up living in the streets, face significant risks to their health and well-being, including poor general health, drug use, HIV, assaults, rape, involvement in crime, and murder, while others may be accidentally injured or killed by exposure to the natural environment. Fortunately, the majority of missing children are found within hours or days by usual law enforcement response (Howard, Broughton, & the Committee on Psychosocial Aspects of Child and Family Health, 2004).

    b. Runaways and throwaways: Most missing children leave of their own accord, usually because of an adverse family situation; others are thrown out of their families, and many of these are not reported. About one third of this group run away from foster care. When these children are gone for prolonged periods of time, they become at risk for medical and psychological problems, as well as crime as they may be subjected to human trafficking (prostitution) and drug trafficking. Runaways are usually 15 to 17 years old, but some are as young as 7 years.

    c. Wanderers and lost children: Children who wander or become lost are also vulnerable to exploitation and abuse, and they may become disoriented and injured (drowning, traffic accidents, dehydration, heat stroke, hypothermia, and falls). A study by Anderson et al. (2012) found that nearly half of children with autistic spectrum disorder (ASD) engaged in elopement behavior, with a sizeable number at risk for bodily harm. Children with autism wander for various reasons: seeking small or enclosed spaces, going to places of special interest to them, or attempting to escape overwhelming stimuli (sights, sounds, activities of others, or surroundings). They often have an attraction to water, and drowning is the leading cause of death resulting from a wandering incident. They are also attracted to other objects and places that can create danger for them, such as roadways, trains, heavy equipment, fire trucks, bright lights, and traffic signals (National Center for Missing and Exploited Children, n.d.). Children with autism may be more vulnerable to stranger abductions because of the social deficits that characterize the disorder; they may not be able to differentiate strangers from known adults, or they may be overly sensitive to the abductor's lures (Gunby, Carr, & Leblanc, 2010).

d.   In response to children going missing after Hurricane Katrina in 2005 and the 2010 Haiti earthquake, the Federal Emergency Management Agency (FEMA) joined with the National Center for Missing and Exploited Children (NCMEC) to launch the Unaccompanied Minors Registry. This is a tool to report children who are missing because of natural and man-made disasters, and allows NCMEC to assist ground emergency personnel in reuniting families. The registry accepts reports of children up to age 18 who have been separated from their parents, other relatives, or legal guardians.

e.   Abductions are categorized as either family or nonfamily. Stranger abductions fall into the latter category; however, the terms stranger and nonfamily tend to be used interchangeably, even though nonfamily abductions also include persons known to the child, including neighbors and babysitters.

- Family abductions: Parental kidnapping is the wrongful removal or retention of a minor child by a parent. However, since child abductions are frequently committed by other family members, the term family abduction is more accurate, and this term is often used interchangeably with the term *custodial interference*. Abductors take or fail to return children from their homes, and deprive them of their other parent, often telling the child that the other parent does not love them or is dead. Family-abducted children frequently live lives of deception, moving often and lacking the stability needed for healthy development. They lose everything, including pets and belongings, receive a new identity, are made to lie about their past and not grieve their loss, and may also be physically harmed. Perpetrators can be male or female. Motivations for family abductions vary: effort to force reconciliation or to continue interaction with the left-behind parent; desire to blame, spite, or punish the other parent; fear of losing legal custody or visitation rights; desire to protect the child from a parent who is perceived to molest, abuse, or neglect the child; delusional thinking; and a total disregard for the law (Daniels & Brennan, 2013). Profiles for family abductors are as follows (Hoff, 2008; Johnston, Sagatun-Edwards, Blomquist, & Girdner, 2001; Miller, Kurlycheck, Hansen, & Wilson, 2008):

- *Profile 1: The parent who has committed a prior credible threat or abduction.* This profile is usually combined with one or more of the others. Other risk factors of flight include: the parent is homeless, unemployed, and without ties to the area; the parent has divulged plans to abduct and has the resources to do so; and the parent has liquidated assets and maxed out credit cards or borrowed from other sources.

- *Profile 2: The parent who suspects or believes that abuse has occurred.* These parents may feel the authorities have not taken their allegations seriously and feel the need to "rescue" the child with help from supporters who concur with their beliefs, including underground networks that help them obtain new identities and safe locations. Risk increases if the parent has a fixed belief that the abuse is occurring, has the support of family or friends, or makes repetitive and increasingly hostile accusations.

- *Profile 3: The parent who is paranoid delusional.* These parents demonstrate paranoid, irrational, and sometimes psychotic beliefs and behaviors toward the other parent. They may claim that the other parent exercises mind control over the child or that the other parent harmed the child. This disorder is rare, but these parents are often dangerous, especially if they have a history of domestic violence, substance abuse, or hospitalization for mental illness.

- *Profile 4: The parent who is severely sociopathic (antisocial).* These parents have contempt for authority, including the legal system, and often have flagrantly violated it. They are self-serving, manipulative, and exploitative, and hold exaggerated beliefs about their own superiority and entitlement. They typically have a history of domestic violence, and, like paranoid abductors, they do not see the child as having separate rights and needs. This profile is also rare.

- *Profile 5: The parent who is a citizen of another country.* The risk is very high at the time of separation when these parents feel cast adrift in a foreign land and desire to reconnect with their ethnic or religious roots. Parents at greatest risk are those who idealize their own family, homeland, and culture, and deprecate the American culture.

- *Profile 6: The parent who feels alienated from the legal system and who has support in another community.* These parents feel alienated and rely on their own networks of kin, who may live in another geographical community, to resolve family problems.

Parental kidnappings may be criminal, civil, or both. The criminal process can enable the arrest of an abducting parent, but does not address the return of the child, and the civil process facilitates the return of the child, but does not address arrest or return of the abductor.

- Nonfamily abductions: Abductions by a complete stranger are rare; however, they tend to be highly dangerous because they can lead to sexual abuse, death, or complete disappearance. Children may also be abducted by neighbors and other acquaintances. Although abduction includes children taken off the street and missing for long periods of time, it also includes cases where children are taken for brief periods but not very far without the consent of or against the will of the parent or guardian. There is no minimum time period for a child to be missing to be considered abduction (Daniels & Brennan, 2013). The most common reasons for nonfamily abductions are: sexual assault, ransom, adoption rings, human trafficking, and domination and control. Persons with mental illness may abduct a child, especially an infant, to make it their own, especially after the loss of their own child, and when a person steals a car with a child inside, it is also considered abduction. Motivation is not usually determined until the abductor is captured. Most nonfamily abductors are male, and most victims are female. Common lures include: offering a child a ride, offering sweets, showing the child an animal, asking the child to help find an animal, offering a child money, and asking a child for directions.

B. Assessment

a.   Wandering children: Assess all vulnerable children for the potential for wandering. Work with parents to identify potential triggers and to determine the child's method of wandering, as well as factors in the home environment that may facilitate wandering, and recognize that these need to be corrected. Wandering types include: goal-directed (wandering to get somewhere, such as a swimming pool or train station); bolting/fleeing (suddenly running, usually to get away from something that caused a negative reaction); and other (boredom, disorientation, transition, nighttime, and becoming lost).

- Family abductions: A high percentage of parental abductions take place between separation and divorce, especially in cases where the separation is acrimonious. Although there is no way to definitely determine which parents or family members may become abductors, there are risk factors related to the potential abductor:
  - Previous abduction of the child by family member
  - Threats to abduct the child
  - Direct/indirect threats of harm to partner, child, or self
  - History of controlling and/or violent behavior

- High levels of hostility, anger, or resentment toward the parent or the family
- Volatile parental relationship with frequent arguments over visitation
- Feeling of alienation from the legal system and support in another community/country
- Child has made comments such as "Dad/Mom says we're going to go live somewhere warm"
- Person has no job, could work anywhere, or is financially independent (not tied to the area for financial reasons)
- Raises irrational concerns about the child's safety and well-being while in the custodial parent's care
- A family court decision creates anger
- Stalking or obsessive behavior
- Engaging in quitting a job; selling a home; terminating a lease; closing a bank account; or applying for passports, birth certificates, or school and medical records; or other activities that may indicate preparation for flight

Children are frequently groomed or even brainwashed by the perpetrator parent prior to the abduction.

- Nonfamily abductions: The health care provider would do best to focus on teaching families and children how to prevent nonfamily abductions. Extra attention should be given to "vulnerable" children, as they are at higher risk for nonfamily abductions.

C. Diagnosis

Identify children at risk for wandering, such as those with autistic spectrum and other developmental disorders.

D. Levels of Prevention/Intervention

a. Primary

For all children, enable families to be prepared for the unthinkable. Teach parents to:

- Create a Child identification kit. NCMEC suggests that the kit include:
  - Complete description of the child: name, nickname, birth date, gender, hair color/style, eye color, height, weight, glasses/braces, and identifying marks including body art.
  - Current color photo that is digital and easily accessible at all times and that really looks like the child. Update every 6 months.

- Fingerprints taken by a trained professional. If needed, these can be entered into the FBI's National Crime Information Center (NCIC) database. Have the child fingerprinted by the local police department, and keep the fingerprint card in a safe place. The police will not keep records themselves.
- DNA sample because DNA has become the "gold standard" for personal identification.

- Record the child's social security number.
- Know where the child's medical records are located and how to access them. Make sure they contain information that can help identify the children.
- Make sure the child has up-to-date dental records and that how to access them.
- Make sure custody documents are in order.
- Never leave young children unattended, not even for a few seconds.

b. Secondary

- Family abductions: For families with risk factors for abduction, inform custodial parent to (Hoff, 2008; U.S. Department of Justice, Office of Juvenile Justice and Delinquency Prevention, 2010):
  - Treat visitation and child support as separate issues.
  - Check for abduction prevention laws in the parent's jurisdiction.
  - Get a court custody determination that defines the rights of both parents, and ensure that the custody order states the basis for the court's jurisdiction and manner in which the opportunity to be heard is given to both parents to facilitate interjurisdictional enforcement if needed.
  - Have the court include prevention measures in the custody order (custodial parent will need to provide the court with tangible evidence of the risk for potential abduction). Measures depend on the level of risk for abduction, potential harm to the child, and potential obstacles in getting the child back if abducted. These may include: supervised visitation, prohibition of unauthorized pickup of the child, restrictions on removing the child from the child's home state, and authorization for the assistance of law enforcement in the event of abduction.
  - Keep certified copies of the court order on hand.
  - Ensure that the child has access to and knows how to use a phone to get help.
  - Notify the child's school or day care.
  - Flag the child's passport applications.

- Nonfamily abductions: Stranger abductions are difficult to predict. However, parents should pay attention to:
    - Strangers who hang around places where children play but who are not supervising a child.
    - Individuals who pay unusual attention to their child.
    - Child telling the parent they met someone live or in cyberspace who makes them feel uncomfortable.
    - News and alerts of child abductions.

    If parents have concerns, they should call the police for advice.

c. Tertiary

- For all children: Ensure that all medical records are up-to-date and easily accessible for the family and law enforcement should the need arise. Assist the family in obtaining emotional support during the crisis, and ensure that family members maintain their own health.
    - Confirm the child is missing. Act immediately. Search your house inside and out, especially places where children can get trapped like old refrigerators and trunks. Check with your neighbors and your child's friends to see if he or she is with them.
    - If you still have not found the child, call law enforcement immediately, and give them as much information about the child as possible. Also provide them with as much information about the abductor as possible, and a certified copy of the custody order.
    - Contact family and friends for support.
    - Utilize resources from the NCMEC: 1-800-THE LOST. Contact the state Missing Children Clearinghouse (every state, the District of Columbia, Puerto Rico, and Canada have one).
    - Family abductions:
        - Get an attorney.
        - Call the child's school, and have them flag the child's records so the custodial parent will know if another school requests the child's records.
        - Consider filing charges.
        - Have the attorney obtain a pickup order.
        - If the abductor may flee the country, contact the U.S Department of State's Office of Children's Issues to complete a *Request Entry into the Children's Passport Issuance Alert Program* form to be notified of any pending passport applications (www.travel.state.gov).
        - Keep a note pad to record thoughts and important information.
        - Keep a cell phone charged at all times.

- Abduction affects the child, parent, siblings, and extended family and friends. There is considerable grief and loss. Children may experience "identity rupture," parentification in caring for the abducting parent, and isolation due to forced hiding. They may also suffer abuse from the abducting parent and problems with their education from being kept from going to school. While the child and custodial parent will need referral for treatment, the nurse practitioner can assist the custodial parent by advising him or her to:

  - Allow the child to reintegrate at his or her own pace.

  - Acknowledge the trauma that the child experienced.

  - Do not personalize rejection; the child needs time to learn how to trust again.

  - Provide structure and clear rules and limits.

  - Do not criticize the abductor in front of the child.

- Nonfamily abductions: Nonfamily abductions are serious crimes in which about three quarters of those murdered by their abductors are dead within 3 hours of abduction; thus, these cases require action.

  - Contact law enforcement immediately, and give them as much information about the child as possible. Also provide them with as much information about the abductor as possible, and a certified copy of the custody order. Since stranger abductions are the most dangerous, they are the primary purpose of an AMBER Alert, which is issued by law enforcement. AMBER alerts are used in all 50 states, the District of Columbia, Puerto Rico, the U.S. Virgin Islands, Indian Country, and the U.S. northern and southern borders. The Department of Justice Recommended Criteria for the issuance of an AMBER alert are:

    - Reasonable belief by law enforcement that abduction has occurred.

    - Law enforcement agency belief that the child is in imminent danger.

    - Presence of enough descriptive information about the child and the abduction for law enforcement to issue the alert.

    - The child is 17 years or younger.

    - The child's critical data elements, including the Child Abduction flag, have been entered into the NCIC system.

  - Have your child identification kit ready, as well as the names and contact information of family and friends. Give them the child's cell phone number and cell service provider. Do not call the child's cell, as it may alert the abductor to discard it—the cell may have GPS tracking that can help locate the child. Police may also ask about social media accounts, especially the child's.

- Police file an incident report. Get the number of the report, the name of the filing officer, and a phone number for follow-up.

- According to the Federal Bureau of Investigation (FBI, n.d.), Congress gave the FBI jurisdiction under the "Lindbergh Law" in 1932 to immediately investigate the kidnapping or mysterious disappearance of a young child, usually age 12 years or younger; there does not have to be a ransom note, nor does the child have to be missing for 24 hours or have crossed state lines for the FBI to get involved.

- Contact family and friends for support and assistance in looking for the child.

- Utilize resources from the NCMEC: 1-800-THE LOST. Contact the state Missing Children Clearinghouse (every state, the District of Columbia, Puerto Rico, and Canada have one). This includes the Missing-Child, Emergency-Response, Quick-Reference Guide (www.missingkids.com/Publications/NC198).

- The media usually get involved in stranger abductions; seek help from law enforcement in how to deal with them.

- Social media may be helpful in locating the child, but seek guidance from law enforcement before proceeding.

- Although it is difficult to think during such a stressful situation, parents should try to consider the following to assist police, per Missing Kids Canada:

  - If an infant is abducted, has there been any contact with someone who is childless and may have a mental health disorder?
  - Has anyone threatened harm against the family?
  - Has anyone been paying extra attention to the missing child, or has someone been around the child's environment lately?
  - Has there been a recent breakup or firing?
  - Is money owed to someone?

- Most abducted children are located quickly; however, parents should be prepared for a long-term search. In these cases, they will need continued support. If the case goes "cold," parents may want to consider contacting a reliable cold case organization for possible assistance. One such agency is the American Investigative Society of Cold Cases (AISOCC; www.aisocc.org). Most agencies require contact from the appropriate law enforcement agency to become involved; however, cold case agencies may be able to help parents make that connection.

E. Parenting Tips

a. Wandering:

Utilize tips from the National Autism Association (www.autismsafety.org/prevention
.php?way=12) and Autism Speaks (www.autismspeaks.org/wandering-resources) to
help prevent wandering and wandering-related tragedies:

- Understand wandering patterns. Know your child's wandering type (goal-directed, non-goal directed, random, sudden runner, etc.). Take steps to identify and manage known triggers for wandering.
- Dress your child in bright clothing, so that he or she is visible.
- Secure your home. Contract a professional locksmith, home improvement professional, or security company to help assess your home for safety. You may need deadbolt locks that require keys on both sides, and alarms. You can also install hook and eye locks and battery-operated door alarms.
- Install a fence.
- Put up "stop" and "do not enter" signs on doors, windows, and gates to provide visual prompts.
- Increase physical activity during the day, and promote sleep hygiene to minimize night wandering.
- Consider a personal tracking device. Talk to your local law enforcement agency about Project Lifesaver (www.projectlifesaver.org) or LoJak SafetyNet services (www.safetynetbylojack.com/). The devices can be worn on the wrist or ankle to help track and locate your child.
- Consider an ID bracelet. An ID bracelet can identify your child, provide your contact information, and note if he or she is nonverbal.
- Teach your child to swim. Autistic children are attracted to water.
- Teach your child about the dangers of wandering.
- Make sure responsible adults monitor the child at all times during times of crises, transitions, or other stressors.
- Watch the news, and take note of how other wandering children absconded, then assess your home and family to see whether these situations may apply to your child. Minimize risk if they do.
- Alert neighbors and first responders that your child wanders, and tell them about your child's method of communication.
- Prevent wandering at school, camp, and other settings. Ask about their wandering policies, including how they minimize risk and respond when a child does wander. Inform the facility of any noticeable breeches.

- Do not develop a false sense of security. Make sure to adapt for your child's developmental growth, and update your child's profile and photo at least annually.

b. Abductions:

- Teach your children about personal safety:
  - Fear tactics do not work; instead, build the child's confidence.
  - Teach children how to make safe decisions and how to recognize potentially dangerous situations (e.g., the luring techniques noted in the Description section).
  - Instruct children not to go anywhere with anyone without parental permission.
  - Encourage the buddy system.
  - Role-play different scenarios, so children can practice what they learned.
  - Teach children Internet safety.
  - Teach active resistance strategies: shouting "NO," screaming, kicking, and biting.
- If it becomes apparent that you need to file for custody of your child, consider the abduction prevention tips recommended by the U.S. Department of State (n.d.):
  - A detailed custody order and good legal advice can go a long way in protecting your parental rights.
  - Detailed custody orders include special provisions on the custody decree such as specifying the beginning and end dates of visits; relocation restrictions; supervised visitation for the potential taking parent; requiring the court's approval to take the child out of the state or country; and asking for the court or a neutral third party to hold passports.
  - Consult your attorney about the drawbacks to joint-custody orders in parental abduction cases, if ordered. Ensure that you clearly specify the child's residential arrangements at all times.
  - Do not ignore any abduction threat. Notify police, and give them copies of any restraining order on your ex-spouse. You may also request restricted locations for visitation rights if you can prove potential harm to your child.
  - Be on the alert for sudden changes in the other parent's life. Changes such as quitting a job, selling a home, or closing a bank account may be signs that the parent may be planning to leave the country.
  - Do not delay action if you think your child has been taken by the other parent. Make sure that if your child is abducted, the police take a detailed

report and that your child is entered into the FBI's NCIC system right away (a warrant is not required).

- Be aware that if one parent is a citizen of another country, your child may have dual nationality. Contact the embassy of that country, and inquire about their passport requirements for minors.

Resources

Association of Missing and Exploited Children's Organizations (AMECO): 1-877-263-2620; www.amecoinc.org

BE REDY Booklet: A wandering prevention resource for the autism community, National Autism Association: http://nationalautismassociation.org/resources/awaare-wandering/be-redy-booklets/

International Parental Child Abduction: http://travel.state.gov/content/childabduction/en.html

National Center for Missing & Exploited Children (NCMEC): 1-800-THE-LOST; www.missingkids.com/home (for both prevention materials and information on what to do if a child is abducted or missing)

Take Root: 1-800-ROOT-ORG; www.takeroot.org

You're Not Alone: The Journey from Abduction to Empowerment: www.ncjrs.gov/pdffiles1/ojjdp/221965.pdf

What About Me? Coping with the Abduction of a Brother or Sister: www.ncjrs.gov/pdffiles1/ojjdp/217714.pdf

References

Anderson, C., Law, J. K., Daniels, A., Rice, C., Mandell, D. S., Hagopian, L., & Law, P. A. (2012). Occurrence and family impact of elopement in children with autistic spectrum disorders. *Pediatrics, 130*(5), 870–877.

Biehal, N., & Wade, J. (2002). *Children who go missing; research, policy and practice*. London, England: Department of Health.

Cornell University Law School. (n.d.). 42 U.S. Code § 5772—Definitions. Retrieved from www.law.cornell.edu/uscode/text/42/5772

Daniels, S., & Brennan, M. (2013). *Missing children: Kidnapped and abducted children and resources available to parents and to the community*. University of Florida IFAS extension, CFCS2256. Retrieved from http://ufdcimages.uflib.ufl.edu/IR/00/00/42/22/00001/FY86700.pdf

Federal Bureau of Investigation. (n.d.). Non-family child abductions. Retrieved from www.fbi.gov/about-us/investigate/vc_majorthefts/cac/non-family-abductions

Gunby, K., Carr, J., & Leblanc, L. (2010). Teaching abduction-prevention skills to children with autism. *Journal of Applied Behavior analysis, 43,* 107–112.

Hoff, R. (2008). *Family abduction: Prevention and response* (6th ed.). Alexandria, VA: National Center for Missing & Exploited Children.

Howard, B., Broughton, D., & the Committee on Psychosocial Aspects of Child and Family Health. (2004). The pediatrician's role in the prevention of missing children. *Pediatrics, 114,* 1100–1105.

Johnston, J., Sagatun-Edwards, I., Blomquist, M., & Girdner, L. (2001). *Early identification of risk factors for parental abduction* (NCJ 185026). Washington, DC: Office of Juvenile Justice and Delinquency Prevention, Juvenile Justice Bulletin.

Miller, J., Kurlycheck, M., Hansen, J., & Wilson, K. (2008). Examining child abduction by offender type patterns. *Justice Quarterly, 25*(3), 523–543.

National Center for Missing and Exploited Children. (n.d.). Missing children with autism. Retrieved from www.missingkids.org/autism

U.S. Department of Justice, Office of Juvenile Justice and Delinquency Prevention. (2010). *The crime of family abduction: A child's and parent's perspective.* Retrieved from www.ncjrs.gov/pdffiles1/ojjdp/229933.pdf

U.S. Department of State. (n.d.). *International parental child abduction.* Retrieved from http://travel.state.gov/content/childabduction/en/preventing/tips.html

CHAPTER 20

Mood Dysregulation

A. Description

Mastering the management of emotions, including frustration and disappointment, is a critical task of childhood. Young children throw tantrums when they do not get what they want, but tantrums diminish with age as children learn to adapt in more socially acceptable ways. However, some children do not progress as expected, and they experience difficulties with their emotional regulation, reacting with irritability, low frustration tolerance, volatile temper, and aggression to minimal provocation (Mendez, Hoy, Sundman-Wheat, & Cunningham, 2011).

a. Self-regulation, which is critical for emotional health, enables one to act in one's best long-term interest, allowing for the ability to calm down when distraught and cheer up when depressed. It also enables one to tolerate frustration, curb aggressive impulses, delay gratification, and express emotions in a socially accepted way. Self-regulation involves multiple domains, and one domain affects another. For example, thinking and emotional self-regulation are not distinct skills—thinking affects emotions, and emotions affect cognitive development. Thus, children who cannot regulate anxiety and discouragement tend to pull away from learning experiences, but when they regulate uncomfortable emotions, they can relax and learn (Florez, 2011; Frankel et al., 2012).

b. Parents play an important role in the development of their child's self-regulation. They act as models for the expression and control of emotions.

c. Problems with mood dysregulation become evident in early childhood, and left unmanaged, can lead to psychopathology and educational issues in later childhood through to adulthood.

B. Assessment (History, Physical, Diagnostic Screening/Testing, Where Appropriate)

a.   Risk factors for mood dysregulation problems include: Having a first-degree relative with a similar disorder; a history of chronic irritability; major life changes; substance abuse; and unstable home environment.

b.   Self-regulation develops during the first 5 years of life, and thus it is crucial that health care providers initiate assessment in infancy. Newborns' emotional arousal is regulated by their biological needs and parental response to those needs; when a newborn cries because of an aversive experience, the cry signals the parents' response to soothe the infant and thus regulate the infant's emotions. Infants begin to self-regulate sensorimotor and arousal responses. Sucking a thumb in response to a loud noise indicates regulation of the environment. Toddlers begin to inhibit response and comply with adults. Once a child reaches the age of 4 years, self-regulation becomes more complex, and children can anticipate appropriate responses and modify responses when circumstances warrant it, such as clapping when a movie is over, but not when a teacher gives directions (Florez, 2011; Frankel et al., 2012).

c.   Irritability, a low threshold to exhibit anger in response to frustration, is a key symptom in mood dysregulation and a clinical manifestation of several disorders. It can present in early life and is a predictor of psychopathology. Episodic irritability during early adolescence is associated with generalized anxiety disorder (GAD), simple phobia, and mania in late adolescence, but only mania in early adulthood. Chronic irritability in early adolescence is associated with disruptive disorders, such as attention deficit hyperactivity disorder (ADHD) and conduct disorder, in late adolescence, but only with major depressive disorder (MDD) in early adulthood (Krieger, Leibenluft, Stringaris, & Polanczyk, 2013).

d.   Negative moods can be attributed to problems such as sleep deprivation, stress overload, overscheduling, and medication side effects (the following table is representative, not all inclusive.)

DEPRESSED MOOD	ELEVATED MOOD	IRRITABLE MOOD
Accutane	Corticosteroids	Pseudoephedrine
Anticonvulsants	Cyclosporine	Atomoxetine
Benzodiazepines	Antidepressants	Some antihistamines
Zorivax	Stimulant drugs for	Albuterol and similar
Norplant (birth	ADHD	antiasthmatics
control)	Some antibiotics (such	Stimulant drugs for
Some antihistamines	as ciprofloxacin)	ADHD
		Corticosteroids

C. Diagnosis, Including Differential Diagnoses, When Appropriate

a. Temper tantrums are a developmental norm in children ages 1 to 3, and typically occur when the toddler is tired, upset, or frustrated. Children may cry, scream, hit, kick, and hold their breath. The underlying rationale is that toddlers cannot verbalize their needs and thus throw tantrums. Tantrums decrease as verbal skills increase. Temper dysregulation, however, is symptomatic of many psychopathologies, including mood and disruptive syndromes, creating the need to differentiate developmentally appropriate tantrums from those that are inappropriate. Signs of temper dysregulation include: worsening of tantrums after the age of 4 years; causing injury to self or others or destroying property during tantrums; breath-holding during tantrums, especially to the point at which it causes fainting; and other symptoms such as nightmares, reversal of toilet training, food or bed refusal, clinging behavior, and somatic complaints (American Academy of Pediatrics, 2009).

b. Disruptive mood dysregulation disorder (DMDD), a new and controversial disorder in the *Diagnostic and Statistical Manual of Mental Disorders, 5th Edition* (*DSM-5*; American Psychiatric Association [APA], 2013), is characterized by the child's having chronic irritability with frequent, severe temper outbursts that are very much out of proportion to the situation that created them. DMDD was developed to more accurately categorize children who had previously been diagnosed with pediatric bipolar disorder (BD) but who do not experience the episodic mania or hypomania characteristic of BD, and who do not typically develop adult BD. As mentioned, there is controversy as to whether DMDD truly represents a distinct disorder. Mayes and colleagues (2015) found that DMDD symptoms were noted in only one child who did not have symptoms characteristic of oppositional defiant disorder (ODD), conduct disorder, ADHD, anxiety, or depression, suggesting that DMDD symptoms are a manifestation of multiple disorders, especially ODD, and do not occur in isolation, thus questioning the validity of DMDD as an independent diagnosis. Saddock, Saddock, and Ruiz (2015) note that DMDD is usually comorbid with the aforementioned disorders and that current evidence does not support DMDD being continuous with emerging BD. For a diagnosis of DMDD, the child must meet the following criteria: severe recurrent verbal or physical temper outbursts that are grossly out of proportion to the triggers that cause them; the outbursts are inconsistent with the child's developmental level; the outbursts occur an average of three or more times per week; the mood between outbursts is persistently irritable or angry most of the day, almost every day; the symptoms have been present for 12 months or more without a remission period of longer than 3 months; the symptoms are present in two or more settings (e.g., at home and school) and are severe in at least one of these settings. A diagnosis of DMDD should not be made before age 6 years or after age 18 years; onset of symptoms usually occurs before age 10. The behaviors do not occur during a depressive episode; there is not more than 1 day during which manic or hypomanic criteria are met; and the symptoms are not better explained by another psychiatric disorder.

c.   Once called manic-depressive disorder, BD demonstrates episodes of depression and mania, with depression usually occurring first. BD cannot be diagnosed until the first manic episode. Strakowski (2015) calls BD a disorder of young people since it has a median onset in the mid to late teens, with most having symptom onset before age 21. It is also lifelong and very disruptive, especially since it interferes with adolescents' process of becoming independent adults. The *DSM-5* does not differentiate between adult and child symptoms of BD; the diagnostic criteria are the same regardless of age at the onset of symptoms. However, "[c]hildren differ from adults in that mixed states are more common, neurovegetative signs may be less common, and onset may be less abrupt and course less episodic" (Strakowski, 2015). Some adult symptoms, such as flight of ideas, can be harder to define in children, and health care providers need to consider developmental status. BDs are viewed as a spectrum, ranging from mild hypomania to extreme mania, which can result in psychosis and life-threatening features. The poor insight and judgment that accompanies mania can result in loss of family and peer ties, school dysfunction, financial ruin, job loss, legal problems, homelessness, and increased risk of suicidality, as well as health consequences that include dehydration, cardiovascular complications, stroke, cancer, and early death. The *DSM-5* (APA, 2013) identifies several behaviors as indicative of mania. The hallmark of a manic episode is a euphoric or irritable mood that lasts at least 1 week. Other characteristics include grandiosity, rapid and pressured speech, decreased need for sleep, reckless behaviors and risk-taking, distractibility, and agitation or increased goal-directed activity. The youth may also experience flight of ideas, disorganized thoughts, delusions of grandeur, poor insight, and poor judgment. Hypomania is similar to mania; it is less severe, but still causes some impairment (Bernstein, 2015).

d.   Emotional dysregulation is the core of borderline personality disorder (BPD), which is also characterized by behavior, relationship, identity, and cognition dysregulation. Linehan (1993) proposed that persons with BPD are emotionally sensitive from birth and that this leads to a tendency to experience negative moods/affect across situations and contexts, making it difficult to learn appropriate emotional regulation. Young adults with BPD have disturbed thinking patterns and always seem to be in crisis. They can be rational and calm one moment, and then explode into inappropriate anger in response to some perceived rejection or criticism the next. Signs and symptoms of BPD may include significant fear of real or imagined abandonment; intense and unstable relationships that vacillate between extreme idealization and devaluation; markedly and persistently unstable self-image; significant and potentially self-damaging impulsivity (spending, sex, binge eating, gambling, substance abuse, and reckless driving); repeated suicidal behavior, gestures, or threats; self-mutilation (carving, burning, cutting, branding, picking and pulling at skin and hair, biting, and excessive tattooing and body piercing); affective instability and significant reactivity of mood (intense dysphoria, irritability, or anxiety that lasts for a few hours or days); persistent feelings of emptiness; inappropriate anger or trouble controlling anger; and temporary, stress-related severe dissociative symptoms or paranoid ideation. Co-morbidities are common with BPD. These disorders, which include mood disorders, substance-related disorders, eating disorders (notably bulimia), posttraumatic stress disorder (PTSD), other anxiety disorders, dissociative identity disorder, and ADHD, can complicate both diagnosis and treatment. Depression is particularly common in patients with BPD. Other personality disorders have also been documented as comorbid with BPD (Carpenter & Trell, 2013; Lubit, 2014; Muscari, 2005).

e. Differential diagnoses include: schizophrenia or schizoaffective disorder, PTSD, substance abuse, anxiety states (e.g., GAD, social nxiety disorder), and traumatic brain injury (Bernstein, 2015). Childhood schizophrenia (onset under age 12 years) is rare, and other causes of psychosis should be considered, including central nervous system disorders such as brain tumors, encephalitis, metabolic disorder, and use of high-dose corticosteroids. Adult schizophrenia can have its onset during the transitional period between ages 18 and 26. In general, schizo-phrenic symptoms are divided into four symptom domains: positive symptoms (include hallucinations, which are usually auditory, delusions, and disorganized speech and behavior); negative symptoms (decreased emotional range, poverty of speech, and loss of interests and volition, tremendous inertia); cognitive symp-toms (neurocognitive deficits in areas such as working memory, attention, and executive functions [e.g., ability to organize and abstract]); difficulty understand-ing nuances and subtleties of interpersonal cues and relationships; and mood symptoms (seem cheerful or sad in a way that is difficult to understand; often depressed; Frankenburg, 2015).

D. Levels of Prevention/Intervention

a. Primary

There are no primary prevention strategies, but health care providers can promote healthy self-regulation in young children by encouraging positive role modeling of emotional regulation, providing hints and cues about how and when to regulate their behavior, and gradually withdraw adult support (Florez, 2011).

b. Secondary

Early identification and intervention may improve long-term management.

c.   Tertiary

- DMDD is treated with medication, psychotherapy, or a combination of the two; however, because the diagnosis is new, researchers are still trying to find which treatments work best. Since it resembles anxiety and unipolar depression in pathophysiology, and is often comorbid with ADHD, selective serotonin reuptake inhibitors (SSRIs) and stimulants would usually be the first drugs of choice. However, if the symptoms are similar to BD, first-line treatment may be antipsychotics and mood stabilizers (Saddock et al., 2015). Applied behavior analysis has all been used, and parents and other caregivers should also be taught specific strategies they can use when responding to a child's disruptive behavior.

- The treatment of BD is complicated and warrants referral to a specialist. Aripiprazole, ziprasidone, risperidone, valproate, and lithium (ages 12 and older) are Food and Drug Administration (FDA) approved for the treatment of pediatric clients. Psychosocial and familial treatments can assist in relapse prevention. Family focused treatment (FFT) may reduce familial stress, conflict, and affective arousal by enhancing communication and problem solving in both client and parent, and cognitive behavioral therapy (CBT) has shown a significant decrease in depressive symptoms, making it reasonable to offer CBT for BD depression (Bernstein, 2015; Krieger & Stringaris, 2013).

- The treatment of BPD is usually psychotherapeutic. Dialectical behavior therapy (DBT), a form of CBT developed in the 1970s by Dr. Marsha Linehan and colleagues, teaches skills to cope with stress, regulate emotions, and improve relationships with others. DBT is founded on four core principles: the primacy of the therapeutic relationship; a nonjudgmental approach; differentiating between effective and ineffective behaviors; and dialectical thinking (viewing issues from multiple perspectives), and moves clients through four phases: mindfulness, distress tolerance, emotion regulation, and interpersonal effectiveness (Linehan, 1993; Saddock et al., 2015). Medication management may be needed; however, clients with BPD tend to be impulsive, which increases their risk of overdosing on their prescribed medication. Antidepressants and mood stabilizers must be prescribed with caution and monitored. Because of their relative safety, SSRIs are the agents of choice for treating anxiety and depression, but antipsychotics may become necessary to manage psychotic symptoms, with monitoring for their potential adverse effects, including tardive dyskinesia or neuroleptic malignant syndrome (Lubit, 2014). When working with youth with BPD, establish a strong therapeutic alliance that includes empathic validation of the patient's experience; coordinate and collaborate with the treatment team; be aware of and manage splitting problems, and assist the youth in integrating both positive and negative aspects of self and others; provide education to the youth and the family on

BPD; manage intense feelings produced by both the client and the health care provider; use supervision and consultation; help the youth take responsibility for his or her own actions, and promote reflective rather than impulsive behaviors (Muscari, 2005).

- Rettew (2015) recommends using the American Academy of Child and Adolescent Psychiatry's guidelines for the use of antipsychotic medications in children (bit.ly/1eat7e9), and notes its key recommendations: regularly check the current literature; antipsychotics are first-line medications for BD, schizophrenia, tic/Tourette's, and autism; antipsychotics are not the first-line medications for other disorders, including ADHD, aggression, eating disorders, and PTSD; antipsychotics are not recommended for preschool-age children; dosing should be as low as possible and not exceed adult maximum; simultaneous treatment with multiple antipsychotics is not recommended; clients should have regular metabolic monitoring before and during treatment. Rettew (2015) further notes that the rigorous guidelines regarding the use of antipsychotics, which include clinical and legal implications of failing to adhere to the guidelines, should give many physicians pause—this should serve for all primary health care providers.

E. Parenting Tips

Parents can help children who have difficulties with self-regulation by (Scholastic, n.d.):

a. Modeling self-control and self-regulation in their own words and actions.

b. Maintaining a structured routine.

c. Keeping the environment as calm as possible, and make it calmer if they suspect their child is getting upset.

d. Being firm when their child has an episode (e.g., do not try to converse with him or her).

e. Helping their child choose his or her friends wisely, and limiting interaction with other impulsive children.

f. Taking time out for themselves if they feel overwhelmed.

g. Getting help when needed.

Resources

American Academy of Child and Adolescent Psychiatry Practice Parameters for the Use of Atypical Antipsychotic Medications in Children and Adolescents: www.aacap.org/App_Themes/AACAP/docs/practice_parameters/Atypical_Antipsychotic_Medications_Web.pdf

Bipolar Disorder in Children and Teens: www.aacap.org/AACAP/Families_and_youth/Facts_for_Families/FFF-Guide/Bipolar-Disorder-in-Children-and-Teens-038.aspx

BPD Central: www.bpdcentral.com/

BPD World: www.bpdworld.org/

Disruptive Mood Dysregulation Disorder (DMDD): www.aacap.org/AACAP/Families_and_Youth/Facts_for_Families/FFF-Guide/Disruptive-Mood-Dysregulation-Disorder-(DMDD)-110.aspx

National Alliance on Mental Illness: www.nami.org/

National Institute of Mental Health: Bipolar Disorder in Children and Teens: www.nimh.nih.gov/health/publications/bipolar-disorder-in-children-and-adolescents/index.shtml

Nemours Foundation KidsHealth: Bipolar Disorder: http://kidshealth.org/teen/your_mind/mental_health/bipolar.html

References

American Academy of Pediatrics. (2009). *Temper tantrums: A normal part of growing up.* Retrieved from http://patiented.solutions.aap.org/handout.aspx?gbosid=156567

American Psychiatric Association. (2013). *Diagnostic and statistical manual of mental disorders* (5th ed.). Washington, DC: Author.

Bernstein, B. (2015). Pediatric bipolar affective disorder treatment and management. *Emedicine Medscape.* Retrieved from http://emedicine.medscape.com/article/913464-treatment#d9

Carpenter, R., & Trull, T. (2013). Components of emotion dysregulation in borderline personality disorder: A review. *Current Psychiatry Reports, 15*(1), 335. doi:10.1007/s11920-012-0335-2

Florez, I. (2011). Developing young children's self-regulation through everyday experiences. *Young Children, 66*(4), 46–51.

Frankel, L., Hughes, S., O'Connor, T., Power, T., Fisher, J., & Hazen, N. (2012). Parental influences on children's self-regulation of energy intake: Insights from developmental literature on emotion regulation. *Journal of Obesity, 2012,* Article ID 327259, 12 pages. doi:10.1155/2012/327259

Frankenburg, F. (2015). Schizophrenia. *Emedicine Medscape.* Retreived from http://emedicine.medscape.com/article/288259-overview

Krieger, F., Leibenluft, E., Stringaris, A., & Polanczyk, G. (2013). Irritability in children and adolescents: Past concepts, current debates, and future opportunities. *Revista Brasileira de Psiquiatria, 35*(Suppl. 1), S32–S39. doi:10.1590/1516-4446-2013-S107

Krieger, F., & Stringaris, A. (2013). Bipolar disorder and disruptive mood dysregulation in children and adolescents. *Evidence Based Mental Health, 16*(4), 93–94.

Linehan, M. (1993). *Cognitive-behavioral treatment of borderline personality disorder.* New York, NY: Guilford.

Lubit, R. (2014). Borderline personality disorder. *Emedicine Medscape.* Retrieved from http://emedicine.medscape.com/article/913575-differential

Mayes, S., Mathiowetz, C., Kokotovich, C., Waxmonsky, J., Baweja, R., Calhoun, S., & Bixler, E. (2015). Stability of disruptive mood dysregulation disorder symptoms (irritable-angry mood and temper outbursts) throughout childhood and adolescence in a general population sample. *Journal of Abnormal Child Psychology, 43*(8), 1543–1549.

Mendez, L., Hoy, B., Sundman-Wheat, A., & Cunningham, J. (2011). Research advances in understanding emotion dysregulation in youth. *Communique: The Newspaper of the National Association of School Psychologists, 40*(3), 1–6.

Muscari, M. (2005). What therapy is recommended for borderline personality disorder in adolescents? *Medscape.* Retrieved from www.medscape.com/viewarticle/508832#vp_4

Rettew, D. (2015, January). Using, and not using, antipsychotics. *Pediatric News, 49*(1), 6.

Saddock, B., Saddock, V., & Ruiz, P. (2015). *Kaplan & Saddock's synopsis of psychiatry* (11th ed.). Philadelphia, PA: Wolters Kluwer.

Scholastic. (n.d.). *Developing self-regulation.* Retrieved from www.scholastic.com/parents/resources/article/social-emotional-skills/developing-self-regulation

Strakowski, S. (2015). What is unique about bipolar disorder in young people? *Medscape.* Retrieved from www.medscape.com/viewarticle/854603

CHAPTER 21

Nonsuicidal Self-Injury

A. Description

Nonsuicidal self-injury (NSSI), also called self-injurious behavior (SIB), is behavior that inflicts injury on one's own body, causing tissue damage and scarring, without the intent to cause suicide, and for purposes not socially sanctioned. The latter implies that tattooing and piercings are not considered NSSI; however, excessive use of either can be considered harmful if done with the same intentions as engaging in NSSI. Cutting (with sharp objects such as razors, knives, and needles) is the most common form of NSSI, but other behaviors include scratching, burning (with lit cigarettes or aggressive rubbing with an eraser), hitting, head banging, hair pulling, preventing wounds from healing, and embedding. Self-mutilation is viewed as a maladaptive form of self-relief from inner pain. While not a suicidal behavior, it does come under the umbrella of deliberate self-harm (DSH), which includes suicide, and parasuicide (suicide attempts and gestures). NSSI is a risk factor for suicidal thoughts and behaviors and a precursor of more serious psychopathology, especially in youths who engage in multiple methods of self-injury. Accidental death and severe injury can occur.

a.   NSSI is different from SIB, which is common and frequently persistent in youth with intellectual disabilities. These youths may engage in SIB because of limitations in cognitive, socioemotional, communicative, personality, and/or sensorimotor and adaptive functioning, as well as pain. Self-injury in this population may not be deliberate and may be learned behavior to communicate with others.

b.   NSSI is a mental health concern among adolescents and transition age youth, with lifetime prevalence rates of 12% to 37.2% and 12% to 20%, respectively (Swannell, Martin, Page, Hasking, & John, 2014). Many of these youths use the Internet to connect with others who self-injure.

c.   Developmental and interpersonal models have been proposed to explain NSSI behaviors, and both examine attachment and relationship variables. Developmental models relate it to adverse childhood experiences (ACEs), while interpersonal models connect NSSI with the person's past relationship history and variables in that person's current relationships. Learning theory holds that the behavior is supported through positive or negative reinforcement. One biochemical model suggests that self-injury increases the production and/or release of endorphins, resulting in an anesthesia-like effect so that the person does not feel any pain during the injury; endorphin release may also provide the person with a euphoria-like feeling (Levesque, Lafontaine, Bureau, Cloutier, & Danurand, 2010).

d.   There is no NSSI "profile." Research results have been mixed, but NSSI behaviors seem to cross both genders and all races and socioeconomic groups. However, sexual minority youth appear to be at higher risk than heterosexual youth, with bisexual and questioning youth having a slightly higher risk than their homosexual and hetero-sexual peers (Whitlock, 2009).

e.   Self-embedding is an extreme form of NSSI, in which adolescents insert objects into their body parts to deliberately hurt themselves or mutilate their bodies. The first professional account of this behavior was in 2008 by William Sheils, DO, Chief of the Department of Radiology at Nationwide Children's Hospital in Columbus, at the annual meeting of the Radiological Society of North America. His findings were based on 10 adolescent females, ages 15 to 18, who had 19 documented episodes of self-embedding injury, and noted the removal of 52 foreign bodies from nine of the females that included metal needles, metal staples, metal paper clips, glass, wood, plastic, graphite, and stone (Young, Shiels, Murakami, Coley, & Hogan, 2010). Consequences from self-embedding can be serious. Wounds can become infected, especially when foreign objects are inserted deep into tissue. Infection can travel to bone or muscle, and further damage can be caused if the youth hits blood vessels, nerves, or tendons. An object can also break, form an embolism, and travel to a vital organ.

f.   Youth injure themselves to express feelings, communicate needs, to feel in control, to minimize psychic pain, and to reenact or try to resolve trauma. Many self-injure to manage their feelings, relieve stress, or experience some feeling when they feel numb. Others self-injure to exert self-control, punish themselves, create a high, gain attention, or join a group. Regardless of the underlying reason, teens who engage in DSH tend to do so in response to a trigger. Mangnall and Yurkovich (2008) describe common triggers:

- Tension and anxiety: Both depression and anxiety are found in persons who self-harm, but anxiety and tension have a unique relationship with it. Self-cutters report more anxiety than those who engage in other forms of self-harm, although the relationship with self-embedding has not been established.

- Hostility and impulsivity: Adolescents may turn to self-harm because of their inability to express anger. They easily become angered, yet they experience self-dislike and guilt, which may result in their directing these feelings against themselves.

- Feelings of derealization and depersonalization: Feelings of unreality or the lack of a feeling state are triggers for DSH. Cutting seems to end these states, returning the adolescent to a sense of realness.

- History of childhood trauma: Self-harmers often have a history of trauma that sometimes begins in childhood. When it does, it may be particularly malignant.

Trigger events can also include problems with boyfriends or girlfriends, friends, school, substances, and bullying (Catledge, Scharer, & Fuller, 2012).

B. Assessment

a.   Risk factors: NSSI is linked to child abuse, especially sexual abuse, and family dysfunction. It is also associated with eating disorders, borderline personality disorder (BPD), depression, anxiety disorders, substance abuse, impulse disorders, and posttraumatic stress disorder (PTSD). The "contagion factor" may play a role in adolescents who mimic peers, social media posts, or celebrities.

b.   Begin assessment in the school-age years. NSSI is typically associated with adolescence. However, research has shown that children as young as 7 years of age engage in NSSI, and that ninth-grade girls reported the greatest rates and did so by cutting themselves (Barrocas, Hankin, Young, & Abela, 2012).

c.   The majority of youths who engage in NSSI do not seek medical attention, and many first disclose to their Internet friends; however, there is a subset of youths who first disclose to their primary care providers. Since NSSI may begin during childhood, it is important to use these same assessment strategies for this population, especially those who have experienced childhood trauma.

- Perform a mental health status exam, especially noting mood and affect.

- Assess for NSSI during routine assessments and when youths present with suspicious symptoms, such as unexplained wounds and infections.

- Although NSSIs are not suicidal behaviors, ask about suicidal ideation and assess lethality if ideation is present.

- Be direct; ask if they have ever deliberately cut or injured themselves.

- Observe skin surfaces, especially on the dorsal side of the forearms, the frontal area of the thighs, and the abdomen for signs of fresh and old injuries. Many choose to cut over the same area, which may minimize the number of traumatic lesions.

- Palpate the skin for embedded objects.

   d.   NSSI can be isolated incidents or repetitive behaviors, and they range in severity. Rao, Sudarshan and Begum (2008) categorized SIB into three groups:

   - Mild and isolated form: Examples are carving a boyfriend's or girlfriend's name into skin; branding self with lit cigarette, match, or candle; scratching wrists; small cut; attempting to burn off tattoo.

   - Moderately severe and repetitive form: Examples are repeatedly cutting self, branding self with hot iron on multiple parts of the body, large cuts, and genital rubbing.

   - Very severe and isolated form: Examples are severe self-inflicted bites, genital mutilation, pulling out eye, and pulling out own teeth.

There is no exhaustive list of NSSI behaviors; however, the majority of adolescents use multiple types.

   e.   Instruments that have been validated to assess for self-injury include the Deliberate Self-Harm Inventory, the Functional Assessment of Self-Mutilation, and the Self-Harm Questionnaire (which addresses other types of self-harm, such as disordered eating). The Brief Non-Suicidal Self-injury Assessment Tool (BNSSI-AT), developed by Janis Whitlock and Amanda Purington, is available via the Cornell Research Program in Self-Injury and Recovery (CRPSIR, www.selfinjury.bctr.cornell.edu). This tool is primarily a research instrument; however, it can be used to evaluate primary NSSI characteristics (form, frequency, and function), as well as secondary characteristics (context for NSSI behaviors, habituation, perceived life impairment, treatment, and impact). The CRPSIR Severity Assessment is also available through their website, and this can easily be used in primary care sites to assess NSSI severity (low, moderate, and high), addressing lifetime number of incidents, number of forms, likeliness of form to cause tissue damage, likelihood of associated disordered eating, suicidality, other mental health challenges, and history of abuse.

   f.   Kerr, Muehlenkamp, and Turner (2010) provided a mnemonic device—"STOPS FIRE"—that can aid primary care providers in knowing what to look for when assessing NSSI:

   - Suicidal ideations during or before self-injury

   - Types of self-injury

   - Onset of self-injury

   - Place (location) on the body that is injured

   - Severity and extent of damage caused by self-injury

   - Functions of the self-injury for the patient

   - Intensity or frequency of self-injury urges

   - Repetition of self-injury

   - Episodic frequency of self-injury

C. Diagnosis, Including Differential Diagnoses, When Appropriate

a. The primary concern is differentiating NSSI from suicidal behavior by determining the goal of the behavior. Since youth who engage in NSSI can also attempt and commit suicide, ascertain if there were any suicide attempts in the past. Some youths will escalate their NSSI behaviors or eventually attempt suicide; thus, ongoing evaluation is critical.

b. Self-mutilating behavior is still listed as a symptom of borderline personality disorder in the *Diagnostic and Statistical Manual of Mental Disorders, 5th Edition* (*DSM-5*), published by the American Psychiatric Association (APA, 2013); however, it has been recognized as a distinct condition seen in other disorders, such as depression, and even appearing with no diagnosable pathology. The *DSM-5* does list NSSI under conditions for further study and notes that the proposed criteria are not intended for clinical use.

c. Differentiate from self-injurious behavior (SIB). SBI has been associated with seizure activity in the frontal and temporal lobes, hypocalciuria, genetic disorders, and pain (Edelson, n.d.; Levesque et al., 2010). It is noted in children with disorders such as Prader–Willi (skin picking), Lesch–Nyhan syndrome (biting around mouth and fingers), and Cornelia de Lange syndrome (self-biting and face hitting; Levesque et al., 2010).

d. Determine whether the self-injurious behaviors stand alone or are symptomatic of another disorder, including depression or BPD. NSSI is usually associated with phases of positive relationships, periods of closeness and collaboration, whereas BPD tends to be associated with aggressive and hostile behaviors (APA, 2013). The *DSM-5* (APA, 2013) identifies several behaviors as indicative of BPD, which is characterized by a pattern of unstable mood, self-image, and interpersonal relationships, as well as marked impulsivity. Manifestations include intense yet unstable relationships, identity disturbance, splitting, impulsivity, labile affect, intense and inappropriate anger, suicidal ideation, and self-mutilating behaviors.

e. Assess for the presence of associated problems, including depression, eating disorders, substance abuse, anxiety, impulse disorder, and PTSD.

D. Levels of Prevention/Intervention

a. Primary

While there are no evidence-based primary prevention strategies, primary care providers can assist children with their ability to identify and cope with developmental and everyday life stressors.

b. Secondary

The CRPSIR notes that little has been written on effective ways of preventing self-injurious practices, but stresses that we can create strategies by acknowledging central reasons for initiating and maintaining self-injurious practices and from lessons in related fields, such as disordered eating:

- Foster the ability to cope and regulate emotional perceptions and impulses. This is one of the elements of dialectical behavior therapy (DBT), an effective treatment approach for SIB.
- Promote social connectedness. Reaching out to others can help at-risk youths to feel meaningfully linked to something larger than themselves and may help give them a more positive view of their self.
- Avoid strategies aimed primarily at raising knowledge of forms and practices of NSSI, which may increase these behaviors.
- Help school personnel and parents in recognizing and responding to signs of SIB.
- Increase students' capacity to recognize distress. Peers are usually the first to know or suspect that a friend is using self-injurious practices, and thus constitute the "front line" in detection and intervention. SIB could be one of many behaviors and perceptions assessed, both positive and negative, such as perceived well-being, eating disorders, life satisfaction, depression, relationships with adults, and suicidality. Students can then be encouraged to seek assistance and be coached on specific strategies for getting help.
- Promote positive norms related to help-seeking and communication. Peers tend to show loyalty to friends rather than to adults, and those with knowledge of a friend's dangerous behavior are unlikely to share that knowledge with an adult without concentrated effort by adults to alter adolescent and adult norms about help-seeking and communication.
- Discuss sources of stress in the environment. The ability to simultaneously manage multiple stressors is especially difficult for children and adolescents. Targeting environmental sources of stress may be a more effective prevention strategy than targeting individual youth deemed to be at risk for self-injurious or other concerning behaviors.
- Educate youth about the role media plays in influencing behavior. Images, songs, and news articles in which SIB is featured have increased significantly over the past decade. Aiding youth in becoming critical consumers of media may lessen their vulnerability to adoption of glamorized but poor coping strategies.

c. Tertiary

- There is no single best strategy for treating NSSI, but the primary concerns are medical and safety issues. Treat the immediate medical problems, and ensure that the youth is not suicidal. Treatment is then based on the youth's individual needs, and tends to be long term.

- Take the behavior seriously, and do not overreact. A caring, trusting therapeutic relationship is critical, with the use of a matter-of-fact approach that is neither overly sympathetic nor critical. These help to engage the youth and promote joint clinical decision making (Catledge et al., 2012).

- Youth who engage in NSSI should be referred for counseling to explore the root of their behavior and to determine whether there is an associated mental health disorder. Strong evidence for NSSI treatment in adolescents is lacking at this point, as many studies focus on adults or both populations, include suicidal behaviors, and vary on their definitions of SIB. However, the literature does show some general efficacy from DBT (the gold standard for treating BPD [linehaninstitute.org]), emotion regulation group therapy, manual-assisted cognitive therapy, problem-solving therapy, developmental group therapy, and individual cognitive behavioral therapy. To date, there are no medications that specifically treat NSSI, although medications may be used for associated disorders (Gonzales & Bergstrom, 2013; Hawton et al., 2015; Rana, Gomez & Varghese, 2013; Turner, Austin, & Chapman, 2014).

- Those who self-embed should also be referred to a radiologist. Using ultrasound diagnosis and ultrasound or fluoroscopic guidance, interventional pediatric radiologists have been able to successfully remove embedded foreign objects found in many parts of the body including the arms, hands, neck, ankles, and feet.

- Many of these youths are in acute emotional distress and want someone to listen to them. They need to know that their primary health care provider is there to listen and support them. Employ reflective listening by paraphrasing the youth's expressed thoughts and nonjudgmentally identifying your own observations. Validate the youth's feelings, demonstrating your understanding of where he or she is coming from and that you are taking the youth seriously.

E. Parenting Tips

The CRPSIR provides the following information for parents:

a.   Know the signs of self-injuring: physical and emotional withdrawal; long periods in their bedroom or bathroom; cuts or burn marks on the arms and legs; finding hidden razors and other sharp objects or rubber bands, used to increase blood flow or numb an area; and wearing long sleeves or other concealing clothing in hot weather.

b.   Validate your own feelings, as many parents experience a wide range of emotions: shock, denial, anger, frustration, sympathy, empathy, sadness, and guilt.

c. Stay calm. Talk with your child as soon as possible. Be constructive and focus on your own concern. Validate your child's feelings, and be reassuring. Ask your child what you can do to help.

d. Avoid lecturing, harsh punishments, threats, and ultimatums.

e. Take your child seriously.

Resources

Berkley Parents Network on Cutting: www.berkeleyparentsnetwork.org/advice/teens/cutting

Challenging Behaviour Foundation Self-Injurious Behaviour Information Sheet: www.challenging-behaviour.org.uk/learning-disability-files/06---SIB-web.pdf

Cornell Research Program on Self-Injury and Recovery: www.selfinjury.bctr.cornell.edu

Cutting: http://kidshealth.org/teen/your_mind/mental_health/cutting.html

How to Understand and Help My Child Who Is Self-Injuring (Online Parent Seminar): http://safealt .evsuite.com/parentseminar7272423175/

International Society for the Study of Self-Injury: http://itriples.org

Safe Alternatives: www.selfinjury.com

Self-Injury in Adolescents: www.aacap.org/AACAP/Families_and_Youth/Facts_for_Families/FFF-Guide/Self-Injury-In-Adolescents-073.aspx

Severe Self-Injury a Threat to Teens WebMD: www.webmd.com/mental-health/news/20081202/ severe-self-injury-a-threat-to-teens

Teens, Cutting and Self-Injury: www.webmd.com/anxiety-panic/cutting-self-injury

Understanding and Responding to Students Who Self-Mutilate: www.naspcenter.org/principals/ nassp_cutting.html

References

American Psychiatric Association. (2013). *Diagnostic and statistical manual of mental disorders* (5th ed.). Washington, DC: Author.

Barrocas, A., Hankin, B., Young, J., & Abela, J. (2012). Rates of nonsuicidal self-injury in youth: Age, sex, and behavioral methods in a community sample. *Pediatrics, 130*(1), 39–45. doi:10.1542/ peds.2011-2094

Catledge, C., Scharer, K., & Fuller, S. (2012). Assessment and identification of deliberate self-harm in adolescents and young adults. *Journal for Nurse Practitioners, 8*(4), 299–305.

Edelson, S. (n.d.). *Self-injurious behavior.* Autism Research Institute. Retrieved from www.autism.com/symptoms_self-injury

Gonzales, A., & Bergstrom, L. (2013). Adolescent non-suicidal self-injury (NSSI) interventions. *Journal of Child and Adolescent Psychiatric Nursing, 26,* 124–130.

Hawton, K., Witt, K. G., Taylor Salisbury, T. L., Arensman, E., Gunnell, D., Hazell, P., . . . van Heeringen K. (2015). Pharmacological interventions for self-harm in adults. *Cochrane Database of Systematic Reviews,* (7), CD011777. doi:10.1002/14651858

Kerr, P., Muehlenkamp, J., & Turner, J. (2010). Nonsuicidal self-injury: A review of current research for family medicine and primary care physicians. *Journal of the American Board of Family Medicine, 23*(2), 240–259.

Levesque, C., Lafontaine, M., Bureau, J., Cloutier, P., & Danurand, C. (2010). The influence of romantic attachment and intimate partner violence on non-suicidal self-injury in young adults. *Journal of Youth Adolescence, 39,* 474–483. doi:10.1007/s10964-009-9471-3

Mangnall, J., & Yurkovich, E. (2008). A literature review of deliberate self-harm. *Perspectives in Psychiatric Care, 44*(3), 175–184.

Rana, F., Gomez, A., & Varghese, S. (2013). Pharmacological interventions for self-injurious behaviour in adults with intellectual disabilities. *Cochrane Database of Systematic Reviews,* (4), CD009084. doi:10.1002/14651858.CD009084.pub2

Rao, K., Sudarshan, C., & Begum, S. (2008). Self-injurious behavior: A clinical appraisal. *Indian Journal of Psychiatry, 50*(4), 288–297. doi:10.4103/0019-5545.44754

Swannell, S., Martin, G. E., Page, A., Hasking, P., & St. John, N. J. (2014). Prevalence of nonsuicidal self-injury in nonclinical samples: Systematic review, meta-analysis and meta-regression. *Suicide and Life-Threatening Behavior, 2,* 1–31.

Turner, B., Austin, S., & Chapman, A. (2014). Treating nonsuicidal self-injury: A systematic review of psychological and pharmacological interventions. *Canadian Journal of Psychiatry, 59*(11), 576–585.

Whitlock, J. (2009, December). The cutting edge: Non-suicidal self-injury in adolescents. *Research Facts and Findings.* Retrieved from www.actforyouth.net/resources/rf/rf_nssi_1209.pdf

Young, A. S., Shiels, W. E., Murakami, J. W., Coley, B. D., & Hogan, M. J. (2010). Self-embedding behavior: Radiologic management of self-inserted soft-tissue foreign bodies. *Radiology, 257,* 233–239.

CHAPTER 22

Sexual Aggression

A. Description

Sexual exploration is a normal part of growing up; however, some children engage in sexual behavior that deviates from the range of normal and that impacts on others. Sexually aggressive children are children age 12 years or younger who sexually act out in an aggressive manner towards persons who are younger or who are perceived as vulnerable, or both (Araji, 1997).

    a.   Most children engage in sexual behaviors before age 13, and most of them engage in behaviors that are developmentally appropriate, such as touching their own genitals. Sexually aggressive children are males and females who perpetrate sexual abuse at or before the age of 12.

    b.   Child sexual behavior is affected by a number of factors, including normal development, parental reaction to their behavior, family stressors, and access to sexual materials. The latter has increased owing to technology, exposing children to sexually explicit materials (Kellogg, 2010). Children are also exposed to new reports of child sexual exploitation, television shows about teenage mothers and young beauty queens, and adultlike child apparel.

    c.   Child sexual aggression is a complex phenomenon, and theories have only partially explained its occurrence. These have included sexual aggression as a response to sexual abuse victimization; learned behavior from exposure to sexuality and/or violence; early exposure to pornography and advertising; substance abuse; heightened sexual arousal to children; and exposure to family violence and aggressive role models (Miranda, Biegler, Davis, Frevert, & Taylor, 2001; Ryan & Lane, 1997). Although many children with sexual behavior problems have a history of sexual victimization, most children who have been sexually abused do not develop problematic sexual behavior (Kellogg, 2010).

    d.   While some jurisdictions also include sexually aggressive children under age 12 in their classification of juvenile sex offenders, the Association for the Treatment of

Sexual Abusers (ATSA; n.d.) recommends that they not be considered sex offenders. There is also a difference between very young children and older children. Preschool children with sexual behavior problems may show more frequent sexual behaviors; they are less likely to live with their biological parents, and have higher rates of general behavior problems, exposure to family violence, and child abuse. Young children have very limited cognitive and coping abilities, and masturbation may become a self-soothing activity when stressed. When compared with older children and adults, sexually aggressive children are also more likely to act impulsively instead of rationally (planned, predatory acts). Their inability to empathize with their victims may be more due to development than pathology. But probably the biggest difference is gender. While adolescent and adult sex offenders are predominantly male, children with sexual behavior problems are chiefly female (Association for the Treatment of Sexual Abusers, n.d.).

e. Juvenile sex offenders (JSOs) are youths between the ages of 12 and 18 who commit illegal sexual behavior as defined by the sex crime statutes of the jurisdiction in which their offense(s) occurred. Juveniles who commit sexual offenses are a diverse group: some are otherwise well-functioning with limited behavioral or psychological problems; some have multiple nonsexual behavior problems or prior nonsexual juvenile offenses; and some have major psychiatric disorders. Many come from well-functioning families; others come from highly chaotic or abusive backgrounds. JSOs also differ according to victim and offense characteristics and a wide range of other variables, including types of offending behaviors, sexual knowledge and experiences, academic and cognitive functioning, and mental health issues. Sexually abusive behaviors range from noncontact offenses to penetrative acts, and their offense characteristics include factors such as the age and sex of the victim, the relationship between victim and offender, and the degree of coercion and violence used for the offense. Many JSOs also engage in nonsexual criminal and antisocial behavior.

f. Female JSOs tend to have backgrounds positive for prior sexual victimization, child maltreatment, family dysfunction, poor social skills, and psychopathology. Some have histories of multiple nonsexual behavior problems or prior nonsexual juvenile offenses, but many are otherwise well-functioning youth with limited behavioral problems. While some female JSOs experience high levels of individual and family psychopathology, others have limited psychological problems and minimal family dysfunction. Female JSOs differ from male JSOs with regard to physical and sexual abuse history. On average, female JSOs have experienced more extensive and severe physical and sexual maltreatment during their childhood than male JSOs. Female JSOs are also sexually victimized at younger ages and are more likely to have had multiple perpetrators. They exhibit greater variability in their sexual arousal and behavior patterns than adult male/female sex offenders, with the most common sexual offenses committed by female adolescents being nonaggressive acts, such as mutual fondling, that occur during a caregiving activity such as babysitting.

Female JSOs rarely commit sex offenses against adults. Their victims are typically young acquaintances or relatives, with male and female children equally at risk for sexual victimization by female adolescents. Female JSOs are similar to male JSOs in the level of diversity that exists within their population. They commit a wide range of illegal sexual behaviors, ranging from limited exploratory behaviors committed largely out of curiosity to repeated aggressive acts, and they can also have co-offenders (Center for Sex Offender Management, 2006; Oliver & Holmes, 2015; Wijkman, Bijeveld, & Hendriks, 2014).

B. Assessment

a. Risk factors for sexual violence, in general, not specific for juvenile sex offending, per the Centers for Disease Control and Prevention (CDC, 2015) are: individual (substance use; delinquency; empathic deficits; general aggressiveness and acceptance of violence; early sexual initiation; coercive sexual fantasies; preference for impersonal sex and sexual risk taking; exposure to sexually explicit media; hostility toward women; adherence to traditional gender role norms; hypermasculinity; suicidal behavior; prior sexual victimization or perpetration; relationship factors); relationships (physical violence and conflict; childhood history of physical, sexual, or emotional abuse; emotionally unsupportive family; poor parent–child relationships, especially with fathers; association with sexually aggressive, hypermasculine, and delinquent peers; involvement in a violent or abusive intimate relationship); community (poverty; lack of job opportunities; lack of institutional support from police and the judicial system; general tolerance of sexual violence within the community; weak community sanctions against sexual violence perpetrators); and societal factors (societal norms that support sexual violence; societal norms that support male superiority and sexual entitlement; and societal norms that maintain women's inferiority and sexual submissiveness; weak laws and policies related to sexual violence and gender equity; high levels of crime and other forms of violence).

b. The CDC also suggests protective factors for sexual offending. These are parental use of reasoning to resolve family conflict, emotional health and connectedness, academic achievement, and empathy and concern for how one's actions affect others.

c. Health care professionals need to obtain detailed sexual histories on all adolescents to ascertain whether they are exhibiting unhealthy sexual behaviors. Harassing behaviors such as repeated obscene phone calls, "flashing," and "peeping" are sex offenses, as are coercive or forcible sexual behaviors, including touching breasts, genitals, and buttocks over one's clothing. Health care professionals should also ask about sexually precocious, coercive, and forcible behavior in younger children who are exhibiting conduct disordered behaviors and/or who have been observed, usually by a parent or teacher, engaging in unusual sexual behavior.

AGE	DEVELOPMENTALLY APPROPRIATE/COMMON SEXUAL BEHAVIORS	UNCOMMON SEXUAL BEHAVIORS THAT MAY INDICATE PROBLEMS	INAPPROPRIATE SEXUAL BEHAVIORS
0–5 years	• Questioning and talking about: differences in gender and private body parts, hygiene, toileting, pregnancy, and birth • Using foul language • Like to be nude • Showing genitals to others • Playing doctor or mommy and daddy • Viewing or touching other's genitals • Touching genitals in private or public • Experiencing pleasure from touching genitals • Exploring • Will explore genitals and can experience pleasure. • Showing and looking at private body parts.	• Having knowledge of specific sexual acts or explicit sexual language • Engaging in adultlike sexual contact with other children • Masturbating persistently • Playing sexually with dolls, stuffed toys • Peeping more than infrequently	• Touching or rubbing self to the exclusion of other activities • Touching self to the point of hurting self • Simulating sex with other children • Forcefully penetrating vagina or anus with objects • Displaying multiple sexual behaviors daily • Displaying other aggressive behaviors as well as sexual ones • Acting on sexual behaviors with children who are 4 or more years apart
6–8 years	• Questioning and talking about: physical development, relationships, sexual behavior, menstruation, pregnancy, personal values • Experimenting with same-age/gender children, usually during games or role-playing, such as "I'll show you mine, if you show me yours"	• Having adultlike sexual interactions with other children • Having knowledge of specific sexual acts	• Touching or rubbing self to the exclusion of other activities • Rubbing other people's genitals • Forcing other children to play sex games • Verbalizing considerable sexual knowledge for age • Displaying multiple sexual behaviors or talking about sex daily

(continued)

	• Self-stimulating in private • Enjoying dirty jokes • Copying observed behaviors such as slapping someone's buttocks	• Behaving sexually in a public place or through the use of phone or Internet	• Displaying other aggressive behaviors as well as sexual ones • Acting on these behaviors with children who are 4 or more years apart • Sexually abusing animals
9–12 years	• Questioning and talking about: sexual materials and information, relationships, sexual behavior • Using sexual words and talking about sexual acts and personal values with peers • Experimenting with same-age/gender children, usually during games or role-playing, such as "I'll show you mine, if you show me yours" • Enjoying dirty jokes • Self-stimulating in private	• Behaving in an adultlike sexual manner regularly • Behaving sexually in a public place • Attempting to expose other people's genitals • Verbalizing considerable sexual knowledge for age • Peeping at others or exposing self once • Simulating intercourse with peers, with clothes on	• Masturbating compulsively • Chronic peeping at others or exposing self • Viewing pornography constantly • Using sexually degrading themes • Threatening in a sexual manner • Forcing sexual activity on others • Simulating intercourse with peers, with clothes off • Penetrating dolls and toys sexually • Sexually abusing animals
13–18 years	• Self-stimulating in private • Talking about sex with peers • Experimenting sexually between adolescents of the same age • Displaying voyeuristic behaviors • Having first sexual intercourse and other sexual activities	• Demonstrating anxiety about or preoccupation with sex • Viewing pornography • Talking about sexual aggression • Invading others' body space	• Masturbating in a public place • Masturbating compulsively anywhere • Displaying/discussing sexual interest in much younger children • Demonstrating preoccupation with sexually aggressive pornography • Viewing child pornography • Verbalizing sexual threats • Forcing sexual activity or sexual touch on others • Sexually abusing animals

Adapted from American Academy of Pediatrics (n.d.); South Eastern CASA (2015); Stop It Now (n.d.); and Wurtele & Miller-Perrin (1992).

d. Differentiate developmentally normal sexual behavior from inappropriate sexual behaviors:

e. Adolescent tools focus on recidivism risk; however, the Child Sexual Behavior Inventory, Version 2 (CSBI-2), a 35-item instrument completed by a parent or caregiver, can determine the presence and intensity of a range of sexual behaviors in children ages 2 to 12 over a 6-month period. This tool assesses the child's sexual behaviors on a continuum ranging from mild to aggressive, providing clinical scores based on the child's age and gender (see www.childwelfare.gov/pubs/usermanuals/sexabuse/sexabusel.cfm).

f. Youths who are disenfranchised from traditional health care services require special attention on immunization status, dental care, developmental and psychosocial issues, and establishing a plan of continued health care. All youth should be evaluated for emergent, acute, and chronic conditions. Since early sexual activity, sexual abuse, and sexual offending are all associated with delinquency, sexually transmitted disease (STD) screening should be performed when appropriate. Young postpubertal females should also be screened for the possibility of pregnancy.

C. Diagnosis

a. Sexually aggressive children of any age may have conduct disorder (CD). These youths usually do not perceive their behavior as a problem; on the contrary, they view others as threatening or the cause of their troubles. They tend to have little guilt or remorse. To be diagnosed with CD, at least three of 15 symptoms must be present in the past 12 months with one symptom having been present in the past 6 months, and the symptoms must cause the youth significant impairment in social, academic, or occupational functioning. These children exhibit negative behaviors against people, animals, and property, characterized as belligerent, destructive, threatening, physically cruel, deceitful, disobedient, or dishonest. The 15 symptoms/criteria are found in Chapter 3.

b. Older adolescents may also have a paraphilic disorder. A diagnosis of a paraphilic disorder requires that the person has intense and persistent sexual arousal in other than genital stimulation or preparatory fondling with phenotypically normal, physically mature, consenting humans; this interest is causing the person significant distress (which includes arrest); this interest involves another person's distress, injury, or death; or this interest results in a desire to engage in sexual behaviors with unwilling persons or those unable to give legal consent (e.g., minor children and unconscious persons). The criteria for pedophilic disorder are that over a period of at least 6 months, the person engages in recurrent, intensely sexually arousing fantasies, sexual urges, or behaviors involving sexual activity with a prepubescent child or children, generally age 13 or younger. The person has acted out on these urges or fantasies, or the urges cause marked distress or interpersonal difficulty. The person is at least 16 years old and at least 5 years older than the child or children. Other listed paraphilic disorders are exhibitionistic disorder, fetishistic disorder, frotteuristic disorder, sexual masochism disorder, sexual sadism disorder, transvestic disorder, and voyeuristic disorder, with other paraphilic disorder criteria-fitting interests/behaviors termed unspecified paraphilic disorder or other specified paraphilic disorder (American Psychiatric Association, 2013).

D. Levels of Prevention/Intervention

a. Primary

ATSA takes the position that primary prevention programs should target modifiable risk factors identified by research. Since it is generally easier to alter developing behaviors as compared with behaviors that are ingrained, ATSA also supports the development of early intervention programs.

b. Secondary

Health care providers need to differentiate unusual sexual behaviors in children from offending behaviors, and should be able to identify early problematic behavior and refer these children for appropriate early interventions. Sexually aggressive children under age 13 require alternate treatment modalities. One suggestion is to target risk factors that predispose a child to sexual behavior problems or that precipitate or perpetuate the problems. Many programs include cognitive behavioral approaches; treatment modalities involving individual, group, pair, and family therapy. Important intervention factors include addressing developmental issues and involving parents and other caregivers. As noted earlier, however, some of these children may be considered and treated as sex offenders in certain jurisdictions.

c. Tertiary

Health care providers should also have an understanding of risk assessment, treatment, and reentry issues (including the sex offender registration laws in their jurisdiction with regard to JSOs) so that they can provide proper health care for these youths and so that they can work with other involved professionals to decrease the chances of recidivism. Most adjudicated JSOs reside at some point in the community, thus requiring a comprehensive and collaborative sex offender management program that combines treatment with supervision to enable the offenders to control their sexually abusive behaviors. The desired outcome of treatment is the prevention of future sexual victimization. In general, most sex offender treatment has the following goals:

- Accept responsibility
- Learn to understand their patterns (cycles) of criminal behavior

- Modify cognitive distortions
- Learn attitudes, cognitive skills, and behaviors needed to live safely in the community
- Develop victim empathy
- Control deviant sexual arousal, interests, preferences, and behaviors
- Improve social competence
- Reduce impulsivity and develop self-regulation
- Manage negative emotions
- Develop healthy relationships and correct intimacy deficits
- Establish supervision conditions and networks
- Develop an effective relapse prevention plan

Treatment is also individualized and aimed at underlying disorders (e.g., conduct disorder) and associated problems (substance abuse, mood disorders center, developmental disability, etc.). Treatment may take place in a detention center, forensic psychiatric unit, or the community. Offenders can be terminated from treatment for noncompliance or failure to make adequate progress in treatment, sexual behavior, assaults and fighting, violating confidentiality of others in the program, or be placed in a high-security category. Special interventions may be warranted for juveniles with intellectual and cognitive impairments since they may not respond well to traditional therapies. Unfortunately, this is a highly understudied area. However, it can be assumed that treatment needs to be tailored to meet the juvenile's cognitive developmental status.

E. Parenting Tips

When your child has sexual behavior problems (ATSA, n.d.; National Center on the Sexual Behavior of Youth, 2012; National Child Traumatic Stress Network, n.d.):

a.   Realize that this is a very stressful situation for parents.

b.   You may experience a range of emotions that include denial, anger, sadness, depression, shame, guilt, disappointment, and confusion.

c.   You may experience nightmares and other trauma reactions, especially if you were sexually abused as a child.

d.   Participate in your child's treatment, as effective treatment needs to address the context of family relationships.

e.   Create and enforce clear and consistent privacy rules for all members of your family. This includes not touching others' private parts or not touching one's private parts in public.

f. Minimize opportunities for sexual acting out. Closely supervise your child around other children, and do not allow your child to share a bed with another child. Use caution or completely avoid high-risk situations, such as sleepovers, contact sports, or camping.

g. Keep your child away from sexually explicit media, print and online, and supervise your child when he or she uses the Internet or cell phone.

h. Use appropriate words for body parts.

i. Teach your child about respecting other people's boundaries and to respect his or her own.

j. Get support—it will help you and your child get through this.

k. Know you are not alone; there are other parents dealing with this same issue.

l. Always remember that your child is still your child; he or she made a very poor decision, but he or she can still learn how to make good ones.

Resources

Center for Sex Offender Management: www.csom.org

The National Guidelines for Sex Offender Registration and Notification: www.ojp.usdoj.gov/smart/pdfs/final_sornaguidelines.pdf

Sexual Development and Behavior in Children: http://nctsn.org/nctsn_assets/pdfs/caring/sexual developmentandbehavior.pdf

References

American Academy of Pediatrics. (n.d.). Sexual behaviors in children. In *Preventing sexual violence: An educational toolkit for health care providers*. Retrieved from www2.aap.org/pubserv/PSVpreview/pages/behaviorchart.html

American Psychiatric Association. (2013). *Diagnostic and statistical manual of mental disorders* (5th ed.). Washington, DC: Author.

Araji, S. (1997). *Sexually aggressive children: Coming to understand them*. Thousand Oaks, CA: Sage Publications.

Association for the Treatment of Sexual Abusers. (n.d.). Children with sexual behavior problems. Retrieved from www.atsa.com/children-sexual-behavior-problems

Association for the Treatment of Sexual Offenders. (n.d.). *Children with sexual behavior problems.* Retrieved from www.atsa.com/children-sexual-behavior-problems

Center for Sex Offender Management. (2006). *Understanding treatment for adults and juveniles who have committed sex offense.* U.S. Department of Justice, Office of Justice Programs. Retrieved from www.csom.org/pubs/treatment_brief.pdf

Centers for Disease Control and Prevention. (2015). *Sexual violence: Risk and protective factors.* Retrieved from www.cdc.gov/ViolencePrevention/sexualviolence/riskprotectivefactors.html

Friederich, W. N., Grambsch, P., Damon, L., Hewitt, S. K., Koverola, C., Lang, R. A., . . . Broughton, D. (1992). Child sexual behavior inventory: Normative and clinical comparisons. *Psychological Assessment, 4,* 303–311.

Kellogg, N. (2010). Sexual behavior in children: Evaluation and management. *American Family Physician, 82*(10), 1233–1238.

Miranda, A., Biegler, B., Davis, K., Frevert, V., & Taylor, J. (2001). Treating sexually aggressive children. *Journal of Offender Rehabilitation, 33*(2), 15–32.

National Center on the Sexual Behavior of Youth. (2012). *Safety planning.* Retrieved from www.ncsby.org/content/safety-planning-0

National Child Traumatic Stress Network. (n.d.). *Understanding and coping with sexual behavior problems in children.* Retrieved from http://nctsn.org/nctsn_assets/pdfs/caring/sexualbehaviorproblems.pdf

Oliver, B., & Holmes, L. (2015). Female juvenile sexual offenders: Understanding who they are and possible steps that may prevent some girls from offending. *Journal of Child Sexual Abuse, 24,* 698–715.

Ryan, G., & Lane, S. (1997). *Juvenile sexual offending: Cause, consequences, and correction.* San Francisco: Jossey-Bass.

South Eastern CASA. (2015). *Age appropriate sexual behavior in children and young people for family, friends, teachers and workers.* Retrieved from www.secasa.com.au/pages/age-appropriate-sexual-behaviour-in-children-and-young-people/

Stop It Now. (n.d.). *What is age-appropriate?* Retrieved from www.stopitnow.org/ohc-content/what-is-age-appropriate

Wijkman, M., Bijeveld, C., & Hendriks, J. (2014). Juvenile female sex offenders: Offender and offence characteristics. *European Journal of Criminology, 11*(1), 23–38.

Wurtele, S.K., & Miller-Perrin, M.C. (1992). *Preventing sexual abuse.* Lincoln, NE: University of Nebraska Press.

CHAPTER 23

Sexual Victimization

A. Description

The U.S. Department of Justice Office on Violence Against Women (2015) defines sexual assault thus: "Sexual assault is any type of sexual contact or behavior that occurs without the explicit consent of the recipient. Falling under the definition of sexual assault are sexual activities such as forced sexual intercourse, forcible sodomy, child molestation, incest, fondling, and attempted rape." Sexual abuse is contact or interaction between a child and an adult when the child is used for sexual stimulation by an adult. The American Academy of Pediatrics defines child sexual abuse as the engaging of a child in sexual activities that the child cannot comprehend, for which the child is developmentally unprepared and cannot give informed consent, and that violate the social taboos of society (American Academy of Pediatrics Committee on Child Abuse and Neglect, 1999). In the United States, minor children cannot consent to any sexual activity, but the legal age of consent varies by state. Sexual activities involving a child may include activities intended for sexual stimulation, categorized as noncontact and contact abuse. Noncontact sexual abuse, which is common, includes exhibitionism, voyeurism, and the involvement of a child in verbal sexual propositions or the making of pornography. Contact sexual abuse ranges from nonpenetrating (sexual kissing and fondling) to penetrating (digital, penile, and object insertion into the vagina, mouth, or anus). Rape is a legal term used to define forced sexual intercourse that occurs because of physical force or psychological coercion. Legal terminology for sex crimes varies among jurisdictions.

a.   Sexual assault victims are at risk for complications that may include unintended pregnancy, sexually transmitted diseases, and mental health problems such as post-traumatic stress syndrome, depression, and anxiety; and child and adolescent victims of sexual abuse are at increased risk for sexual victimization in adulthood.

b.   Children are often targets of poly-victimization; those who are physically assaulted in the past year are five times more likely to be sexually victimized (Finkelhor, Turner, Hamby, & Ormrod, 2011). Sexually abused children may present in primary care with a variety of manifestations, some of which may be nonspecific, such as sleep disturbances, abdominal pain, enuresis, encopresis, or phobias, often causing these symptoms to be mistaken for other physical or emotional problems. Children may also be coerced into secrecy by the perpetrator who may even threaten to harm or kill the child or the child's family if he or she discloses the abuse. Disclosure can be difficult for a child, especially if a case goes through the criminal justice system, as the child must first be believed by the first confidant (parent, teacher, friend, or primary care provider), then by the police and/or social services, a prosecutor (Connolly, Coburn, & Yin, 2015), and, finally, a judge and/or jury. Thus, the primary care provider should maintain a level of suspicion and carefully and appropriately question the child to detect sexual abuse when nonspecific symptoms are present (Muscari & Brown, 2010).

c.   Adolescents and young adults have the highest rates of sexual assaults of any age group (Kaufman & American Academy of Pediatrics Committee on Adolescence, 2008), and adolescents are less likely to report sexual assault than adult victims. Just less than half of both adolescent victims and offenders use alcohol or drugs before sexual assault, and drug-facilitated sexual assault is not unusual. The rate of perpetration by a known offender is similar for males and females, but forced oral sex, the use of weapons, and multiple assailants are more common in males (Kaufman & American Academy of Pediatrics Committee on Adolescence, 2008). Adolescents may also be victims of sexual assault when they agree to sexual contact with persons aged 18 and older, including older peers. Although this may be perceived as a "relationship scenario," it is still considered sexual assault when the minor is under the legal age of consent; however, the adolescent may be very reluctant to discuss it because he or she may not want to get their partner in trouble. Disclosure is difficult in general, and it may be voluntary (those who choose to disclose through the help-seeking process), involuntary (those encouraged and assisted by friends to tell an adult), or situational (those who were unconscious at the time of the assault and whose friends sought help for them). Those who do disclose usually do so to a friend or to their mother, but those who disclose to their mothers are more likely to report to law enforcement (Campbell, Greeson, Fehler-Cabral, & Kennedy, 2015). Adults tend to be the last ones in the disclosure cycle, making it more critical for health care providers to assess for sexual assault.

d.   Reports of campus sexual assault vary, with one showing that 19% of undergraduate women experienced attempted or completed sexual assault after entering college, and another finding lifetime prevalence base-rates of completed or attempted rape of more than half of college women reporting unwanted sexual experiences that included sexual contact, sexual coercion, attempted rape, and rape (Cleere & Lynn, 2013; Sable, Danis, Mauzy, & Gallagher, 2006). As noted in the following section, males can also be victims of sexual assault, and both male and female victims might be reluctant to report it. Barriers to reporting include shame, embarrassment, not wanting others to know, concerns about confidentiality, and fear of not being believed; both males and females also report fear of perpetrator retaliation and male victims being judged as gay (Finkelhor et al., 2011). Some students may also "underreport" and label their assaultive experiences in benign terms, such as "a serious miscommunication" (Muscari & Brown, 2010).

e.   Approximately 28% of men were age 10 or younger at the time of their first sexual victimization (Black et al., 2011), and in one study of clients at a child advocacy center, boys ages 6 to 10 years were the largest group in the male sample (Carlson, Grassley, Reis, & Davis, 2015). Fears of doubts about their sexuality, disbelief, blame, and other negative reactions may prevent male victims from coming forward (Davies, 2002). Some males may experience sexual assault at higher rates than others, including males who are gay or bisexual; males who have mental health disorders, physical disabilities or cognitive impairment; veterans; and males who are detained or incarcerated. In prison and detention culture, once a youth is raped for the first time, that youth is "turned out" and "fair game" for further abuse (Beck, Guerino, & Harrison, 2010). The perpetrator is usually another male who is known to the victim. Male victims of sexual assault may suffer from depression, anxiety, posttraumatic stress disorder, and dysfunctional sexual behavior, and may exhibit self-mutilation, angry outbursts, risk-taking behaviors, and suicidal threats that may be presenting complaints in primary care (Du Mont, Macdonald, White, & Turner, 2013).

f.   Studies on sexual victimization among individuals who identify as gay, lesbian, or bisexual (GLB) showed significant rates of child, adult, intimate partner, and hate-related sexual assault, suggesting that individuals who identify themselves as GLB may face a higher risk of sexual violence than the general population (Rothman, Exner, & Baughman, 2011). There is also a relationship between sexual assault victimization and high-risk sexual behaviors, mood disorders, and suicide attempts among individuals who identify as LGBTQ (lesbian, gay, bisexual, transgender, and queer), as well as barriers to post-trauma services owing to homophobia and transphobia (National Sexual Violence Resource Center, 2012).

g.   Health care providers who work with young adult active military or veterans should be aware of military sexual assault/trauma (MST). MST is a prevalent problem among active and reserve duty in the five branches of the U.S. military. Although it is typically associated with female service personnel, males are also victims, usually in the form of hazing or punishment. Reporting is hampered by fear of retaliation by other soldiers and the chain of command, and many bases and Veteran's Affairs are outdated, understaffed, and underfunded, and thus not equipped to handle sexual assault victims (Sable et al., 2006).

h.   Drug-facilitated sexual assault (DFSA) is an increasing problem among older adolescents and young adults at social parties, clubs, bars, and rave clubs. Some perpetrators may merely coax victims into ingesting drugs or alcohol, while others covertly use prescription and nonprescription drugs to induce sedation, disinhibition, and amnesia in order to facilitate sexual assault. Substances used include alcohol, alprazolam, chloral hydrate, gamma-hydroxybutyrate, flunitrazepam (Rohypnol, known as the "date rape drug"), ketamine, lorazepam, tetrahydrocannabinol (THC), and zopiclone. Regardless of how drugs are administered, the goal is to render the victim defenseless, and the amnesic effect of some of these drugs results in delayed reporting of the sexual assault for days, weeks, or longer. Victims of DFSA may have multiple symptoms, including impaired memory and judgment, drowsiness, confusion, partial or total amnesia, dizziness, reduced inhibition, feeling of having blacked out, nausea, vomiting, impaired motor skills, "rubbery legs," and weakness. They may also report a strange sensation of being paralyzed and powerless, disassociation, as well as unexplained genital and/or other injuries, unexplained bodily fluids found on their body, and a vague sensation that "something happened" (Du Mont et al., 2009; Schwartz, Milteer, & LeBeau, 2000).

i. Child sexual exploitation is a complex problem that involves: possession, manufacture, and distribution of child pornography; online enticement of children for sexual acts; child prostitution; and trafficking.

- Federal law defines child pornography as any visual depiction, including any photograph, film, video, picture, or computer or computer-generated image or picture, whether made or produced by electronic, mechanical, or other means, of sexually explicit conduct, where: the production of the visual depiction involves the use of a minor engaging in sexually explicit conduct; or the visual depiction is a digital image, computer image, or computer-generated image that is, or is indistinguishable from, that of a minor engaging in sexually explicit conduct; or the visual depiction has been created, adapted, or modified to appear as though an identifiable minor is engaging in sexually explicit conduct. Federal law also criminalizes knowingly producing, distributing, receiving, or possessing with intent to distribute, a visual depiction of any kind, including a drawing, cartoon, sculpture, or painting, of a child that: depicts a minor engaging in sexually explicit conduct and is obscene, or depicts an image that is, or appears to be, of a minor engaging in graphic bestiality, sadistic or masochistic abuse, or sexual intercourse, including genital–genital, oral–genital, anal–genital, or oral–anal, whether between persons of the same or opposite sex and such depiction lacks serious literary, artistic, political, or scientific value. Sexually explicit conduct is defined under federal law as actual or simulated sexual intercourse (including genital–genital, oral–genital, anal–genital, or oral–anal, whether between persons of the same or opposite sex), bestiality, masturbation, sadistic or masochistic abuse, or lascivious exhibition of the genitals or pubic area of any person.

- Most online sex offenders target teens and groom their victims into sexual relationships, usually under the guise of romance. Online offenders typically target vulnerable youths, those with histories of abuse, family problems, and high-risk behaviors.

- Prostitution is illegal in most places in the United States, and minors who take money for sex are usually taking part in that illegal activity; however, they are also victims of crime. Most minors who become involved in prostitution are runaway or thrown away children from abusive or otherwise dysfunctional homes. They are usually lured into prostitution by sophisticated criminals (frequently pimps), who convince them that they will earn money to survive and will be taken care of in a secure loving environment that they lacked at home. However, the pimps take the child's money and often engage in severe physical abuse to build a relationship of dependency.

- Human trafficking is modern-day slavery. It is the recruitment, harboring, transportation, provision, or obtaining of a person for labor or services through the use of force, fraud, or coercion for the purpose of involuntary servitude, debt bondage (peonage), or slavery. Trafficking is different from smuggling, which is the crime of getting paid to assist another in illegally crossing a border. However, if the smuggler sells or brokers the smuggled individual into a condition of servitude, or if the smuggled individual is forced to work the debt off, the crime turns from smuggling into human trafficking. Contrary to a common assumption, human trafficking is not just a problem in other countries—cases have been reported in all 50 states, Washington, DC, and some U.S. territories.

j.   Health care providers avoid screening for sexual assault for a variety of reasons, including lack of training, fear of approaching sensitive subjects, and lack of time to screen or private facilities for screening. However, most do not screen because they do not know how to ask questions and/or how to respond when the victim discloses (National Sexual Violence Resource Center, 2011a). Health care providers may also have experienced sexual violence in their own lives, either directly or in a family member. In such cases, the health care provider should seek counseling to resolve his or her own distress to avoid a countertransference response (provider transfers his or her own emotions to a client). However, when properly screened, victims can disclose their abuse and receive the care and services they need. The "telling" alone provides meaning to their experience and helps to better manage emotions, and not asking reinforces the victims' silence.

B. Assessment (History, Physical, Diagnostic Screening/Testing, Where Appropriate)

a.   Risk factors: Sexually abused children may present to medical settings with a variety of symptoms and signs. Since they are often coerced into secrecy by the perpetrator, the health care provider needs a high level of suspicion and may need to carefully and appropriately question the child to detect sexual abuse in these situations. Presenting symptoms may be so general or nonspecific (such as sleep disturbances, abdominal pain, enuresis, encopresis, or phobias) that caution must be exercised when the pediatrician considers sexual abuse, because the symptoms may indicate physical or emotional abuse or other stressors unrelated to sexual abuse.

b.   Behavior indicators of sexual abuse by age group may include the following:

- Under age 5: regression, feeding or toileting disturbances, temper tantrums, requests for frequent panty changes, and seductive behavior. Ages 5 to 10: school problems, night terrors, sleep problems, anxieties, withdrawal, refusal of physical activity, and inappropriate behaviors. Adolescence: school problems, running away, delinquency, promiscuity, drug and alcohol abuse, eating disorders, depression, and other significant psychological problems, such as suicide attempts.

c.   The medical history and exam differ from the forensic exam. Should a separate, follow-up medical evaluation be warranted in acute sexual assault cases, the primary health care provider should proceed as usual in obtaining a complete history and physical assessment.

d.   Screening should take place during routine wellness exams and during episodic illness exams when symptoms are suspicious for sexual assault. Victims vary in response to sexual assault, ranging from showing no emotional response to showing significant emotional or physical symptoms. The National Sexual Violence Resource Center (2011a) recommends the following:

- Normalize the questioning by integrating it into the history.
- Provide context by connecting the history to the youth's health and well-being.
- Be nonjudgmental.
- Be direct, but avoid using terms like rape and sexual assault.
- Validate the youth's responses.
- Ask about experiences that were uncomfortable or unwanted, and use those that are developmentally appropriate for the child/adolescent:
  - Have you been touched without your consent?
  - Have you ever been pressured or forced to have sexual contact?
  - Do you feel that you have control over your sexual relationships?
  - Allow the youth to verbalize and be heard.

Health care providers can develop a protocol to ensure that all youths are screened adequately and consistently. Protocols should ensure privacy in both the interview, which should take place when victims have their clothing on, and the documentation. For example, the SAVE (a screening protocol developed by the Florida Council Against Sexual Violence in 2003) screening all clients, asking direct questions, validating responses, and evaluating, educating, and referring (Council Against Sexual Violence, 2003). Some youths will not disclose when first asked. Thus, screening should take place with each visit. Some may also not be sure whether what happened to them was sexual violence, giving the health care provider an opportunity to discuss it further. Some patients, including males who were abused by other males, may not want to talk to a male provider and may need referral to a female provider.

C. Diagnosis

As with other forms of child abuse, certain conditions and disorders can mimic sexual abuse, and thus health care providers need to carefully consider possible differential diagnoses:

a.   Crohn's disease can result in anal/rectal lesions that may be mistaken for abuse.

b.   Foul-smelling discharge may indicate a foreign body.

c.   Lichen sclerosis, a dermatological condition that is manifested by genital soreness and subpendymal hemorrhages, usually affects the vulva and perianal regions and has an hourglass appearance.

d.   Nonsexually transmitted organisms, such as *Candida*, can cause discharge.

e.   Poor hygiene and pinworm infestation can both cause redness and pruritus.

f.   Streptococcal infection can yield marked redness and vaginal discharge.

g.   Symptoms may be nonspecific, such as erythema of the vulva.

h.   Widespread bruising can indicate a bleeding disorder.

D. Levels of Prevention/Intervention

a.   Primary

Teach families about healthy relationships and how to identify potentially abusive situations. Encourage parents to talk to you if they suspect their child is at risk of being abused. Strive to change social structures or norms that support the occurrence of child sexual abuse (National Sexual Violence Resource Center, 2011b).

b.   Secondary

- Assess for and intervene with risk factors: parent abused as a child; multiple caretakers for the child; caretaker or parent who has multiple sexual partners; drug and/or alcohol abuse; stress associated with poverty; social isolation and family secrecy; child with poor self-esteem or other vulnerable state; other family members abused; and gang member associations (National Sexual Violence Resource Center, 2011b).

- Teach parents how to watch for grooming behaviors (Bennett & O'Donohue, 2014; Maryland Coalition Against Sexual Assault, n.d.; Pennsylvania Coalition Against Rape, 2015); the offender may:
  - Target the child victim by testing for vulnerability and looking for isolation, and low self-confidence, emotional neediness, as well as little parental attention.
  - Gain the trust of the child's family, and even community—a process that can take years.
  - Target a specific child; may want that child to stay home with him or her, while the other children leave the house.
  - Engage youth on social media.
  - Prefer to be with children rather than adults.
  - Engage in voyeuristic behaviors, such as watching children who are in bathing suits or pajamas.
  - Gain the child's trust by getting to know their victims and their needs, including how to fulfill them. They build trust with secrecy and parental distancing, usually by allowing the child to do something that is disallowed by the parents.
  - Provide students with special rewards (educator sex offenders).
  - Fill the child's needs with affection, attention, money, cigarettes, alcohol, drugs, gifts, or special privileges for no apparent reason. Predators take on an important role in the child's life.
  - Engage in regular roughhousing behavior with children, and/or insist on touching, hugging, kissing, or wrestling with the child, even if the child does not want the behavior.
  - Touch the child "accidentally."
  - Repeatedly offer to babysit for free or do favors or enjoyable activities to get time alone with the child without adult interruptions. Unfortunately, parents may unknowingly encourage this by appreciating these activities.
  - Dress inappropriately when around children (e.g., tight pants that outline genital area).
  - "Accidentally" expose self to child (e.g., offender walks out of shower naked except for bath towel covering lower torso, drops bath towel to the floor, exposing genitalia).
  - Talk about inappropriate topics with children.

- Sexualize the interaction, first with nonsexual touching, such as accidental or playful touches that desensitize the child so the child does not resist increased sexualized touching. The offender next exploits the child's curiosity to advance the sexual interaction. The offender may also show the child pornography.

- Maintain control with threats (harm/kill child or child's family) and guilt to enforce secrecy and force the child's continued participation and silence. The offender may also blame the child for allowing the abuse to happen, fostering even more guilt.

c. Tertiary

- Jenny and Crawford-Jakubiak (2013) note five critical issues that should be addressed in primary care settings: the child's safety; reporting the abuse to the proper authorities; the child's mental health; the need for an exam to rule out injury, especially if the child reports bleeding or pain; and the need for a forensic evaluation, especially if the abuse occurred in the past 72 to 96 hours, dependent upon local jurisdiction.

- Appropriate interventions depend on whether the sexual assault was recent or in the past. If the assault was recent, a forensic examination may be warranted. Young adult victims can decide whether or not to have the exam and usually may do so without reporting the incident to the police, depending upon the jurisdiction. For all ages, exams are best conducted by Sexual Assault Forensic Examiners/Sexual Assault Nurse Examiners (SAFE/SANE), usually in emergency departments or specialized centers (such as a Children's Advocacy Center). Overall, clients have positive experiences with SANEs. One study of adolescent sexual assault victims found that the adolescents viewed the SANEs as sensitive to their physical and emotional needs, compassionate, caring and personable, but they mostly appreciated that the SANEs believed and validated their accounts of the assault (Campbell, Greeson, & Fehler-Cabral, 2013). Youths may also have needs regarding emergency contraception, antibiotics for sexually transmitted diseases, and/or physical injuries (National Sexual Violence Resource Center, 2011a).

- Counseling is recommended to prevent or minimize the complications of sexual abuse. Sexually abused children and adolescents can suffer a range of short- and long-term problems that include depression, anxiety, guilt, fear, sexual dysfunction, withdrawal, eating disorders, substance abuse, promiscuity, and acting out. Many of these problems can continue into adulthood. Revictimization is also a common phenomenon among adults abused as children, and studies have shown that they are more likely to be the victims of rape or to be involved in physically abusive relationships than adults with no history of abuse. Some victims and their families may need crisis intervention, legal services, or support groups. Young adults may need housing, if going home means imminent danger. Clinicians should develop, maintain, and update a list of community resources for ready access, and family patients should receive a copy of appropriate resources with their contact information. Since child sexual abuse can result in either toxic or traumatic stress, refer to those sections for additional information.

E. Parenting Tips

Although you can never completely protect your child from sexual abuse, you can do your best to drastically minimize his or her chances of being abused:

a. Preschoolers:

- Teach the child the proper name for body parts, including genitals and breasts.
- Tell the child that no one—strangers, friends, or relatives—has the right to touch his or her private parts (parts covered by a bathing suit) or hurt him or her.
- Tell the child it is okay to say "NO" to people who make him or her feel scared, uncomfortable, or embarrassed.
- Instruct the child to tell you if adults ask him or her to keep secrets.

b. School-age children:

- Give the child straightforward information about sex.
- Emphasize that the child's body belongs to the child and that no one has the right to touch his or her private parts.
- Explain that some grown-ups have problems and are confused about sex and that these adults may try to do things that make the child feel uncomfortable.
- Teach the child personal safety and to get away from those adults who make him or her feel uncomfortable.
- Tell the child her to come to you immediately if such an adult bothers him or her.

c. Teenagers:

- Explain that unwanted sex is an act of violence, not an act of love.
- Discuss rape, date/acquaintance rape.
- Reinforce the teen's right to say "NO."
- But remember, sexual abuse can occur under your own roof—family members, babysitters—so keep the lines of communication open at all times. Listen to your children, and be alert for unusual behaviors from them and others in your household.

Resources

American Academy of Child & Adolescent Psychiatry Child Sexual Abuse Resource Center: www.aacap.org/AACAP/Families_and_Youth/Resource_Centers/Child_Abuse_Resource_Center/Home.aspx

Florida Council Against Sexual Violence. (2012). How to Screen Your Patients for Sexual Assault: A Guide for Health Care Professionals: www.fcasv.org/sites/default/files/SAVE%202012.pdf

MedLine Plus Child Sexual Abuse: www.nlm.nih.gov/medlineplus/childsexualabuse.html

National Center for Victims of Crime: https://victimsofcrime.org/

National Children's Advocacy Center: www.nationalcac.org

National Plan to Prevent the Sexual Abuse and Exploitation of Children: www.preventtogether.org/Resources/Documents/NationalPlan2012FINAL.pdf

Rape, Abuse & Incest National Network: www.rainn.org

References

American Academy of Pediatrics Committee on Child Abuse and Neglect. (1999) Guidelines for the evaluation of sexual abuse of children: Subject review. *Pediatrics, 103*(1), 186–191.

Beck, A., Guerino, P., & Harrison, P. (2010). *Sexual victimization in juvenile facilities reported by youth, 2008–09* (Bureau of Justice Statistics, NCJ 228416). Retrieved from www.bjs.gov/index.cfm?ty=pbdetail&iid=2113

Black, M. C., Basile, K. C., Breiding, M. J., Smith, S .G., Walters, M. L., Merrick, M. T., ... Stevens, M. R. (2011). *The National Intimate Partner and Sexual Violence Survey: 2010 summary report*. Retrieved from http://www.cdc.gov/ViolencePrevention/pdf/NISVS_Report2010-a.pdf

Bennett, N., & O'Donohue, W. (2014). The construct of grooming in child sexual abuse: Conceptual and measurement issues. *Journal of Child Sexual Abuse, 23*, 957–976. doi:10.1080/10538712.2014.960632

Campbell, R., Greeson, M.R., & Fehler-Cabral, G. (2013). With care and compassion: Adolescent sexual assault victims' experiences in sexual assault nurse examiner programs. *Journal of Forensic Nursing, 9*(2), 68–75.

Campbell, R., Greeson, M., Fehler-Cabral, G., & Kennedy, A. (2015). Pathways to help: Adolescent sexual assault victims' disclosure and help-seeking experiences. *Violence against Women, 21*(7), 824–847. doi:10.1177/1077801215584071

220CHILD BEHAVIORAL AND PARENTING CHALLENGES

Carlson, F., Grassley, J., Reis, J., & Davis, K. (2015). Characteristics of child sexual assault within a child advocacy center client population. *Journal of Forensic Nursing, 11*(2), 15–21.

Cleere, C., & Lynn, S. (2013). Acknowledged versus unacknowledged sexual assault among college women. *Journal of Interpersonal Violence, 28,* 2593–2611.

Connolly, D. A., Coburn, P. I., & Yiu, A. (2015). Potential motive to fabricate and the assessment of child witnesses in sexual assault cases. *Journal of Police and Criminal Psychology, 30*(2), 63–70. doi:10.1007/s11896-014-9146-1

Council Against Sexual Violence. (2003). *SAVE: Screening your patients for sexual assault.* Tallahassee, FL: Author.

Davies, M. (2002). Male sexual assault victims: A selective review of the literature and implications for support services. *Aggressive and Violent Behavior, 7,* 203–214.

Du Mont, J., Macdonald, S., Rotbard, N., Asllani, E., Bainbridge, D., & Cohen, M. (2009). Factors associated with suspected drug-facilitated sexual assault. *Canadian Medical Association Journal, 180,* 513–519.

Du Mont, J., Macdonald, S., White, M., & Turner, L. (2013). Male victims of adult sexual assault: A descriptive study of survivors' use of sexual assault treatment services. *Journal of Interpersonal Violence, 28,* 2676–2694.

Finkelhor, D., Turner, H., Hamby, S., & Ormrod, R. (2011). Polyvictimization: Children's exposure to multiple types of violence, crime, and abuse. *U.S. Department of Justice Office of Juvenile Justice and Delinquency Prevention National Survey of Children's Exposure to Violence Bulletin.* Retrieved from www.ncjrs.gov/pdffiles1/ojjdp/235504.pdf

Kaufman, M., & American Academy of Pediatrics Committee on Adolescence. (2008). Care of the adolescent sexual assault victim. *Pediatrics, 122,* 462–470.

Jenny, C. & Crawford-Jakubiak, J.E. (2013). The evaluation of children in the primary care setting when sexual abuse is suspected. *Pediatrics, 132*(2), e558–e567.

Maryland Coalition Against Sexual Assault. (n.d.). *Behaviors of sexual predators: Grooming.* Retrieved from www.mcasa.org/_mcasaWeb/wp-content/uploads/2013/12/Behaviors-of-Sexual-Predators-Grooming.pdf

Muscari, M., & Brown, K. (2010). *Quick reference to child & adolescent forensics.* New York, NY: Springer.

National Sexual Violence Resource Center. (2011a). *Assessing patients for sexual violence: A guide for health care providers.* Retrieved from www.nsvrc.org/sites/default/files/Publications_NSVRC_Guides_Assessing-patients-for-sexual-violence.pdf

National Sexual Violence Resource Center. (2011b). *Child sexual abuse prevention.* Retrieved from www.nsvrc.org/sites/default/files/Publications_NSVRC_Bulletin-Child-sexual-abuse-prevention.pdf

National Sexual Violence Resource Center. (2012). *Research brief: Sexual violence and individuals who identify as LGBTQ.* Retrieved from http://nsvrc.org/publications/nsvrc-publications-information-packets-research-briefs/LGBTQ

Pennsylvania Coalition Against Rape. (2015). *What behaviors might a person who sexually abuses children use to gain trust?* Retrieved from www.pcar.org/behaviors-to-gain-trust

Rothman, E., Exner, D., & Baughman, A. (2011). The prevalence of sexual assault against people who identify as gay, lesbian, or bisexual in the United States: A systematic review. *Trauma, Violence, and Abuse, 12,* 55–66.

Sable, M. R., Danis, F., Mauzy, D. L., & Gallagher, S. K. (2006). Barriers to reporting sexual assault for women and men: Perspectives of college students. *Journal of American College Health, 55,* 157–162.

Schwartz, R. H., Milteer, R., & LeBeau, M. A. (2000). Drug-facilitated sexual assault ("date rape"). *Southern Medical Journal, 93,* 558–561.

U.S. Department of Justice Office on Violence Against Women. (2015). *Sexual assault.* Retrieved from www.justice.gov/ovw/sexual-assault

CHAPTER 24

Stalking

A. Description

The word stalking usually describes a pattern of overtly criminal and/or apparently innocent behaviors whereby an individual inflicts repeated, unwanted communications and intrusions upon another. Stalking has also been referred to as a pattern of behavior directed at a specific person that would cause a reasonable person to feel fear. It can be distinguished from other crimes in two ways: Stalking involves repeated victimization, and it is partly defined by its impact on the victim. The first stalking law was passed in California in 1990. Increasing awareness has since made stalking a crime, in many cases a felony, under the law of all 50 states, the District of Columbia, the federal government, and Tribal codes.

    a. A literature review by McCann (2003) revealed that empirical literature on children and stalking is limited. However, he found that stalking behaviors, such as dating violence, spying, and leaving unwanted notes or photos, were found in young populations. McCann also noted that a small study of 13 juvenile stalkers found patterns consistent with adult perpetrators. Most adolescent stalking is perpetrated by current or former dating partners, and most occur during midadolescence; other perpetrators are classmates, acquaintances, friends, and coworkers. Unfortunately, many adolescents are inexperienced with relationships and view the stalking as normal and even flattering (Garcia, 2008).

    b. Like adults, adolescents can be stalked by or stalk acquaintances, past or current friends or paramours, and strangers. Adolescent relationship abusers commonly use stalking to monitor their partner's activities during and even after the relationship. Teen stalking behaviors include: knowing the victim's schedule; showing up at places the victim goes to; sending persistent unwanted or threatening mail, e-mail, and pictures; calling or texting repeatedly; contacting or posting about the victim on social networking sites; writing letters; damaging the victim's property; creating a website about the victim; sending gifts; stealing the victim's things; and any other actions to contact (unwanted), harass, track, or frighten the victim. Electronic stalking is referred to as cyberstalking, which also includes using tracking apps to monitor victims (more information on this is in Chapter 8). While some of these behaviors may seem harmless, they are designed to intimidate the victim and exert control over him or her (National Centers for Victims of Crime, n.d.).

c.   Stalking behavior can be found in youth with autistic spectrum disorder (ASD) who unintentionally stalk without realizing the implications of their behaviors. Persons with ASD have difficulty reading social cues and understanding the viewpoint of others, and they are at risk for inappropriate courtship behaviors. Their behaviors are also easily misunderstood by others (Post, Haymes, Storey, Loughrey, & Campbell, 2014).

d.   College students are at high risk for stalking, since the highest rates of stalking are in emerging adults, ages 18 to 24. However, this group is less likely to report it.

Stalking is a pattern of conduct that may involve criminal activities and/or seemingly nonthreatening acts. According to the National Centers for Victims of Crime (2012), stalking often includes: assaulting the victim; violating protective orders; sexually assaulting the victim; vandalizing the victim's property; burglarizing the victim's home or otherwise stealing from the victim; threatening the victim; and killing the victim's pet. Other common stalking behaviors include: sending unwanted cards or gifts; leaving phone and/or e-mail messages; voyeurism; identity theft; disclosing to the victim personal information the offender has uncovered about the said victim; disseminating personal information about the victim; following the victim; visiting the victim at the latter's workplace; workplace violence; waiting outside the victim's home; sending the victim photographs taken of the victim without consent; monitoring the victim's computer usage; using technology to gather images of or information about the victim; and violating protective orders. Stalking is often a feature of domestic violence, and like domestic violence, it is often not taken sufficiently seriously because it involves acts that health care and law enforcement professionals may perceive as everyday courtship. However, when gestures are part of a course of conduct that instills fear in the victim, they are being used to terrorize.

B. Assessment (History, Physical, Diagnostic Screening/Testing, Where Appropriate)

a.   Risk factors for violence in stalking perpetration include prior intimate partner, threats, presence of psychosis, presence of personality disorder, substance abuse, criminal history, violence history, and stalker gender (Churcher & Nesca, 2013).

b.   Victim impact is critical in stalking cases, not only for health care intervention, but also for potential evidence since the legal definition of stalking includes its effect on the victim. Many victims feel constantly hypervigilant, vulnerable, out of control, and anxious. Stalking can rob them of their energy, leaving them with a loss of trust, long-term emotional distress, and significant disruption in everyday living. Symptoms may worsen with each new incident, and may be compounded by the victims' concerns about the effects on their children and other secondary victims. Victims may experience: anxiety, fear, and/or depression; post-traumatic stress disorder (PTSD); altered thought or perceptual processes (lowered self-esteem, confusion, irrational beliefs); impaired physical health (eating disorders, sleep disorders, digestive distress); financial changes (job loss, investing in home security); altered normal routines to avoid detection by the offender; changing phone numbers, e-mail addresses, driver's license, social security number; relocating (temporarily or permanently); changing identity, uprooting themselves and their immediate families, while leaving behind friends and other relatives. Some victims may experience resilience through stronger relationships with family and friends and a heightened sense of personal safety. However, these positive aspects are unlikely to outweigh the detriments caused by the victimization.

c.   When assessing children and adolescents, differentiate developmentally normal behaviors from stalking. It is not unusual for children to have crushes on teachers (writing notes, giving small gifts) or for older children to idolize celebrities (sending letters and e-mails, posting on social network sites). They may also experience intense romantic feelings toward peers and follow them around, call them repeatedly, send multiple e-mails or texts, frequently contact them via social media, or wait in areas where the admired person is likely to show up; however, these behaviors are rarely seen as threatening. Contact becomes intrusive when it is unwelcome in the other person's life and consists of multiple behaviors (Garcia, 2008).

d.   Stalking typology is based on adults and may be helpful for understanding college student stalking. Mullen (2003) provides a typology that describes five types of stalkers, based on those perpetrators who exhibit stalking behaviors for more than 2 weeks. This classification is based on a multiaxial approach, whereby the primary axis is a typology relating to the stalker's predominant motivation in commencing and sustaining the stalking. Mullen notes that the five types can overlap and that in practice it is difficult to consign the vast majority of stalkers to a single type (Knoll & Resnick, 2007; Mullen, 2003):

- Rejected stalkers usually stalk former intimate partners and are motivated by a desire for reconciliation and/or revenge. Their stalking becomes a substitute for the lost relationship. Some derive satisfaction from inflicting pain. They often have personality disorders and are among the most persistent, intrusive, and dangerous stalkers.

- Intimacy seekers see their victims as their true love and endow their victims with unique qualities. Some imagine that the persons they are stalking reciprocate such feelings. They may be completely oblivious to the victims' response to them or be enraged by their sought-after partners' indifference. Many intimacy seekers have significant mental illnesses such as delusional disorders and need psychiatric intervention. Many "celebrity stalkers" fall into this category.

- Incompetent suitors tend to stalk particular persons for only a short time. They are aware of their victims' disinterest; however, these perpetrators, who are often intellectually limited and socially impaired, are unable or unwilling to appreciate the negative responses to their approaches, and may then pursue others. Incompetent suitors are probably the most common type of stalker in the community.

- Resentful stalkers feel humiliated or treated unfairly. They desire to carry out a vendetta against a specific person or choose someone at random as representative of those they believe harmed them. Resentful stalkers are primarily motivated by the desire to frighten and distress their victims, and the majority are paranoid, oversensitive personalities with a tendency to be obsessive and to ruminate.

- Predatory stalkers stalk in preparation for a physical or sexual assault. Many have paraphilias, particularly sexual sadism, and prior convictions for sexual offenses. The very process of stalking alone may provide satisfaction because it gives the stalker a sense of power and control. This may be heightened by the stalkers leaving the victims subtle hints that they are being observed (silent phone calls, entering their homes to move the furniture), causing unease and confusion in the victims. However, there may also be no warning before the attack.

The RECON (relationship and context-based) typology (Mohandie, Meloy, McGowan, & Williams, 2006) focuses on the relationship, or lack of it, between the stalker and the victim, the behavior, and the context in which the stalking occurs:

- Intimate stalkers, who have had prior relationships with their victims, are the most malignant. They have violent criminal records and a history of alcohol and/or stimulant abuse, are rarely psychotic, but may be suicidal. Many were abusive during the relationship, and most reoffend. Most do not have major psychiatric disorders, other than depression.

- Acquaintance stalkers are usually women who are motivated by the desire to establish a relationship, but who are also resentful about rejection. They tend to threaten repeatedly and may assault their victims or destroy the victims' property. Their pursuit patterns are usually indirect and sporadic, but relentless. Psychiatric disorders vary, and borderline personality disorder is common.

- Public figure stalkers target celebrities and are more likely to have a diagnosable mental illness. They are usually older, with less criminal histories and a greater chance of being psychotic than the other types. Most do not threaten their target.

- Private stranger stalkers tend to be men with mental illness, and the risk of violence is real. This is the smallest group of stalkers, who are usually mentally ill, but who do not abuse substances or have criminal records. They are direct, close, and frequent followers.

- Despite the plots of mystery television shows, stalkers are unlikely to fit this profile. Many are men with mental illness, and the risk of violence is real.

C. Diagnosis, Including Differential Diagnoses, When Appropriate

There is no one specific mental health disorder. While some stalkers have substance abuse disorders, depression, psychosis, or borderline personality disorder, it is important to discern whether and how the disorder relates to stalking behavior.

D. Levels of Prevention/Intervention

a. Primary

Thus far there are no specific prevention measures other than those to keep victims safe.

b. Secondary

Similar to the primary level, there are no specific prevention measures other than those to keep victims safe.

c. Tertiary

Health care professionals need to be knowledgeable of this crime, the behaviors, and the impact it has on victims. To better assist victims:

- Ascertain why a victim believes he or she is being stalked—assess for stalking behaviors.
- Do not challenge or belittle the victim's concerns.
- Assess for and intervene with physiological and psychological consequences, such as eating and sleep disorders, posttraumatic stress disorder, anxiety, and depression.
- Refer victims for counseling.
- Enable the victim to access victims' resource services, both local resources and web-based resources. Local victim groups can also assist victims in coping with the legal process if the case comes to trial.
- Encourage the victim to report his or her concerns to the proper authorities (usually local or state police).

- Encourage the victim to obtain a protective/restraining order. These orders are not "bulletproof"; therefore, victims must also take other measures to protect their safety:
  - Obtain an unlisted telephone number, caller ID, voice mail, and cell phone.
  - Install and utilize quality deadbolt locks, solid core doors, and security systems.
  - Install adequate outdoor lighting; trim bushes and shrubs to eliminate hiding places.
  - Notify family, friends, and trusted neighbors of stalking. Provide them with a photo and the vehicle information of the stalker, if possible.
  - Create a contingency plan should going to or staying home not be possible; keep a suitcase packed with necessary supplies.
  - Stay alert, and be aware of surroundings.
  - Vary routes of travel to and from work.
  - Park in secure and well-lit areas. Ask a trusted person for an escort to the car.
  - Do not dismiss threats. Report them immediately to the authorities.
- Encourage the victim to collect evidence of stalking:
  - Document all incidents.
    - Keep a stalking journal or log (the Stalking Resource Center has a Stalking Incident and Behavior Log that can be downloaded from its website: www.ncvc.org/src). Since this information can possibly be used as evidence or inadvertently shared with the stalker at a future time, encourage the victim not to include any information that they do not want the offender to see.
    - Take photographs.
    - Obtain affidavits from witnesses.
    - Videotape.
    - Keep phone answering machine messages.
    - Keep a list of potential witnesses.
  - Carefully preserve all evidence.
    - Letters, notes, e-mails
    - Gifts
    - Damaged property

In view of the incidence of stalking against health care professionals, providers should assist health care facilities in developing workplace violence policies that address stalking and its management. Forensic professionals prove invaluable in implementing these policies by working with the risk management department to create safety measures to minimize stalking incidents and to intervene should one occur.

E. Parenting Tips

The following are modified from the University of North Alabama (2015) for parents of stalking victims:

a.   Learn about stalking and its consequences.

b.   Encourage your child and do not disbelieve what your child tells you; stalking is hard to prove, and your child may vocalize self-doubt or a loss of a sense of reality.

c.   Obtain pictures and other information about the stalker from your child so that you can warn your child and help keep track of the stalker's behavior.

d.   Screen all visitors and calls for the victim.

e.   Do not provide your child's personal information unless necessary.

f.   Do not confront the stalker; this can be more dangerous than helpful.

g.   Be cautious of your own safety, as well as that of other family members and pets.

h.   Talk to the parents of your child's friends so that they are mindful of your child's safety, as well as their own.

Resources

Penn State Resources for Stalking Victims: http://studentaffairs.psu.edu/womenscenter/awareness/stalking.shtml

Stalking: A Handbook for Victims: www.victimsofcrime.org/docs/src/stalking-a-handbook-for-victims.pdf?sfvrsn=2

Stalking Incident and Behavior Log: www.victimsofcrime.org/docs/src/stalking-incident-log_pdf.pdf?sfvrsn=4

Stalking Laws: www.victimsofcrime.org/our-programs/stalking-resource-center/stalking-laws

Stalking Resource Center National Center for Victims of Crime: www.ncvc.org/src

References

Churcher, F., & Nesca. (2013). Risk factors for violence in stalking perpetration: A meta-analysis. *FWU Journal of Social Sciences, 7*(2), 100–112.

Garcia, M. (2008, December 11–13). *Stalking and teens.* 11th National Indian Nations Conference: Justice for Victims of Crime Strengthening the Heartbeat of All Our Relations. Retrieved from www.tribal-institute.org/2008/Handouts%20for%20Conferece/PowerPoints/E7_TeensAndStalking.pdf

Knoll, J., & Resnick, P. (2007). Stalking intervention: Know the 5 stalker types, safety strategies for victims. *Current Psychiatry, 6*(5), 31–38.

McCann, J. (2003). Stalking and obsessional forms of harassment in children and adolescents. *Psychiatric Annals, 33*(10), 637–640.

Mohandie, K., Meloy, J. R., McGowan, M. G., & Williams, J. (2006). The RECON typology of stalking: Reliability and validity based upon a large sample of North American stalkers. *Journal of Forensic Sciences, 51,* 147–155.

Mullen, P. (2003). Multiple classifications of stalkers and stalking behavior available to clinicians. *Psychiatric Annals, 33,* 650–658.

National Centers for Victims of Crime. (2012). *Stalking Resource Center.* Retreived from http://victimsofcrime.org/our-programs/stalking-resource-center

National Centers for Victims of Crime. (n.d.). *Bulletins for teens: Stalking.* Retrieved from www.victimsofcrime.org/help-for-crime-victims/get-help-bulletins-for-crime-victims/bulletins-for-teens/stalking

Post, M., Haymes, L., Storey, K., Loughrey, T., & Campbell, C. (2014). Understanding stalking behaviors by individuals with autism spectrum disorders and recommended prevention strategies for school settings. *Journal of Autism and Developmental Disorders, 44*(11), 2698-706. doi: 10.1007/s10803-012-1712-8.

University of North Alabama. (2015). Stalking: Safety and resistance. Retrieved from www.una.edu/assault/stalking-safety-and-resistance.html

CHAPTER 25

Status Offense Behaviors

A. Description

Status offenses are those acts considered criminal only when committed by a juvenile. These acts include truancy, running away from home, underage drinking, disobeying parents, and even purchasing tobacco products. Although some states have decriminalized some of these behaviors, other jurisdictions still consider status offenses delinquent acts. In states where these acts have been decriminalized, juveniles can be classified as dependent children (i.e., children dependent on the court for safeguarding), giving child protective services the primary responsibility for responding to this population. This may seem immaterial to health care, but status offenses are anything but irrelevant, and should be of significance to primary care providers who work with children and adolescents because status offense behaviors can lead to more serious offending and continuous psychosocial consequences.

a.   The juvenile court's formal status offense caseload increased 6% between 1995 and 2010. In 2010, juvenile courts formally processed an estimated 137,000 status offense cases, which accounted for about 16% of the court's formal delinquency and status offense caseload that year. These included: 14,800 runaway cases, 49,100 truancy cases, 14,200 curfew cases, 16,100 ungovernability cases, 30,100 status liquor law violation cases, and 12,600 other status offense cases, such as smoking tobacco and violations of a valid court order.

b.   Status offense cases tend to be referred to the courts less frequently than delinquency cases. However, females make up a disproportionate number of status offense charges. While females were charged in only 28% of the delinquency cases formally processed in 2010, they were involved in 43% of status offense cases (Sickmund & Puzzanchera, 2014). With the exception of prostitution, running away is the only instance in which the percentage of female juvenile offenders outnumbers that of males (Kendall, 2007).

c.   States vary in how they respond to adolescent noncriminal behavior. Some require alleged offenders and their families to receive precourt treatment and diversion services to improve family functioning and avoid court involvement; others do not provide precourt interventions. Some place youth in secure facilities regardless of circumstances, and others use the court's contempt powers to confine them (Kendall, 2007). Youth were adjudicated in 56% of the formally processed status offense cases in 2010, with 8% of these youth placed out of the home; 53% received formal probation, and 39% (chiefly curfew violations) resulted in other sanctions, such as fines, community service, restitution, or referrals to other agencies for services (Sickmund & Puzzanchera, 2014). Terminology also varies per jurisdiction, and many states do not use the term status offense. For example, New York state uses the designation of Person in Need of Supervision (PINS) for children under age 18 who do not attend school; behave in a way that is out of control or dangerous; or disobey their parents, guardians, or authorities (New York City Family Court, 2014). Other terms include: Undisciplined Juvenile, Unruly Child, Dependent Child, Incorrigible Child, Ward of the Court, Child (or Family) in Need of Services, and Minor Requiring Authoritative Intervention (Coalition for Juvenile Justice/SOS Project, n.d.).

d.   The placement of youth who commit status offenses in locked detention facilities jeopardizes their safety and well-being and may increase the likelihood of their committing delinquent or later adult criminal behavior. Removing them from their families and communities prevents them from developing the strong social networks and support systems needed to successfully transition to adulthood.

e.   The National Standards for the Care of Youth Charged with Status Offenses (www.juvjustice.org) aims to promote practices based on research and social service approaches to better engage and support youth and families in need of assistance. The Standards call for prohibition of the detention of status offenders and divergence from the delinquency system by promoting the most appropriate services for families and the least restrictive placement options for status offending youth. The Standards also promote uniform policy and practice across states and high-quality, equitable services and representation for status offending youth and their families.

f.   The more common petitioned (formally handled cases) status offenses include:

- Curfew violation: A curfew violation is committed when a juvenile is in a public place after a specified time. Towns pass curfews to get potential troublemakers and potential victims off the streets at night. Although curfews are generally supported by the public, they have not been shown to be effective in decreasing juvenile crime and victimization.

- Underage drinking: U.S. federal law essentially established 21 as the national minimum drinking age. The rationales for prohibiting minors from using alcohol are considerable: According to statistics compiled by the National Institute on Alcohol Abuse and Alcoholism (n.d.), 4,358 young people under the age of 21 die as a result of alcohol-related accidents, homicides, and suicides. Alcohol results in youths making poor decisions that can result in risky behavior including drinking and driving, violence, and sexual activity.

- Truancy: Truancy is a defined period of school absenteeism. Chronic absenteeism can lead to poor school performance, dropout, expulsion, substance abuse, and delinquency and crime. It can also result in youth being less likely to be employed 6 months after schooling, which impacts their lifetime earning ability (Vaughn, Mayndar, Salas-Wright, Perron & Abdon, 2013).

- Disobedience: Disobeying parents (also known as incorrigibility, ungovernability, unruliness, and being beyond the control of one's parents): According to Benton et al. (2010), incorrigible behaviors range from a child refusing to consistently follow a parent-imposed curfew or physically abusing a parent. Most of these cases involve dysfunctional family dynamics that may feel unmanageable to the petitioner, who is usually the parent. The petitioner may request removing the child from the home to have a break from the behavior, or they may hope that additional threats or punishment will cause their child to be "scared straight."

- Running away from home: Fortunately, several states define a runaway youth as one who has been neglected. However, some states still consider this a status offense. Runaway youth are vulnerable to numerous negative experiences including victimization and exploitation. They can become homeless and engage in substance abuse and delinquent behaviors. Risk factors for running away include being female, neighborhood victimization, personal victimization, school suspension, and delinquency (Tyler & Bersani, 2008).

B. Assessment

a.   Risk factors: Developmentally, adolescence is a time of emotional upheaval and risk-taking behavior. While redefining their self-concepts, they may experiment with illegal behaviors including underage drinking, driving while intoxicated (or texting while driving), and vandalism. However, Bartol and Bartol (2012) note that normal development can be adversely affected by a number of risk factors that place the adolescent at increased risk for status—and more serious behaviors:

- Poverty
- Chronic illness
- Negative peers or peer rejection
- School failure and/or lack of parental involvement in school
- Neglecting parental style
- Poor parental monitoring
- Family dysfunction
- Close relationship with older siblings who engage in criminal behavior

- Parental psychopathology (depression, alcoholism, and aggression [especially parental intimate partner violence])
- Lack of attachment
- Lack of empathy
- Cognitive and language deficiencies
- Psychiatric disorders in the youth (untreated attention deficit hyperactivity disorder [ADHD], conduct disorder, oppositional defiant disorder, mood disorders [depression and bipolar disorder], borderline personality disorder, and substance abuse)
- Sexual abuse of the youth

b. Conduct a psychosocial assessment that includes a history of:

- Interactions with parents/guardians and authority figures
- School attendance
- Activities, including the times that the youth comes home at night (school nights, non-school nights, and special occasion nights)
- Substance use

c. Ask at-risk youths if they ever thought of running away from home. If so, ask about their plan and reason for thinking about running away.

C. Diagnosis

While one incident of status offense behavior may not be indicative of an underlying problem, multiple incidents may indicate that the youth is experiencing mental illness or family dysfunction, including child abuse and neglect. Truant and runaway youth may also be experiencing teen pregnancy or parenthood, home and/or community violence, school problems, and substance abuse.

D. Levels of Prevention/Intervention

a. Primary

While there are no specific interventions, health care providers can encourage positive parenting skills, especially parents becoming active in their child's schooling, to minimize the risk of status offending behaviors.

b. Secondary

Since status offenses can act as the gateway to more serious offending and many of these youth come from dysfunctional families, primary care providers are instrumental in identifying youth at risk for committing status offenses.

c. Tertiary

- Most interventions are already familiar to primary care providers. Youth with other risk factors, and those who have committed status offenses, warrant proper referrals that may include psychiatric evaluation and counseling, substance abuse treatment, educational support, and family therapy.

- The parents or guardians may have been the ones who turned their child in, especially in cases of runway and ungovernability, so, although family engagement is critical, it can be challenging. One strategy is family group decision making (FGDM), which recognizes the importance of having the family lead the decision making and actively participate in viable solutions. Assessment of family needs and strengths will identify: the current level of family functioning; youth, family, and community strengths; risks related to the youth's offending behavior; current risk for re-offense status; safety issues; and services needed.

- Those who have been victimized by sexual and other abuse should be treated as victims, and may require forensic evaluation and further intervention from law enforcement.

- Recommend that the parents obtain legal counsel (attorney) for their child to ensure that the child receives due process.

E. Parenting Tips

Primary care providers can encourage family members to stay actively involved in the youth's treatment. Also foster their participation in parenting classes, and family therapy and support groups.

Resources

American Humane Association Guidelines for Family Group Decision Making in Child Welfare: www.americanhumane.org/assets/pdfs/children/fgdm/guidelines.pdf

Juvenile Status Offenses Fact Sheet: http://act4jj.org/sites/default/files/ckfinder/files/factsheet_17.pdf

Pennsylvania Family Group Decision Making Toolkit: A Resource Guide and Support Best Practice Implementation: http://pacwcbt.pitt.edu/Organizational%20Effectiveness/FGDM%20Evaluation%20 PDFs/FGDM%20Toolkit.pdf

Right to Counsel in Status Offense Cases: www.americanbar.org/content/dam/aba/migrated/child/ PublicDocuments/right_to_counsel_factsheet.authcheckdam.pdf

University of Colorado National Center on Family Group Decision Making: www.ucdenver.edu/ academics/colleges/medicalschool/departments/pediatrics/subs/can/FGDM/Pages/FGDM.aspx

References

Bartol, C., & Bartol, A. (2012). *Criminal behavior: A psychological approach*. Boston, MA: Prentice Hall.

Benton, H., Bilchik, S., Heyd, J., Pinheiro, E., Shubik, C., Smith, T., . . . Tulman, J. (2010). *Representing juvenile status offenders*. American Bar Association. Retrieved from www.abanet.org/child/rjso_final.pdf

Coalition for Juvenile Justice/SOS Project. (n.d.). *Status offenses: A national survey*. Author. Retrieved from www.americanbar.org/content/dam/aba/events/aba-day/StatusOffensesANationalSurveyWEB.authcheckdam.pdf

Kendall, J. (2007). *Juvenile status offenses: Treatment and early intervention* (Technical Assistance Bulletin No. 29). Chicago, IL: American Bar Association Division for Public Education. Retrieved from www.americanbar.org/content/dam/aba/migrated/publiced/tab29.authcheckdam.pdf

National Institute on Alcohol Abuse and Alcoholism. (n.d.). *Underage drinking*. Retrieved from http://niaaa.nih.gov/alcohol-health/special-populations-co-occurring-disorders/underage-drinking

New York City Family Court. (2014). *Persons in Need of Supervision (PINS)*. New York State Unified Court System. Retrieved from www.nycourts.gov/courts/nyc/family/faqs_pins.shtml

Sickmund, M., & Puzzanchera, C. (Eds.). (2014). *Juvenile offenders and victims: 2014 national report*. Pittsburgh, PA: National Center for Juvenile Justice. Retrieved from www.ojjdp.gov/ojstatbb/nr2014/downloads/NR2014.pdf

Tyler, K., & Bersani, B. (2008). A longitudinal study of early adolescent precursors to running away. *The Journal of Early Adolescence, 28*(2), 230–251. doi:10.1177/0272431607313592

Vaughn, M., Mayndar, B., Salas-Wright, C., Perron, B., & Abdon, A. (2013). Prevalence and correlates of truancy in the U.S.: Results from a national sample. *Journal of Adolescence, 36*, 767–776.

CHAPTER 26

Substance Abuse

A. Description

Substance abuse and dependence are among the most prevalent disorders diagnosed in the United States. The prevalence rates of substance abuse are difficult to determine because of the secrecy and illegality of the behaviors associated with the use of illicit substances. *Substance abuse* is the excessive use of a substance that persists despite negative consequences that include being arrested for driving under the influence, poor work performance, and marital problems. *Substance dependence* indicates the presence of problems such as tolerance (increased amounts of the substance are needed to produce a desired effect), withdrawal (physiological symptoms develop when substance use is discontinued abruptly), and giving up pleasurable or important activities because of substances. In substance dependence, the substance dominates the user's life. While there is a difference in terminology, the term substance abuse will be used here to stand for both problems. The *Diagnostic and Statistical Manual of Mental Disorders, 5th Edition (DSM-5)*, published by the American Psychiatric Association (APA, 2013) combined abuse and dependence into one disorder.

a. There are five scientific categories of substances:

- Depressants include alcohol, sedatives, hypnotics, and anxiolytics, and result in behavioral sedation. They are used to induce relaxation in the individual.

- Stimulants result in mood elevations and cause the individual to become more alert and active. These include amphetamines, cocaine, nicotine, and caffeine.

- Opioids produce analgesic effects, as well as euphoria.

- Hallucinogens change the sensory perceptions of the user and can result in delusions, paranoia, and hallucinations. Substances in this class are cannabis and other hallucinogens.

- Other drugs of abuse are those that do not fit neatly into one of the previous categories, including inhalants, steroids, designer drugs, and some over-the-counter medications. These substances produce a wide variety of effects on the brain and body that may span more than one of the previously discussed classes.

b.   Most youths limit their experimentation to tobacco, alcohol, and marijuana, but a small number try other drugs. The majority of adolescents who use drugs and alcohol will, when they assume adult roles and responsibilities, spontaneously quit using drugs and develop controlled patterns of alcohol use. However, some will be seriously affected by substance abuse and its associated consequences, including addiction, withdrawal, school failure, diseases such as HIV/AIDS, unwanted and unprotected sex, motor vehicle accidents, violence, and suicide. The younger a child is when using drugs, the more likely he or she is to develop a drug problem, and more than 90% of people with substance addiction began using substances before age 18 (National Center on Addiction and Substance Abuse at Columbia University [CASA], n.d.).

c.   Drugs, including alcohol, depress the cerebral cortex of the brain (a still-immature intellectual and reasoning center in teens) and release inhibitions in the limbic system, the center of pleasure, anger, and other emotions. The limbic system craves instant and constant gratification and contributes to the teen's sense of boredom. Thus, some adolescents go to extremes in seeking alcohol, hard drugs, and aggressive outlets.

d.   Nicotine is a drug; thus cigarettes, cigars, smokeless tobacco, e-cigarettes, hookahs, and other forms of nicotine use should be considered substance use/abuse in youth.

e.   New drugs, such as designer drugs and newer herbs, make their appearance regularly, and thus health care providers need to keep current.

f.   The increase in heroin use and overdose deaths has warranted Food and Drug Administration (FDA) approval of intranasal naloxone hydrochloride (Narcan), to reverse opioid overdose. The nasal form allows for easier use by first responders and others, and also eliminates the threat of contaminated needle sticks. The product can be used for both children and adults, and can be repeated, if needed. Recipients still require additional emergency treatment (Brown, 2015).

g.   Anabolic steroids are used by teens and adults interested in body building because they believe that these drugs contribute to body weight and muscle strength. They want to run faster, jump higher, hit farther, lift heavier weights, or have more endurance. The drugs are taken orally or by injection, usually in cycles of weeks or months (cycling), rather than continuously. Users typically take different types of steroids to maximize their effectiveness and minimize the side effects (stacking). Steroid abuse can cause serious side effects, including hair loss, jaundice (yellowing of the skin), severe acne, fluid retention, high blood pressure, increased LDL (bad cholesterol) and decreased HDL (good cholesterol), trembling, heart enlargement, heart attacks, strokes, kidney tumors, and liver tumors or cancer. Other side effects are gender or age related:

Males: baldness, breast enlargement, withering testicles, sterility, impotence, and an increased risk for prostate cancer. Females: facial hair growth, male-pattern baldness, deepened voice, breast shrinkage, clitoral enlargement, and changes in or cessation of the menstrual cycle. Teenagers: Premature halting of growth through early skeletal maturation and accelerated puberty. Thus, teens risk being short for life if they take anabolic steroids prior to their growth spurt. Youths who inject steroids also run the risk of contracting and transmitting hepatitis and HIV/AIDS. Aggression and other psychiatric side effects can develop. Psychological effects include depression and the occurrence of very aggressive behavior labeled "roid rage," which affects both sexes. Many users also suffer from paranoid jealousy, extreme irritability, delusions, and impaired judgment stemming from feelings of invincibility. Other users turn to other drugs to alleviate the negative effects of steroids, including opioids to counteract irritability and insomnia.

h. According to CASA (2003), girls use cigarettes, alcohol, and other drugs for reasons different than boys, and they are more vulnerable to substance abuse, addiction, and the consequences that come with these problems. The risks and consequences of smoking, alcohol, and other drug use identified by CASA are:

- Girls who experience early puberty have a higher risk of using substances more frequently and in greater quantities than later maturing peers.
- Girls are more likely to be sexually abused and to have eating disorders and depression than boys, and all of these factors put them at higher risk for substance abuse.
- Girls become addicted quicker than boys.
- Girls who use alcohol and other drugs are more likely to commit suicide than those who do not use substances.
- Girls are more likely to experience adverse health effects (greater lung damage from cigarettes, higher likelihood of getting alcohol-induced brain, heart, and liver damage).
- Girls are more likely to abuse prescription medications than boys.
- Transition times—from elementary to middle school, from middle school to high school, and from high school to college—mark times of increased substance abuse risk for girls.
- Girls are more likely to be offered substances from other girls or a boyfriend and in private settings, whereas boys are more likely to be offered substances from other boys, a parent, or a stranger and in public settings.

- Religion provides more protection for girls than boys.
- Girls who drink coffee are more likely to smoke and drink, and to do so at earlier ages.

i.   Alcohol abuse, particularly binge drinking, has become an increasing problem on college campuses, with consequences rising in destructiveness and cost. These consequences can affect virtually all college students, whether they drink or not: death from alcohol-related injuries; assault; sexual abuse; unsafe sex; unintentional injuries while under the influence; academic problems; alcohol-related health problems; property damage; arrest; and suicide. The first 6 weeks of freshman year are particularly vulnerable for heavy drinking and its consequences because of academic and social pressures (National Institute on Alcohol Abuse and Alcoholism, 2015).

B. Assessment (History, Physical, Diagnostic Screening/Testing, Where Appropriate)

a.   Risk factors: Adolescents use and abuse drugs for a number of reasons, including curiosity, peer pressure, need for acceptance, imitation of family members, rebellion, escape, unhappy home life, feelings of alienation, and attempts at sophistication. No single factor determines who will use drugs and who will not, but there are some predictors: poor school performance, aggressive and rebellious behaviors, excessive influence by peers, lack of parental support and guidance, substance-abusing family members or friends, and behavior problems at an early age.

b.   Crocker (2015) notes that drug and alcohol screening is frequently overlooked in the primary care setting, and that when it does occur, providers rarely use evidence-based tools, thus missing the opportunity for these adolescents to receive appropriate care. The American Academy of Pediatrics Committee on Substance Abuse (2011) recommends routine screening for alcohol and drug abuse for all adolescents.

c.   The following suggest substance abuse; however, some may indicate a behavioral or psychological problem other than drug use.

- Demonstrates changes in personality, especially if sudden: lack of empathy, less affectionate, apathetic, withdrawn, sullen, less attentive, depressed, irritable, uncooperative, unpredictable, easily provoked, hostile.
- Becomes irresponsible. Forgets important occasions, does not do chores or homework, frequently late for school.
- Exhibits secretive behaviors about personal possessions such as dresser drawers, pocketbook, or backpack.

- Develops loss of interest in usual hobbies or activities. No longer participates in family activities, school or church functions, sports, or organizational activities.

- Changes personal appearance; becomes deteriorated or imitates drug-related music stars. Dresses in tee-shirts, belt buckles, jewelry, or other apparel with drug logos, or has magazines or bumper stickers with drug logos.

- Changes vocabulary or music tastes to resemble drug culture.

- Has irregular school attendance and/or decreased school performance without a valid reason. Claims that school performance is poor because of boredom, not caring about school, or disliking his or her teacher. Be suspicious if the child is unconcerned that his or her grades drop dramatically.

- Becomes difficult to communicate with; refuses to talk about friends, school, or activities. Changes conversations to talk about adult bad habits, and/or defends rights of youths and/or use of drugs.

- Changes friends, and new friends are unkempt and/or abrasive. Secretive about friends.

- Behaves irrationally, drives recklessly, and has explosive rage episodes.

- Engages in rebellious behavior; shows disrespect for authority, lies persistently; demonstrates antisocial behaviors without remorse.

- Cannot or will not account for where all their money goes.

- Finding that household money is missing; credit cards, checks, jewelry, heirlooms, and other items of value.

- Finding drug paraphernalia: whiskey/beer bottles, marijuana plants or seeds, rolling papers, clips, hemostats, pipes (homemade pipes can even be made out of a glass jar with some aluminum foil on top), drug buttons, mirrors, small medicine bottles, eye droppers, butane lighters, and razor blades.

- Shows physical signs: pale face, red eyes, dilated pupils; chews heavily scented gum; uses heavy cologne, aftershave, or perfumes; hypersensitive to touch, taste, or smell; weight loss alone or despite increased appetite.

- Shows mental signs: disordered or illogical thinking, decreased ability to remember things, severe lack of motivation, rapid thought pattern.

d.   Use evidence-based screening tools:

- The CRAFFT screen (www.ceasar-boston.org/CRAFFT/index.php) has been the instrument with the best evidence for use in primary care. It consists of sex questions, can be used effectively in children under age 21, and is recommended by the American Academy of Pediatrics Committee on Substance Abuse.

- The Adolescent Screening, Brief Intervention, Referral for Treatment (SBIRT; massclearinghouse.ehs.state.ma.us/BSASPRO/SA3542.html) tool, which was developed at Boston Children's Hospital, informs brief interventions with teens and their families. The tool obtains usage information for tobacco, alcohol, marijuana, prescription drugs not prescribed for youth, illegal drugs such as cocaine or Ecstasy, inhalants such as nitrous oxide, and herbs or synthetic drugs including salvia, K2, and bath salts, with the following scale: never, once or twice, monthly, and weekly or more.

e.   Assess for comorbid mental health disorders.

f.   Assess for signs of chronic substance abuse, including hypertension; poor hygiene; weight loss; needle marks; nasal irritation/excoriation; arrhythmias; gynecomastia; testicular atrophy.

g.   Assess for physical consequences of substance abuse, such as sexually transmitted infections, including HIV/AIDS, pregnancy, signs of unintentional and intentional injuries, brain damage, and effects of anabolic steroids as noted earlier.

C. Diagnosis

a.   The *DSM-5* (APA, 2013) combined abuse and dependence into one disorder that utilizes a continuum from mild to severe. Specific alcohol- or drug-related disorders are each addressed as separate entities, but require a pattern of substantial impairment or distress within a 12-month period. This impairment or distress may result in health problems, disability, and failure to meet home, school, or work responsibilities. The most common substance abuse disorders in the United States are alcohol use disorder, tobacco use disorder, cannabis use disorder, stimulant use disorder, hallucinogen use disorder, and opioid use disorder (Substance Abuse and Mental Health Services Administration, 2015).

b.   Substance abuse is associated with a number of other psychiatric disorders, including depression, bipolar disorder, eating disorders, attention deficit hyperactivity disorder (ADHD), and conduct disorder, sometimes in an attempt to self-medicate the underlying disorder.

D. Levels of Prevention/Intervention

Prevention/interventions are from the American Academy of Pediatrics substance abuse policy (American Academy of Pediatrics Committee on Substance Abuse, 2011). Brief alcohol interventions are efficacious in improving alcohol consumption issues in low-severity alcohol problems, but there is a lack of evidence that they have any efficacy in increasing the receipt of alcohol-related services (Glass et al., 2015).

a. Primary

- Abstinence, the time before the youth has ever used substances beyond more than a few sips of alcohol, is the time for primary prevention.
- These adolescents report no use and answer "no" to the CRAFFT car question, or "never" (green) on the SBIRT.
- Promote the prevention or delayed initiation of substance use through parent and child education and positive reinforcement.
- Praise and encouragement for making healthy choices and smart decisions are important and can delay the initiation of substance use.
- Include guidance regarding avoidance of riding in a vehicle whose driver has been drinking or using drugs.

b. Secondary

- Secondary prevention is aimed at at-risk youth and those who are at the level of experimentation or limited use, and who scored negative on the CRAFFT (0–1) or "once or twice" on the SBIRT.
- Experimentation is the stage when substances are used for the first and second time because the youth wants to know what the drug effects or intoxication feels like, while limited use is when youths are using substances with one or more friends in relatively low-risk situations, usually on weekends, and without any related problems.
- Promote client strengths, and encourage cessation through education and counseling.

c. Tertiary

Tertiary prevention aims at youth in the categories of problematic use, abuse, or addition. These youth score 2 or more on the CRAFFT and monthly or more on the SBIRT.

- Youths who engage in problematic use are those who use substances in high-risk situations, including babysitting and driving; whose use results in problems such as fighting, school suspension, or arrest; or whose use is for emotional regulation. These clients warrant a specific change plan, complete with a change plan worksheet and brief intervention (outcome-responsive discussion) to enhance motivation for behavioral change, as well as close follow-up and consideration of breaking confidentiality. Address the accompanying issues, such as driving under the influence (see Chapter 10), and consider using the Contract for Life developed by Students Against Destructive Decisions (SADD; www.sadd.org).
- Youth who abuse substances are those whose drug use is connected to recurrent problems or for whom substance abuse interferes with their functioning, as per the *DSM-5*. Treatment continues for these youths, as it does for those

with problematic use, with exploration of ambivalence and triggering. Youth should be monitored closely for progression to addiction, and confidentiality breaching is again considered.

- Addiction is loss of control or compulsive drug use, as defined in the *DSM-5*. Treatment continues with enhanced motivation to accept referral to subspecialty treatment, if necessary. Specialized treatment options are:

  - Group therapy is a pillar of treatment for adolescents with substance use disorders. It is cost-effective and involves congregating with peers; however, group therapy has not been extensively evaluated as a therapeutic modality for adolescents.

  - Family-directed therapies are the best validated methods for treating adolescent substance abuse. Family therapy targets family conflict, communication, parental monitoring, discipline, child abuse/neglect, and parental substance use disorders.

  - Intensive outpatient programs (IOPs) are an intermediate level for youth whose needs are between outpatient treatment and inpatient services. They allow youth to continue with their daily routine and practice their new recovery skills both at home and at school, using a combination of supportive group therapy, educational groups, family therapy, individual therapy, relapse prevention and life skills, 12-step recovery, case management, and aftercare planning.

  - Partial hospital is a short-term outpatient program affiliated with a hospital designed to treat substance use disorders. The services are structured throughout the entire day and offer medical monitoring in addition to individual and group therapy.

  - Detoxification centers manage the medical care of symptoms of withdrawal. Medically supervised detoxification is indicated for any adolescent who is at risk of withdrawing from alcohol or benzodiazepines and might also be helpful for adolescents withdrawing from opioids, cocaine, or other substances. Detoxification is a first step, not definitive treatment, and clients are discharged from outpatient or residential substance abuse treatment programs.

  - Acute residential treatment, which typically targets adolescents with comorbidities, is a short-term placement designed to stabilize patients in crisis, usually before beginning longer-term residential treatment program.

  - Residential treatment programs are highly structured live-in environments that provide therapy for those with severe substance abuse, mental illness, or behavioral problems that require 24-hour care. These are short-term, and the youth is released to another outpatient facility or other form of care.

- Address comorbidities and psychosocial issues (such as family dysfunction, association with substance abusing peers). Problem persistence can trigger relapse of substance abuse.

E. Parenting Tips (Muscari, 2004)

a.   Drug Proof Your Child

No one is immune to alcohol and drug problems. You may be the best parent in the world with the world's greatest kid. But circumstances can put your child in the wrong place at the wrong time. You are your child's most important source of information when it comes to drugs and alcohol. To prevent your child from abusing alcohol and drugs, start at an early age, and continue open communication throughout his or her development.

- Get the facts. You need to know about drugs and alcohol so that you can provide your child with correct and current information. Know what is out there, and know their effects on the body. Get familiar with the street names of drugs and drug using. Know what drugs look like. Learn the signs of alcohol and drug use, and know how to get help if you suspect that your child is using drugs.

- Set family standards and rules on drug and alcohol use. Be specific. Explain the rules, what behavior is expected, and what the consequences will be if your child breaks them. Be consistent; keep the rules the same at all times—at home, in school, at friends' houses, anywhere he or she goes. Be reasonable; "the punishment should fit the crime" if rules are broken. Make sure to state the rules early in grade school, and repeat them often.

- Set an example. Actions speak louder than words, and you will not be too effective telling him or her not to use tobacco and alcohol when you sit there with a cigarette in one hand and a beer in the other. Follow your own rules, and demonstrate your attitude toward drugs and alcohol. Do not use illicit drugs. Use prescription drugs and other pharmaceuticals properly. Avoid alcohol, but if you do drink, drink responsibly.

- Let your child know that there are consequences for breaking the rules, and be sure to set up and clarify the consequences before rules are broken.

- Foster his or her self-esteem. Strong self-esteem minimizes the chances of your child abusing substances. Help your child to set realistic goals for his or her academic, athletic, social, and other activities. Praise your child when he or she does well, and get excited about the things your child cares about.

- Do things as a family. Have family meetings to discuss important family issues, and let your child have a say. Discuss responsibilities, the child's and yours. Make your home a happy, safe, positive place.

- Keep the lines of communication open, and create a warm, caring environment that tells your child you are available whenever your child has questions or wants to talk about his or her feelings. Make time every day to talk to your children about their lives, how their day went, their feelings, and what they think. Talk to them about the future. Make sure to listen and show them that you care.

- Be nosey. Get to know their friends. Ask questions. Know where they are, who they are with, and what they are doing. Make sure they know that you ask questions because you love them, not because you do not trust them. Limit the time they spend without adult supervision, and realize that the hours between 4 and 6 p.m. are the most dangerous times for them to be on their own. Peer pressure and boredom can too easily lead to an after-school drug habit.

- Get involved. Know what your child learns in school about drugs and alcohol. If they have an antidrug program, join it. Know your neighborhood. Different communities have different trends in drug use.

b.   Talk to your child about drugs and alcohol. Be open and straightforward. Remember that more than half of all children try alcohol by the time they reach the eighth grade. Start your discussions early.

- Under 4 years old: Attitudes and habits that form during the preschool years may greatly influence your child later on. Little ones may not understand statistics, but they can develop the baseline for the problem-solving and decision-making skills they will have when they get older.

  - Allow your child to make small decisions, such as what he or she wants to wear. Do not worry if those choices do not match; just let your child know that he or she is able to make good decisions.

  - Encourage your child to help around the house as best he or she can, and express your appreciation for the help your child provides.

  - Be careful about the messages you send. Do not ask your child to get you a beer and then praise him or her for it. You do not want them to associate drinking with praise.

- 4 to 6 years old: At this age your child still thinks and learns primarily from experience, and does not understand things that will happen in the future. Focus on the present and people and places he or she knows.

  - Talk to your child about how he or she has to take medicine when ill because the doctor said so, and therefore, your child should take only the medicine that the doctor prescribes.

  - Instruct your child to refuse offers of candy from a stranger and to tell you or another adult he or she trusts about it. Role-play scenarios with you being the stranger to allow your child to practice this skill.

  - Watch for teachable moments, such as when you both see someone smoking or drinking on television. Bring up the topic about these chemicals, and that they can harm the child's body.

- 6 to 9 years old: Your child loves school and the new opportunities that it provides. He or she loves to learn, but still learns by experiences and still lives in the present. Keep discussions in the here and now.

  - Your child will be interested in how his or her body works, so discuss ways to maintain good health (brushing teeth, washing hands before eating, and eating nutritious food) and to avoid things that may be harmful (smoking, drugs, drinking to excess).

  - Adults are important role models, and your child is generally trusting, believing that all decisions adults make for him or her are right. Talk to them about the adults your child can trust. Create a file of people your child can rely on with their phone numbers: relatives, family friends, neighbors, teachers, religious leaders, the police, and the fire department. Remind your child not to talk to strangers.

  - Discuss how advertisers try to persuade children to buy their products, such as toys and candy bars. This will prepare your child to face the advertising pressures for tobacco and alcohol when he or she gets older.

  - Talk about the differences between medicine and illicit drugs. Medicine helps one to get better, illicit drugs make one sick. However, your child should also know that medicines are drugs that can be harmful if misused.

  - Ask whether your child knows anyone in school who smokes or uses alcohol or other drugs. Launch into a basic discussion of the effects of these products, especially tobacco, inhalants, and alcohol. Talk about incidents in the news. For example, in Media, Pennsylvania, five girls were killed when their car plowed off the road into a utility pole. The girls had been huffing a commercial spray duster used for cleaning keyboards. When tragic events like this happen, use them to start a discussion with your child.

- Practice ways for your child to say no. Describe simple situations that would make him or her uncomfortable, such as eating live worms. Practice the following steps to make it easier for your child to turn down an offer of alcohol or drugs. Tell your child to:

  - Ask questions when something is offered. "What is it, and where did you get it?"

  - Say no—no arguments or discussions. Say no, and show them that you mean it.

  - Give a reason if the person persists. The old "My parents would kill me if I did" line still works today.

  - Suggest other things to do when a friend offers alcohol or drugs. Propose going to the movies, working on a project, going to the mall,

> playing a game or sport. This way your child rejects the drugs, not the friend.
>
> – When all else fails, leave. Get out of the situation. Go home. Go to school. Join a group of friends, or talk to someone else.

- 10 to 12 years old: Even more energy goes into learning at this age. Your child loves to learn facts, especially weird ones, and wants to know how things work and what sources of information are available. Friends become very important, and your child's interests will be greatly influenced by what his or her peer group thinks. A child's self-image is partly determined by the extent to which he or she is accepted by friends. Because of this, if your child is a follower, he or she may be unable to make independent decisions and choices. Keep him or her out of the follower position by teaching decision-making skills.

Preadolescence is the most important time to focus on drug and alcohol prevention. Crucial decisions about drugs and alcohol crop up at this age. Your child is at the greatest risk of starting to smoke in the sixth or seventh grade, and research shows that the earlier children start to use alcohol or drugs, the more likely they are to have a real problem.

- Give your child a clear no-use message, factual information, and strong motivation to resist the pressures to use drugs and alcohol. Provide the following information:
  - How to identify specific drugs, including alcohol, tobacco, inhalants, marijuana, and cocaine, all in their various forms.
  - The short- and long-term effects of substances and the consequences of their use, including criminal prosecution since drugs are illegal, as is drinking alcohol under the age of 21.
  - The effects of drugs on the growing body.
  - The effects of drug and alcohol abuse on the family and society.
- Encourage your child to participate in positive activities. Limit "free-time," which often leads to experimentation with alcohol and other drugs.
- Discuss the advertising pressures of drugs and alcohol, not forgetting TV shows and song lyrics that glorify their use. Separate the myths from the realities.
- Continue to practice ways of saying no. Sixth graders are offered cigarettes and beer, and most of them know other children who smoke and drink.
- Encourage your child to join a school or local antidrug group, or peer assistance group that encourages drug-free activities.
- Scan the newspaper or news with your child, and discuss drug-related crime. Talk about the influence it has on society and individuals.
- Get together with your child's friends' parents so that you can reinforce each other's efforts to teach good personal and social habits.

- 13 to 14 years old: Your young teen begins to deal with abstractions and the future. He or she understands that actions have consequences, and knows that his or her behaviors affect others. Your teen still has a shaky self-image that is strongly influenced by friends, causing self-doubt as to whether he or she is normal. Your teen is often in conflict with you, is not sure where he or she is heading, and tends to see himself or herself as "not okay." This rocky ground paves the way for experimentation. Young people who use drugs including alcohol typically begin during this age.

  - Emphasize the immediate effects of drug use, not what will happen over time. Instead of talking about lung cancer, tell him or her about bad breath, yellow teeth, and burned clothes.

  - Bring up the topic of steroids. You can start by discussing their use by professional sports players. Talk about their negative effects, and discuss body image issues.

  - Offset peer influence with parent influence. Reinforce your no-use rules. When counterattacked with "but everyone else does it," inform him or her that everyone does not do it. Emphasize how unpredictable drug use can be, that even though some users appear to function properly, drug use remains risky and that their effects may not always be readily apparent.

  - Make sure he or she knows the following:
    - The characteristics of specific drugs and drug interactions (such as the deadly effects of mixing sedatives and alcohol).
    - The effects of drugs on the cardiac, respiratory, nervous, and reproductive systems.
    - The stages of chemical dependency and how they vary from person to person.
    - The way drugs affect daily activities such as driving and sports participation.
    - Your family history, especially if alcoholism or drug addiction is a problem.

  - Monitor his or her whereabouts.

  - Role-play several variations on how to say no until you are confident your teen knows how.

  - Continue to allow your teen to discuss his or her fears and feelings.

  - Review and revise household rules on issues such as chores and curfews. Reinforce the rules on drugs and alcohol.

  - Plan supervised no-alcohol parties for your child in your home. Similar adult parties set good examples.

  - Discuss friendships, and emphasize that real friends do not ask each other to do things that are wrong or harmful.

- 14 to 17 years old: Peer influence remains strong, but your child develops an increasingly realistic understanding of adults, begins to develop a broader outlook on life, and becomes more interested in the welfare of others.

  - Focus on the long-term effects of alcohol and other drugs during these years. They can ruin your child's chance of getting into college, being hired for certain jobs, and being accepted into the military.

  - Remind your child that he or she serves as a role model for your younger children.

  - Minimize his or her unsupervised hours at home. Lunchtime and after school (3–6 p.m.) are times that teens are likely to experiment.

  - Encourage your child to volunteer to help out at a drug prevention program or a hotline call service, or to volunteer as a peer counselor.

  - Keep him or her busy with school, sports, clubs, volunteer work, religious activities, trips to museums and the library, film festivals, work, arts and crafts—anything constructive. Plan activities for vacation and holiday times. A busy routine will minimize your child's chances of getting bored and seeking an outlet in drugs.

  - Cooperate with other parents to keep get-togethers and parties drug- and alcohol-free.

  - Discuss drinking and driving. Chances are your child will drive or have friends who drive, and will know other kids who use alcohol and other drugs. Talk about the legal issues, and highlight the possibility of an accident where someone, including your child, may get killed.

  - Draw up a written contract on the conditions of using the car, and have him or her sign it. Promise to pick up your child, no questions asked, at any time when he or she or the person who is driving is under the influence. Promise not to scream or yell, and say that you will talk about it the next day.

  - Set consequences for substance use in your car—regardless of who it is, your child or his or her friends.

  - If your child is giving a party or going to a party, follow the suggestions of the American Academy of Pediatrics:

    - If your child is planning a party, let him or her plan the guest list activities, but go over them and ensure it is small, no more than 10 to 15 teens, and provide adult supervision without being intrusive. Set a time limit, restrict attendance to invited guests only, and do not allow people to leave the party and then return. Make rules—no tobacco, alcohol, or other drugs; lights on at all times; certain rooms are off limits—and stick to them. Realize that you are legally responsible for anything that happens to a minor who is served alcohol or other drugs at your home, and discuss this with your teen. If any teen arrives at the party intoxicated, call him or her or the parents to ensure the child returns home safe.

- If your child is going to a party, call the host's parents to verify they know about it. Ascertain that there will be no tobacco, alcohol, or other drugs at the party, and that a supervising adult will be present. Know where your child is going; have the phone number and address handy, and ask him or her to call you if the location changes. Make sure you let your child know where you will be during the party in case he or she needs to contact you. Be sure he or she has a way to get home. Tell your child you are available for a ride at any time, and *never* to ride with someone who has been drinking alcohol or using other drugs. Finally, make sure you greet your child on arrival home so you can check the time, note his or her sobriety level, and talk about the evening.

• 18 to 21 years old: At this point, your child should be thinking more like an adult and looking forward to a productive lifestyle. However, he or she still needs your direction. Continue to discourage drug use, and promote responsible attitudes toward alcohol. Your budding young adult can enjoy his or her leisure time without alcohol or drugs. Discuss the consequences of drugs and alcohol, especially binge drinking. Encourage responsible drinking for when your child reaches 21. Tell him or her to eat before drinking and never drink on an empty stomach; food slows alcohol absorption. Also advise your child to drink slowly, sip rather than gulp, and absolutely avoid binge drinking. Carbonated mixers are to be avoided because these drinks are more likely to be gulped, especially when one is thirsty. At parties, your child should drink nonalcoholic drinks or alternate alcoholic beverages with nonalcoholic ones. Most importantly, your child should know his or her limit.

Resources

Alcohol Screening and Brief Intervention for Youth: A Practitioner's Guide (CME/CE Program): www.medscape.org/viewarticle/806556

National Institute on Alcohol Abuse and Alcoholism: http://niaaa.nih.gov/

National Institute on Drug Abuse: www.drugabuse.gov/

Substance Abuse and Mental Health Services Administration: www.samhsa.gov/

References

American Academy of Pediatrics Committee on Substance Abuse. (2011). Substance use screening, brief intervention, and referral to treatment for pediatricians. *Pediatrics, 128*(5), e1330–e1340.

American Psychiatric Association. (2013). *Diagnostic and statistical manual of mental disorders* (5th ed.). Washington, DC: Author.

Brown, T. (2015). FDA approves Narcan nasal spray to treat opioid overdose. *Medscape Medical News.* Retrieved from www.medscape.com/viewarticle/854716

Crocker, K. (2015). Adolescent substance abuse: How to interview and assess in the primary care setting. *Journal for Nurse Practitioners, 11*(4), 471–472.

Glass, J., Hamilton, A., Powell, B., Perron, B., Brown, R., & Ilgen, M. (2015). Specialty substance use disorder services following brief alcohol intervention: A meta-analysis of randomized controlled trials. *Addiction, 110*(9), 1404–1415.

Muscari, M. (2004). *Not my kids 2: The 21 threats of the 21st century.* Scranton, PA: University of Scranton Press.

National Center on Addiction and Substance Abuse at Columbia University. (2003). *The formative years: Pathways to substance abuse among girls and young women ages 8–22.* Retrieved from www .casacolumbia.org/addiction-research/reports/formative-years-pathways-substance-abuse-among-girls-and-young-women-ages

National Institute on Alcohol Abuse and Alcoholism. (2015). *College drinking.* Retrieved from http:// niaaa.nih.gov/alcohol-health/special-populations-co-occurring-disorders/college-drinking

Substance Abuse and Mental Health Services Administration. (SAMHSA, 2015). Substance abuse disorders. Retrieved from www.samhsa.gov/disorders/substance-use

CHAPTER 27

Technology Dependence

A. Description

Technology is in a constant state of evolution in terms of access and engagement; what is current and hot today can become outdated and cold by tomorrow (Allison et al., 2012), and its use has significantly increased among children, adolescents, and young adults. In fact, youth use massive amounts of media. Social media alone allows youths to extend friendships, receive support they lack in traditional relationships, and obtain information—including information about their health concerns. However, for some, technology can affect physical and mental well-being,

a.   Technology is an agent of social change because it facilitates the swift diffusion of information, the establishment and maintenance of social networks, and the acceleration of the process of autonomy from parents for adolescents, and socialization via technology begins during early childhood (Mesch, 2012; Plowman & McPake, 2013):

- Nearly all young children watch television and DVDs, but vary in their enthusiasm for video games and web surfing; play preferences vary.

- Parents consider it important to balance technology-based activity with more traditional games, outdoor play, and books. Some parents worry that cell phones endanger heath, while others worry about their children becoming addicted to video gaming, but do not feel that technology is having a detrimental effect on their children's behavior, health, or learning.

- Not all young children are digital natives, a term coined by Prensky (2001) for college students who were born into the technology era. Some feel overwhelmed, at least initially, especially with computers designed for adults. Children need support through guided interaction (showing interest, asking questions, making suggestions) until they develop familiarity with their devices.

- Three- and 4-year-olds are adept at ignoring the television, but had favorite programs and DVDs they watch repeatedly, usually intermingled with other activities. Some young children are also proficient with electronic devices, such as using cell phones for taking photos. With help, they engage in video calls, enabling them to engage in communication with relatives they never met. Thus, technology could enhance rather than hinder social interaction.

- Technology is an important feature in family life, and most children use some form of screen device every day.

- Online communication is now the main channel for youth interaction with friends and family, and it expands adolescents' social circle to include more diverse members, thus decreasing social homophily (bonding with those who are similar) of adolescent peer groups.

- Introverted teens report that the Internet offers more freedom of expression, and they are more likely than extroverts to choose online communications. Socially anxious adolescents report higher friendship quality in online contact.

- Online and cell communication foster close friendships because youth can: discuss issues that create discomfort face to face; disclose intimate information; and feel a sense of togetherness anytime, anywhere.

- Online and cell communication allow youth to stay in contact without the strict control of parents.

- Online communication provides a sense of empowerment and expanded autonomy.

- Family conflict may ensue when there is a hierarchical change because the adolescent may be the family computer expert and other members rely on the teen for technical guidance. This is more likely to happen in homes of lower socioeconomic status and little parental education. Conflicts can also happen because of adolescents' frequent use of the Internet.

- The expansion of adolescents' networks allows greater awareness of vocational opportunities.

- The online environment increases the spheres of adolescent intimacy, identity formation, peer pressure, and autonomy, but also bullying, harassment, and racism.

b.   Media and technology have been shown to have a negative impact on child and adolescent health, particularly in the areas of psychological well-being, sleep, school function, and weight. Rosen and colleagues (2014) investigated the impact of technology on psychological issues, behavioral problems, attention problems, and physical health in children ages 4 to 18, and found some type of impact in all ages.

c.   More children and adolescents are preoccupied with Internet gaming, with multiplayer online role-playing games (MORPGs), such as "World of Warcraft" and "League of Legends," being the most popular. Children and adolescents gravitate to online games for several reasons including opportunities to achieve goals, immerse oneself in a fantasy world, and socialize with other players. However, some children develop problematic online gaming, demonstrating compulsivity to the games and exclusion of other activities to the point of significant distress or impairment.

B. Assessment (History, Physical, Diagnostic Screening/Testing, Where Appropriate)

a. Risk factors are unknown. Problems that contribute to problem online gaming include: preference for online socialization (individuals with poorer psychosocial well-being may see online interaction as safer); mood regulation; deficient self-regulation; escape from conflict; salience/distorted cognition (viewing gaming as the most important thing in their life); and existing psychosocial problems (such as depression, loneliness, social anxiety, and deficient social skills; Bass, 2015; Haagsma, Caplan, Peters, & Pieterse, 2012). The American Psychiatric Association (2013) notes that adolescents and Asian males may be at increased risk for gaming disorder, but it does note an abundance of literature from Asian countries on this problem, and few from North America and Europe.

b. The American Academy of Pediatrics (AAP), Council of Communications and Media (2013) recommends that providers ask two media questions at all well-child visits:

- "How much recreational screen time does your child or teenager consume daily?"
- "Is there a television set or Internet-connected device in the child's bedroom?"

They further recommend (AAP, 2013) obtaining a more detailed media history on children and adolescents who have difficulty in school; are aggressive; are overweight or obese; and who use tobacco, alcohol, and other drugs.

c. Youth with problem Internet gaming may develop consequences that include decreased sleep, verbal memory or attention, increased aggression and hostility, school problems, loneliness, and psychosomatic complaints (Bass, 2015; Kuss, 2013).

C. Diagnosis

a. Internet "addiction" is the excessive or poorly controlled preoccupation, urges, or behaviors regarding Internet access to the point of distress or impairment. Psychiatric comorbidity is common, especially mood, anxiety, impulse control, and substance abuse disorders (Shaw & Black, 2008). This is not a *Diagnostic and Statistical Manual of Mental Disorders, 5th Edition (DSM-5)* diagnosis.

b. Modern technology has also brought about new "syndromes," such as *phantom vibration syndrome* and *Facebook depression*. Phantom vibration syndrome, also called perceived vibrations, arises when a person senses vibrations from a device that is not really vibrating. However, research suggests that, although the phenomenon exists, it may not be a syndrome, and noted that those afflicted did not seem bothered by it (Drouin, Kaiser, & Miller, 2012; Rothberg et al., 2010). Facebook depression is a condition that develops when youth spend considerable time on social media sites, such as Facebook, and then show signs of depression. The AAP (O'Keeffe, Clarke-Pearson, & AAP, Council on Communications and Media, 2011) cited six articles and notes that researchers have proposed this phenomenon, and at least one study was in disagreement. Jelenchick, Eickhoff, and Moreno (2012) found no evidence for a relationship between social network sites and depression, stating that counseling about the risk of Facebook depression may be premature.

c. Gambling disorder is the only nonsubstance-related disorder included as an addictive disorder in the *DSM-5*. However, Internet gambling is included in the *DSM-5* as a condition that requires more research. Petry and O'Brien (2013) note that further research is needed to understand the identifying features, prevalence rates, biological features, and epidemiology of Internet gaming disorder. Refer to Chapter 14 for further information in gambling disorder.

D. Levels of Prevention/Intervention

a. Primary

The AAP Council of Communications and Media (2013) and the American Academy of Family Physicians (2004–2015) recommend: encouraging parents and youth to participate in media education and literacy programs; limiting entertainment screen time to less than 1 to 2 hours per day; discouraging any screen media exposure before age 2 years; removing all media (television, computers/laptops, tablets, cell phones, video games, DVDs, etc.) from children's bedrooms; establishing and enforcing reasonable rules about technology use; developing and enforcing mealtime and bedtime curfews for all media devices, including cell phones; using technology that turns off the television or computer after a set amount of time and that locks out specific channels; monitoring the media and websites that children are using; coviewing movies, television, and videos as a way to discuss family values; alternatives to technology-based entertainment, especially books.

a. Secondary

Screen youth at greater risk for issues related to technology, those with problems related to psychological well-being, sleep, school function, and weight, and provide early intervention.

b. Tertiary

There are no recommended treatments at this time for problem gaming; however, cognitive behavioral therapy (CBT) has been suggested for Internet addiction (Bass, 2015).

E. Parenting Tips

Make technology use more positive (APA, 2013; Muscari, 2002; Nemours Foundation, 2014):

a. Do not use technology as a babysitter.

b. Do not use technology as a reward or punishment: Both make it more important to children.

c. Set limits on nonproductive tech time.

d. Turn the devices off during conversations and mealtimes. Do not arrange family/living room furniture with the TV as the focal point.

e. Try a weekday nonproductive technology ban to increase family time using alternative activities.

f. Ban the use of entertainment technology before homework completion.

g. Plan viewing together in advance. Use the television rating system to determine which shows are appropriate. Discuss reasons for both approving and disapproving shows.

h. Preview programs first whenever possible. Screen new shows intended for children; forbid shows with graphic violence.

i. Watch programs with children to help them interpret what they see. Observe children as they watch, and make note of their mood, that is, whether they are sad, confused, worried, happy, or bored. Discuss their reactions, and foster critical thinking skills.

j. Use current technology to block children from watching inappropriate material on TV.

k. Set an example. Children will not learn self-discipline if parents do not exhibit it in their technology use.

Resources

Kids and Technology: Tips for Parents in a High-Tech World: www.cdc.gov/media/subtopic/matte/pdf/CDCElectronicRegression.pdf

Pew Research Center (multiple papers on youth and technology): www.pewinternet.org/

Tech Guide for Parents: www.techguide4parents.com/

References

Allison, S., Bauermeister, J., Bull, S., Lightfoot, M., Mustanski, B., Shegog, R., & Levine D. (2012). The intersection of youth, technology, and new media with sexual health: Moving the research agenda forward. *Journal of Adolescent Health, 51*(3), 207–212.

American Academy of Family Physicians. (2004–2015). *Violence in the media and entertainment.* Retrieved from www.aafp.org/about/policies/all/violence-media.html

American Academy of Pediatrics, Council of Communications and Media. (2013). Children, adolescents, and the media. *Pediatrics, 132*(5), 958–961. doi:10.1542/peds.2013-2656

American Psychiatric Association. (2013). *Diagnostic and statistical manual of mental disorders* (5th ed.). Washington, DC: Author.

Bass, P. (2015, November). Gaming addiction. *Contemporary Pediatrics.* Retrieved from http://contemporarypediatrics.modernmedicine.com/contemporary-pediatrics/news/gaming-addiction

Drouin, M., Kaiser, D., & Miller, D. (2012). Phantom vibrations among undergraduates: Prevalence and associated psychological characteristics. *Computers in Human Behavior, 28,* 1490–1496.

Haagsma, M., Caplan, S., Peters, O., & Pieterse, M. (2012). A cognitive-behavioral model of problematic online gaming in adolescents aged 12–22 years. *Computers in Human Behavior, 29,* 202–209.

Jelenchick, L., Eickhoff, J., & Moreno, M. (2012). "Facebook depression?" Social networking site use and depression in older adolescents. *Journal of Adolescent Health, 52,* 128–130.

Kuss, D. (2013). Internet gaming addiction: Current perspectives. *Psychology Research Behavior Management, 6,* 125–137.

Mesch, G. (2012). Technology and youth. *New Directions for Youth Development, 135,* 97–105.

Muscari, M. (2002). *Not my kid: 21 steps to raising a nonviolent child.* Scranton, PA: University of Scranton Press.

Nemours Foundation. (2014). Healthy habits for TV, video games, and the internet. Retrieved from https://kidshealth.org/en/parents/tv-habits.html?ref=search

O'Keeffe, G., Clarke-Pearson, K., & American Academy of Pediatrics, Council on Communications and Media. (2011). The impact of social media on children, adolescents, and families. *Pediatrics, 127*(4), 800–804. doi:10.1542/peds.2011-0054

Petry, N.M. and O'Brien, C.P. (2013). Internet gaming disorder and the DSM-5. *Addiction,* 108, 1186–1187. doi:10.1111/add.12162

Prensky, M. (2001). Digital natives, digital immigrants. *On the Horizon, 9*(5), 1-6.

Plowman, L., & McPake, J. (2013). Seven myths about young children and technology. *Childhood Education, 89*(1), 27–33.

Rosen, L., Lim, A., Felt, J., Carrier, L., Cheever, N., Lara-Ruiz, J., . . . Rokkum J. (2014). Media and technology use predicts ill-being among children, preteens and teenagers independent of the negative health impacts of exercise and eating habits. *Computers in Human Behavior, 35,* 364–375.

Rothberg, M., Arora, A., Hermann, J., Kleppel, R., St Marie, P., & Visintainer, P. (2010). Phantom vibration syndrome among medical staff: A cross sectional survey. *BMJ, 341,* c6914. Retrieved from http://dx.doi.org.proxy.binghamton.edu/10.1136/bmj.c6914

Shaw, M., & Black, D. (2008). Internet addiction: Definition, assessment, epidemiology and clinical management. *CNS Drugs, 22*(5), 353–365.

CHAPTER 28

Toxic Stress

A. Description

The first 5 years of life lay the foundation for the sound mental and physical status, economic productivity, and responsible citizenship of a healthy adulthood. Children learn to cope with this stress through the modeling and support of their families. But when stressors are severe, or when parents and caretakers have insufficient abilities, this stress becomes toxic. Toxic stress is the negative effect of the environment on the stress systems of young children who lack the buffering influence of secure adult relationships. It disrupts the structure of the developing brain and can result in permanent changes that have long-term consequences on future education, vocational abilities, and health outcomes (Rushton & Kraft, 2013).

POSITIVE STRESS RESPONSE	TOLERABLE STRESS RESPONSE	TOXIC STRESS RESPONSE
• Normal, essential part of healthy development	• More significant stressors	• Intense, prolonged, or frequent stressor(s)
• Brief duration	• Longer duration	• Prolonged duration
• Brief increase in heart rate and mild elevations of hormone levels	• Brain and other organs recover, if time limited and buffered by supportive adults	• Potential disruption of brain architecture development and other organ/systems with increased risk for stress-related disease and cognitive impairment into the adult years
• Example: first day of school	• Example: death of a loved one	• Example: abuse victimization; exposure to violence

Adapted from the Center on the Developing Child, Harvard University (n.d.).

a.   Toxic stress differs from positive and tolerable stress:

Toxic stress can begin as early as infancy, when infants' needs are not met adequately and consistently (e.g., not feeding the baby when hungry; low levels of human affection, and allowing the infant to cry without parental attention). Infants exposed to high levels of cortisol, the "stress hormone," are more likely to develop adult stress-related diseases later in life, as well as altered brain growth and shortened life spans (Asok, Bernard, Roth, Rosen, & Dozier, 2013; Luby et al., 2013).

b.   Exposure to toxic stress, including poverty and violence, during early childhood increases the risk for a number of negative health outcomes as adults, including depression, cardiovascular disease, cancers, and asthma (Johnson, Riley, Granger, & Riis, 2013). Toxic stress can also be caused by homelessness, bullying victimization, and witnessing community violence.

c.   Toxic stress can arise from adverse childhood experiences (ACE), which are of three types: abuse (physical, emotional, and sexual), neglect (physical and emotional), and household dysfunction (mental illness, mother treated violently, divorce, incarcerated relative, and substance abuse). The ACE study (Felitti et al., 1998) was a collaboration between the Centers for Disease Control and Prevention (CDC) and Kaiser Permanente's Seattle Health Appraisal Clinic that showed that adults, regardless of race, socioeconomic, and other demographic factors, were at a much higher risk for long-term health problems that included: adolescent pregnancy; risk for intimate partner violence; alcoholism and alcohol abuse; chronic obstructive pulmonary disease (COPD); depression; early initiation of sexual activity; early initiation of smoking; fetal death; health-related quality of life; illicit drug use; ischemic heart disease (IHD); liver disease; multiple sexual partners; sexually transmitted diseases (STDs); smoking; suicide attempts; and unintended pregnancies. A systematic literature review by DeVenter, Demyttenaere, and Bruffaerts (2013) found that child abuse, substance abuse, and parental divorce were very frequent risk factors; the occurrence of child abuse was the most important risk factor for the development of depression, while sexual child abuse and family violence were the greatest risk factors for anxiety disorders; and, finally, strong correlations were noted between family violence or physical neglect and substance abuse. A history of childhood adversity was even found to be significant in new onset depression, though not posttraumatic stress disorder, among National Guard soldiers (Rudenstine et al., 2015).

d.   The risk for these long-term problems increases as the ACE score increases. However, a surveillance of ACE prevalence in Minnesota showed that while the risk for anxiety, depression, and smoking increases as the numbers of ACEs increase, there was no correlation between ACEs and obesity or diabetes (Minnesota Department of Health, 2013). The ACE score also does not take positive experiences into account, and these can help build resilience and protect children from the effects of trauma—there are people who do well despite high ACE scores.

e. Stress does not have to be toxic to create concerns for health care providers. Childhood is filled with normal stressors, including developmental stressors, such as toilet training and puberty, and situational stressors, such as moving and going to a new school. The way children cope with these stressors can also affect their development and the way they handle subsequent life events. Some stressors, like illness, are universal to all children; others are age specific.

- Infants: Infants do feel stress, including that of their parents. They become distressed when their parents are angry, when they are unresponsive, and when they exhibit other negative emotions. Other infant stressors are:

    - Uncomfortable temperatures; young infants cannot regulate their body temperature
    - Pain
    - Short-term separation from mother
    - Overstimulation
    - Strangers (between 4 and 8 months)

- Toddlers: The normal demands of growing up accompanied by the day-to-day strains most families experience disallow a stress-free existence for most young children. Small stressors are beneficial because they teach toddlers to cope, but excessive stress is harmful, and toddlers are especially vulnerable because of their limited coping abilities. Sources of stress for a toddler include:

    - Fear of losing his or her newly developed skills
    - Having his or her rituals taken away; change in daily structure or disruption of family routines
    - Separation from parents or parental loss (divorce, death, jail)
    - New sibling
    - Strangers
    - Bedtime (can be viewed as separation from parents)
    - Loss of security object (favorite blanket, doll)
    - Overstimulation (too much commotion at once, such as a family reunion)

- Preschoolers: Preschoolers face many unique stressors because of the magical thinking of this stage. Some stressors are due to their own distinctive understanding of the world, such as fears; others are imposed, including preschool. Preschool-age stressors include:

    - Separation from parents, which creates less stress than it did when he or she was a toddler, but it still persists, and seems to increase for a while around age 6.

- Being mocked or insulted by others. Despite the fact that they may like to insult others to boost their own self-image, preschoolers do not like to be on the receiving end of such comments.

- Having their questions go unanswered. Enterprising preschoolers ask constant questions, especially "why," and they can become upset if adults do not respond or know the answer.

- Decreased attention. Preschoolers like to talk, and they can become frustrated if ignored or put off.

- School-age children: Today's school-age children face more stressors than ever. They are pressured by friends to be like them and do what they do, and by parents to excel in school and extracurricular activities. Extracurricular activities (sports, clubs, scouts, dance classes, karate) themselves can be stressful, especially if they take up much of children's free time. Being out in the world more than when they were younger exposes them to more stress. The school environment creates stress to their self-image as they compete for grades and teacher recognition, as well as temptations to smoke cigarettes, drink alcohol, take drugs, or steal. School-age children may be pressured to think, feel, and behave at a level of maturity far beyond what should be expected of them. They may have adult responsibilities, such as watching young siblings or cooking meals, or they may be making decisions that they are not really capable of making. They may have little time for being a child and enjoying the spontaneous activities of childhood. General sources of stress for school-age children are:

  - Starting school. This may be their first experience with being away from home all day. They may be fearful of getting lost or making an embarrassing social mistake.

  - Long vacations mean extended time away from peers. Friends are important at this age, and your child may fear losing them by his or her absence.

  - Moving signifies changes in both school and peer group, both of which are very stressful. They need to adjust to both losing old friends and making new ones.

  - Change in family structure (divorce, remarriage) is an all-too-common stressor. A child's ability to cope with this depends on a number of factors.

  - Major holidays, such as Christmas.

  - Puberty. Preteens, especially girls, may become self-conscious regarding obvious signs of sexual development.

- Adolescents: Adolescence itself is stressful because of all its physical and psychological changes. Add the stresses of relationships, school, competition, and the uncertainty of what lies ahead, and it becomes easy to understand adolescent angst. Adolescents also need to become less dependent on their parents and learn to make their own decisions. Sources of adolescent stress include:

- Pregnancy
- Peer loss
- Breakup with boyfriend/girlfriend
- Parental loss (divorce, death, jail), or death of other loved ones
- School demands or frustrations
- Changes in the adolescent's body and/or negative thoughts or feelings about him or herself
- Having too many activities or having too high expectations

B. Assessment

a.   Risk factors for toxic stress are intense, prolonged, or frequent stressors, including poverty, abuse, family member incarceration, witnessing violence, parental divorce, parental substance abuse, or mental illness.

b.   Differentiate toxic stress from positive and tolerable stress, but do not ignore the latter two.

c.   Chronic stress leads to feelings of being "stressed out" or "burned out." Stress may not be easy to recognize because it often affects the body, leading to the impression that the child is ill rather than stressed out. General signs of chronic stress include:

- Headaches, backaches, chest pain, stomachaches, indigestion, nausea, or diarrhea
- Rashes
- Overeating or undereating
- Sleep disturbances (too much sleep, restless sleep, difficulty falling asleep, difficulty staying asleep, waking up early)
- Twitching
- Having trouble concentrating or with school work
- Feeling anxious or worried
- Feeling inadequate, frustrated, helpless, or overwhelmed
- Feeling bored or dissatisfied
- Feeling pressured, tense, irritable, angry, or hostile
- Aggressive behavior
- Substance abuse

- Excessive or inappropriate crying
- Avoiding others

d. Age-specific signs of stress include:

- Ages 1 to 5: Excessive clinging or crying; regressed behavior (goes back to wanting his or her bottle); severe sensitivity to loud noises; irritability; trembling
- Ages 5 to 12: Vague physical complaints; refusal to go to school; easily distractible; poor school performance
- Ages 12 to 14: Isolates from family and friends; feels sad or depressed; turns aggressive
- Ages 14 to 18: Same as ages 12 to 14; antisocial behavior (fights, stealing); night fears

e. Use screening tools to assess for risk factors. The forms and instructions for each of these tools are available at the associated weblink:

- The Family Psychosocial Screen (Kemper & Kelleher, 1996): www.pedstest.com/Portals/0/TheBook/FPSinEnglish.pdf
- The Bright Futures Pediatric Intake Form: https://brightfutures.org/mental health/pdf/professionals/ped_intake_form.pdf

C. Diagnosis

Potential diagnoses include depression, anxiety, and substance abuse.

D. Levels of Prevention/Intervention

a. Primary

- The most effective way to engage parents in the primary care setting is to talk with them about parenting. Health care providers need to be proactive and ask, since parents may be hesitant to bring up concerns.
- Wellness visits have time constraints; however, other models can be used. The medical home model allows for the use of case managers and other supportive staff to assess and promote parenting skills, connect families with resources, and evaluate the response to the interventions (O'Connell, Davis, & Bauer, 2015).
- The Tennessee Chapter of the American Academy of Pediatrics (n.d.) recommends the following:
  - Since more than 60% of people report at least one ACE, encourage parents to talk about their own childhood experiences to better understand what they have learned about how to overcome adversity and protect themselves.

They can use what they learn to build resiliency and protect their children from the effects of ACEs.

- Encourage parents to expose children to awesome childhood experiences: spend time with them, tell them that they are loved and that they have a purpose in life, and tell them that they have people to talk to if bad things happen.

- Build resiliency by further encouraging parents to: be strong, loving, and supportive; talk and read to their children; nurture healthy relationships with parents, other family members, and friends; and teach good communication skills, as well as how and why to make good choices.

- Foster age-appropriate coping skills (see the section Parenting Tips). Coping mechanisms vary, depending on a child's developmental level, helpful resources, situation, style, and previous experience with stressful events.

b. Secondary

- In healthy homes, children can rely on support from a parent or other adult to relieve their stress. However, in some situations, there is no supportive adult, leaving the child in a persistent state of elevated stress—toxic stress. The Nurse Family Partnership (NFP), which sends nurses to the homes of at-risk new parents to help them learn about child development and development skills, has consistently been proven to mitigate risks (Shonkoff, 2014). NFP provides home visits from registered nurses to first-time, low-income mothers to support their attainment of a healthy pregnancy, responsible and competent childcare, and greater economic self-sufficiency.

- Parental support is critical in the prevention of toxic stress; however, many parents are dealing with their own problems, including mental illness, poverty, and their negative childhood experiences. Medical homes provide an avenue for reaching the whole family. Health care providers can screen parents to better ascertain their risks and strengths, promote positive parenting, and connect families to services in their communities (Kuehn, 2014).

- Wherever possible, utilize the NFP.

c. Tertiary
- Franke (2014) recommends an individualized, yet integrated, approach that decreases stressors and increases resiliency. Possible interventions include relaxation techniques, such as breathing exercises, guided imagery, and biofeedback, which may be taught by health care providers experienced in these techniques or through referral. Referral may also be necessary for children who would benefit from psychotherapy, including cognitive behavioral therapy, trauma-focused therapy and parent–child interaction therapy. Health care providers may need to provide parenting education, or in the case of significant dysfunction, refer the family to social services.

E. Parenting Tips

Foster positive coping skills:

a. Your toddler may cope with stress by using infantile motor activities (rocking, restlessness, changing positions to move away from stressor) until he or she begins to use other strategies, such as play. Play serves as a stress relief method for toddlers. He or she can release frustrations and anxieties by banging on drums, working with a play hammer and nails, or molding clay dough. Your toddler will also hug a favorite toy, throw tantrums, suck his or her thumb, and even withdraw and become quiet.

b. Your preschooler may attempt to handle stress in a variety of ways, including occasionally lapsing into babyish behaviors such as thumb-sucking or bedwetting. He or she may also develop unsightly nervous habits such as nail biting, hair pulling, nose picking, or masturbation.

c. Your school-aged child uses a number of coping mechanisms to deal with stress. Some of these are unconscious, such as denial and reaction formation. Denial temporarily allows your child to deny that the stressor occurred in the first place. Reaction formation allows your child to act or say the opposite of how he or she actually feels. For example, if your child is afraid, he or she may say something like, "I'm not afraid of anything. I'm the bravest one in this whole room." These mechanisms are healthy and normal, but help your child learn more age-appropriate coping mechanisms, such as communication and problem solving when he or she is ready.

d. Adolescents have a variety of coping mechanisms. One is cognitive mastery, whereby teenagers attempt to learn as much as possible about the situation. They can then use their problem solving skills to work through the situation. By using conformity, teens attempt to mirror the actions and appearance of their friends. Controlling behavior allows them to be in charge of some aspects of their lives, and they will not accept parental or school rules without questioning them. Young teens use fantasy, and teens of all ages rely on motor activities, such as sports, dancing, or other high-energy activities—all very effective tension-relieving strategies. Adolescents may react negatively to stress by acting out, blaming others for their mistakes or problems, or by using drugs and alcohol. Therefore, it is helpful to teach your teen healthy stress management techniques before he or she feels overwhelmed by stress.

Resources

American Academy of Pediatrics Resilience Project: www.aap.org/en-us/advocacy-and-policy/ aap-health-initiatives/resilience/Pages/default.aspx

American Academy of Pediatrics Trauma Toolbox for Primary Care: www.aap.org/en-us/advocacy-and-policy/aap-health-initiatives/healthy-foster-care-america/Pages/Trauma-Guide.aspx#trauma

ACE Study: www.acestudy.org/home

Adverse Childhood Experiences: www.rwjf.org/en/library/collections/aces.html

Bright Futures (A strengths-based approach to well-child supervision): https://brightfutures.aap.org/Pages/default.aspx

Early Brain and Child Development: www.aap.org/en-us/advocacy-and-policy/aap-health-initiatives/EBCD/Pages/Public-Health-Approach.aspx

Get Your ACE Score: http://acestoohigh.com/got-your-ace-score/

Nurse Family Partnership: www.nursefamilypartnership.org/

Protecting Your Child's Health From Toxic Stress: http://tnaap.org/pdf/toxic_stress_ace/ACEs_Handout.pdf

References

Asok, A., Bernard, K., Roth, T., Rosen, J. B., & Dozier, M. (2013). Parental responsiveness moderates the association between early-life stress and reduced telomere length. *Developmental Psychopathy, 25*(3), 577–585.

Center on the Developing Child, Harvard University. (n.d.). *Toxic stress.* Retrieved from http://developingchild.harvard.edu/science/key-concepts/toxic-stress

DeVenter, M., Demyttenaere, K., & Bruffaerts, R. (2013). The relationship between adverse childhood experiences and mental health in adulthood. A systematic literature review. *Tijdschrift Voor Psychiatrie, 55*(4), 259–268.

Felitti, V. J., Anda, R. F., Nordenberg, D., Williamson, D. F., Spitz, A. M., Edwards, V., . . . Marks, J. S. (1998). Relationship of childhood abuse and household dysfunction to many of the leading causes of death in adults. The adverse childhood experiences (ACE) study. *American Journal of Preventative Medicine, 14*, 245–258.

Franke, H. (2014). Toxic stress: Effects, prevention and treatment. *Children, 1*, 390–402. doi:10.3390/children1030390

Johnson, S., Riley, A., Granger, D., & Riis, J. (2013). The science of early life toxic stress for pediatric practice and advocacy. *Pediatrics, 131*, 319–327.

Kemper, K., & Kelleher, K. (1996). Family psychosocial screening: Instruments and techniques. *Ambulatory Child Health, 1,* 325–329.

Kuehn, B. (2014). AAP: Toxic stress threatens kids' long-term health. *JAMA, 312,* 585–586.

Luby, J., Belden, A., Botteron, K., Marrus, N., Harms, M. P., Babb, C., . . . Barch D. (2013). The effects of poverty on childhood brain development: The mediating effect of caregiving and stressful life events. *JAMA Pediatrics, 167*(12), 1135–1142. doi:10.1001/jamapediatrics.2013.3139

Minnesota Department of Health. (2013). *Adverse childhood experiences in Minnesota: Findings and recommendations based on the 2011 Minnesota behavioral risk factor surveillance system.* Retrieved from www.health.state.mn.us/divs/chs/brfss/ACE_ExecutiveSummary.pdf

O'Connell, L., Davis, M., & Bauer, N. (2015). Assessing parenting behaviors to improve child outcomes. *Pediatrics, 135*(2), e286–e288. doi:10.1542/peds.2014-2497

Rudenstine, S., Cohen, G., Prescott, M., Sampson, L., Liberzon, I., Tamburrino, M., . . . Galea, S. (2015). Adverse childhood events and the risk for new-onset depression and post-traumatic stress disorder among U.S. National Guard soldiers. *Military Medicine, 180*(9), 972–978.

Rushton, F., & Kraft, C. (2013). Family support in the family-centered medical home: An opportunity for preventing toxic stress and its impact in young children. *Child Abuse and Neglect, 37*(Suppl.), 41–50.

Shonkoff, J. (2014). Changing the narrative for early childhood investment. *JAMA Pediatrics, 168*(2), 105–106. doi:10.1001/jamapediatrics

Tennessee Chapter of the American Academy of Pediatrics. (n.d.). *Protecting your child's health from toxic stress.* Retrieved from http://tnaap.org/pdf/toxic_stress_ace/ACEs_Handout.pdf

CHAPTER 29

Transition Age Youth

A. Description

Transition age youth (TAY) are persons ages 16 through 25, with youth ages 16 to 17 considered older adolescents, and those 18 to 25, young adults. They are neither children nor adults. Their development, functioning, and service needs differ from those of children and adults.

a. Transitioning from adolescence to adulthood can be challenging, as youth must develop and refine the adult skills they need to finish school, acquire rewarding work, create a stable domicile, engage in long-term romantic relationships/marriage and raise children with effective parenting skills. To accomplish all this, they need: bio-physiological maturation, including the ability to think abstractly; a moral structure based on the greater good; complex processing of social signals, behaviors, and rules; a mature concept of self in society; and physical sexual maturity. Today's youth must also be self-sufficient in a job market that demands higher academic degrees and provides fewer opportunities to those without degrees. Many are not achieving these milestones until age 30 or later (Davis, 2006). Most youth have successful transitions into adulthood, but for those who do not enjoy that success, failure to accomplish the transition milestones can result in dissatisfaction, anxiety, and depression.

b. The challenges can be even greater for youth with disabilities, youth with mental health disorders, youth leaving foster care or juvenile detention facilities, youth who have run away from home or dropped out of school, and youth who are homeless. For example, TAY with disabilities consistently lag behind their nondisabled peers in rates for high school graduation, employment, postsecondary education, and independent living (Wagner, Newman, Cameto, Levine, & Garza, 2006).

c. In a 1995 study of young people ages 18 to 29, Arnett (2004) noted common themes that transcended socioeconomic backgrounds. He named this period "emerging adulthood" and discussed the five features of this "age." The first is identity exploration, whereby youth decide who they are and what they want out of work, school, and love. The second is instability as this stage is marked by residence changes, as youth go to college, enter the military, or live with friends or a romantic partner. These frequent moves usually end when families and careers are established in their 30s. The third is self-focus as youth try to decide what they want to do now that they are free from parental and school direction. They also choose where they want to go and whom they want to be with until these choices are limited by the limitations of marriage, family, and career. The fourth is the feeling in between, where many emerging adults say that they are taking responsibility for themselves yet still do not fully feel like adults. The last is the age of possibilities. Most are optimistic and believe they have good chances of living lives better than their parents'.

d.   The major issues during this period are: residential stability; education; health care insurance coverage; delinquency and criminal activity; mental illness; transition from foster care; being LGBTQI2; homelessness; and rurality.

B. Assessment

a.   Risk factors: Youth who are more likely to have a difficult transition are those who: have mental health issues or other disabilities; are homeless; are runaways; and who are released from juvenile detention facilities or foster care during their transition years. Not having a high school diploma or general equivalency diploma (GED) can also interfere with transition and diminish the youth's lifelong earning potential.

b.   Assess for the warning signs of mental illness (or instability/worsening in those TAY who are already diagnosed with mental illness):

- Suicidal or homicidal ideation
- Sudden changes in behavior
- Extreme moods
- Decreased motivation
- Difficulty concentrating
- Distorted body image
- Disorganized or rapid speech
- Marked decline in academic performance
- Inattention to or inability to care for basic needs
- Withdrawal from family and friends
- Changes in eating habits as well as marked changes in weight
- Sleep problems

- Loss of pleasure
- Persistent anxiety
- Excessive activities
- Development of strange thoughts and/or behaviors
- Confusing thoughts or speech
- Hallucinations
- Delusions

c. College-bound TAY with previously diagnosed psychiatric disabilities face normal college stress along with illness-related challenges, including medication management, therapy appointments, academic accommodations, emotional variability, and sleep difficulties. Students with higher rates of stress may have lower academic motivation and demonstrate ineffective use of learning strategies, resulting in impaired information-processing skills, poor academic performance, reduced confidence, less effective time management, less effective use of study resources, and higher test anxiety. Specific disorders can create specific issues. Students with impulse-control disorders and substance-use disorders are at high risk of quitting college, as are those with panic disorder or bipolar disorder and the co-occurrence of three or more psychiatric disorders (Muscari, 2012).

C. Diagnosis

a. The transition period is when the start of mental illness peaks, as the vast majority of mental health disorders have onset by the early 20s, and 3.9% of all young adults had a serious mental illness in the past year (Substance Abuse and Mental Health Services Administration [SAMHSA], 2014). This transition age also has the highest rates of onset of problematic substance use and substance-use disorders (i.e., abuse, dependence).

b. TAY is a heterogeneous group of individuals between the ages of 16 and 25 years with severe emotional disorders (SED; under age 18 years) or serious mental illness (SMI; over age 18 years; Clark & Unruh, 2009). These serious mental health conditions (SMHC) result in significant functional impairment, and do not include developmental disorders, substance use disorders, or mental disorders caused by medical conditions.

c. SEDs include: anxiety disorder, major depression bipolar disorder, learning disorders, conduct disorders, eating disorders, autistic spectrum disorders, and schizophrenia. Criteria are:

- Inability to learn that cannot be explained by intellectual, sensory, or health factors

- Inability to build or maintain satisfactory interpersonal relationships with peers and teachers
- Inappropriate types of behavior or feelings under normal circumstances
- General pervasive mood of unhappiness or depression
- Tendency to develop physical symptoms or fears associated with personal or school problems

d. SMIs include major depression, bipolar disorder, schizophrenia, obsessive compulsive disorder, panic disorder, post-traumatic stress disorder (PTSD), and borderline personality disorder. Criteria are:

- Established *Diagnostic and Statistical Manual of Mental Disorders, 5th Edition* (*DSM-5*; American Psychiatric Association [APA], 2013) diagnosis, exclusive of dementia, developmental disorder, or substance abuse as the principal diagnosis
- Persistence of the disorder for a period of time sufficient to meet the *DSM-5* diagnostic criteria
- Significant and persistent impairment in one or more life roles/functions

  SMI has a detrimental effect on thought, mood, perception, orientation, or memory; thus, it significantly impairs the youth's judgment, behavior, capacity to recognize reality, and/or ability to meet the ordinary demands of life.

e. Consequences of mental illness during the transition phase include (SAMHSA, 2014):

- Education: More than half of youth with mental health needs will drop out of school, and only 5% to 20% will enter postsecondary education.
- Employment: Youth with disabilities experience high unemployment as well as insufficient opportunities to obtain competitive employment with potential career growth.
- Military: Of the roughly 31.2 million Americans aged 17 to 24, 35% are unqualified for military service because of physical and medical issues. Within this group, 18% are ineligible because of illegal drug use, 5% because of a criminal record, and 6% because they have too many dependents under age 18. All branches of the armed forces require members to be high school graduates or have equivalent credentials such as the GED.
- Crime: The most common mental health disorders among youth in the juvenile justice system are disruptive behavior disorders (e.g., attention deficit hyperactivity disorder [ADHD], conduct disorder), anxiety disorders (e.g., PTSD [now classified as a trauma disorder], generalized anxiety disorder), and mood disorders (e.g., major depression, bipolar disorder).

f. There is an important distinction between disruptive behavior disorders and other mental health problems for TAY. A disruptive behavior disorder diagnosis allows minors to access mental health services, but adults presenting solely with a disruptive behavior disorder can be denied coverage (Zajac, Sheidow, & Davis, 2013); however, the Affordable Care Act supports state-based programs to improve mental health outcomes for persons ages 16 to 25 (Munoz, 2013). Thus, TAY with primarily behavioral disorders are often in the position of losing access to mental health services as they age out of child mental health systems.

D. Levels of Prevention/Intervention

a. Primary

- Primary prevention works best before youth graduate high school. Assess fears about their upcoming graduation and teach them how to best manage transition stress. Counseling includes general stress-management techniques and specific strategies designed to minimize the occurrence of the health-risk behaviors common in the transition years, including substance abuse.

- TAY need an array of healthy coping strategies. Conduct a coping-skills inventory and assist them in developing healthy coping mechanisms that fit in with their lifestyles. Encourage them to set priorities, schedule tasks for peak efficiency, set and visualize realistic goals, budget enough time for projects, avoid procrastinating, learn to say "no" when necessary, and take breaks when needed.

- College students should discover and use the resources available to them on campus, which include the wellness center, counseling, campus safety, academic support services, financial aid, and career services, as well as specific programs, such as drug- and alcohol-use prevention and interpersonal-violence prevention. Most colleges also have services for specific populations, including LGBTQI2, international, and graduate students.

b. Secondary

- Identify TAY at risk, and encourage early intervention. Find programs that focus on effective principles for this population. If unavailable, utilize the principles of effective programs to work with these youth in the primary care practice. Researchers have identified common characteristics of effective programs for teens (Hall, Israel, & Shortt, 2004):
  - Youth develop a sense of independence through participation in the program, including financial independence via wages or stipends.
  - Programs offer job skills/preparation/training and provide employment opportunities.
  - Schools are active partners.

- Youth continue to receive support in navigating life after they finish high school.
- Youth are involved in decision making, and all feel that the time they have dedicated counts.
- Youth interact with peers and adults, including community and business leaders.
- Youth are exposed to life outside of their immediate neighborhood.
- Programs are flexible.
- The Transition to Independence Process (TIP; Clark & Deschenes, n.d.) approach is an evidence-based model that promotes the importance of engaging young adults in their own future planning process, providing access to appropriate services, and using services that focus on individual strengths:
  - Engaging young people through relationship development, person-centered planning, and a focus on their futures; providing tailored supports that are accessible, coordinated, and developmentally appropriate.
  - Ensuring a safety net of support by involving a young person's parents, family members, and other informal and formal key players; focusing on acknowledging and developing personal choice and social responsibility with young people.
  - Enhancing a person's competencies.
  - Maintaining an outcome focus.
  - Involving young people, parents, and other community partners in the TIP system at the practice, program, and community levels.

c. Tertiary

When prospective students have preexisting disorders, set up ongoing collaboration with the college health and counseling centers to ensure that the student's needs are met once in college. College stressors can exacerbate symptoms, warranting medication adjustment and more intensive counseling. Even if this is not the case, students may need additional support to ensure that they successfully complete their studies and graduate at their optimum level of health (Muscari, 2012).

E. Parenting Tips

a. TAY need to plan their living arrangements, career/schooling/military enlistment, long-term relationships, community involvement, and free time, and planning should include parents/guardians, school personnel, health care provider, and other services as needed.

b. Plan for life. Many TAY do not know what they want to do with the rest of their lives; however, they can make a smooth transition with some help and access to resources. Create a plan to assist them in identifying the following:

- Support persons: Who are the family members and friends they can count on for advice and support, including emotional, physical, and financial needs.

- Career goals: TAY may still need assistance in deciding a career path. Have them begin with an Internet search. The Bureau of Labor Statistics (www.bls.gov) provides the occupational outlook for numerous careers, including median pay, typical entry-level education, on-the-job training, number of jobs, job outlook, and employment change.

- Career planning: College, vocational school, work, or military—living off parents should not be an option. A college education is required for many, but not all, careers, and families need to consider future career goals, loan burden, and other factors when making this critical decision. Get assistance from a career counselor.

- Living arrangements: If the youth does not go away to college, where will he or she live? If the youth moves to his or her own place, what can the youth take with him or her (e.g., is the bedroom furniture the youth's or the parents')?

- Transportation: If the youth has a car, how will he or she pay for fuel, maintenance, repairs, and insurance?

- Health care needs: Is a change of providers needed? If the youth has a pediatrician, he or she will need to transition to an adult provider. Regardless of provider, the health care provider should be a good source of information for the youth's wellness care and health promotion needs. The health care provider can also recommend community agency resources, especially for TAY with disabilities.

Resources

Building a COMMUNITY OF PRACTICE to Support Young Adults With Serious Mental Health Conditions: http://labs.umassmed.edu/transitionsRTC/Resources/publications/Tipsheet9.pdf

College Health and Safety: www.cdc.gov/family/college

College Survival Guide: http://psychcentral.com/college/

Going to College—A Resource for Teens With Disabilities: www.going-to-college.org/

NYSOMH Transition Age Youth Resources: www.omh.ny.gov/omhweb/consumer_affairs/transition_youth/resources/

Society for the Study of Emerging Adulthood: http://ssea.org/ Your Future Now: A Transition Planning & Resource Guide for

Transitions RTC: www.umassmed.edu/transitionsrtc

Transition Age Youth With Mental Health Challenges in the Juvenile Justice System: www.tapartnership .org/docs/TransitionAgeYouthWithMentalHealthChallengesJJ_10-17-13.pdf

Transition and Aging Out: http://youth.gov/youth-topics/transition-age-youth

Your Future Now: A Transition Planning & Resource Guide for Youth With Special Needs & Their Families: www.mcf.gov.bc.ca/spec_needs/pdf/your_future_now.pdf

References

American Psychiatric Association. (2013). *Diagnostic and statistical manual of mental disorders* (5th ed.). Washington, DC: Author.

Arnett, J. (2004). *Emerging adulthood: The winding road from the late teens though the twenties.* New York, NY: Oxford University Press.

Clark, H., & Unruh, D. (2009). *Transition of youth and young adult with emotional or behavioral difficulties: An evidence-supported handbook.* Baltimore, MD: Brookes Publishing.

Davis, M. (2006). The path from adolescence to adulthood. *NAMI Beginnings, 8,* 3–6.

Hall, G., Israel, L., & Shortt, J. (2004). *It's about time! A look at out of school time for urban teens.* Wellesley, MA: The National Institute on Out-of-School Time.

Munoz, C. (2013). The affordable care act and expanding mental health coverage. *The White House Blog.* Retrieved from www.whitehouse.gov/blog/2013/08/21/affordable-care-act-and-expanding-mental-health-coverage

Muscari, M. (2012). *How should I assess college-bound students for mental health issues?* Retrieved from www.medscape.com/viewarticle/771197

Substance Abuse and Mental Health Services Administration. (2014, May). *Serious mental health challenges among older adolescents and young adults.* The CBHSQ Report. Retrieved from http:// archive.samhsa.gov/data/2k14/CBHSQ173/sr173-mh-challenges-young-adults-2014.htm

Wagner, M., Newman, L., Cameto, R., Levine, P., & Garza, N. (2006). *An overview of findings from wave 2 of the National Longitudinal Transition Study-2 (NLTS2)* (NCSER 2006–3004). Menlo Park, CA: SRI International.

Zajac, K., Sheidow, A. J., & Davis, M. (2013). *Transition age youth with mental health challenges in the juvenile justice system.* Washington, DC: Technical Assistance Partnership for Child and Family Mental Health.

CHAPTER 30

Traumatic Stress

A. Description

A traumatic event is an experience that threatens injury, death, or the physical integrity of self or others and also causes horror, terror, or helplessness at the time it occurs (American Psychological Association, 2008). The level of psychological distress following exposure to trauma is variable, and most children handle trauma well. However, severe trauma can have significant effects on children's development that undermine their sense of security, as well as cause them to believe that their parents cannot protect them from harm. Premature destruction of these beliefs can have profound negative consequences on childhood development. Traumatized youth tend to be preoccupied with danger and vulnerability, which can sometimes lead to misperceptions of danger, even in situations that are not threatening. Several studies have shown that once posttraumatic stress symptoms emerge, posttraumatic stress disorder (PTSD) leads to neurophysiological correlates that impact brain function in developing children and adolescents.

a. The National Child Traumatic Stress Network (n.d.) describes different types of childhood trauma: community violence (neighborhood violence in which involved persons are not family members); child neglect; physical abuse; sexual abuse; complex trauma (chronic exposure to multiple or prolonged traumatic events); intimate partner violence; early childhood trauma (accidents); school violence; medical trauma (serious illness, invasive procedures, or treatments); traumatic grief (due to sudden, unexpected death of someone important to the child); disasters (natural and man-made); terrorism; and refugee and war zone trauma.

b. PTSD can affect children as young as 3 years as a result of a child's exposure to one or more traumatic events that were life-threatening or perceived to be likely to cause serious injury to self or others. The incidence of PTSD in children varies according to several factors, including the type of trauma, how close the child was to the trauma, and the reaction of the child's parents. The prevalence of PTSD is considerable among high-risk children who have experienced specific traumatic events, such as abuse or natural disasters. PTSD can have a considerably negative impact on life, particularly for children. Besides the symptoms of numbing, hyperarousal, and recollections of the event that adults experience, children can suffer from a decreased ability to participate in normal academic and social activities.

c.   Complex PTSD: The term complex PTSD was developed by Dr. Judith Herman to describe symptoms experienced by survivors of significant long-term (months to years) trauma. Dr. Herman notes that the victim is generally held in a state of captivity, physically or emotionally, for a prolonged period of time. The victim is under the control of the perpetrator and unable to flee. Examples of such traumatic situations include: concentration camps, prisoner of war camps, prostitution brothels, long-term domestic violence, long-term child physical abuse, long-term child sexual abuse, and organized child exploitation rings. Treatment of complex PTSD usually takes much longer, may progress at a much slower rate, and requires a highly structured treatment program delivered by a team of trauma specialists. Sometimes called "Disorder of Extreme Stress," complex PTSD is a form of PTSD that can be very debilitating with a more pervasive pattern of symptoms. People with complex PTSD often have been diagnosed with a personality or dissociative disorder, and may exhibit behavior problems (impulsivity, aggression, eating disorders, sexual acting out, drug abuse, and other self-destructive behaviors), extreme emotional difficulties (intense rage, depression, panic, or suicidal thoughts), relationship difficulties (isolation, distrust, and repeated search for a rescuer), and altered consciousness (fragmented thoughts, dissociation, amnesia). They may have distorted views of their perpetrator, such as attributing total power to him or her, being preoccupied with the relationship to the perpetrator, being preoccupied with revenge. Persons with complex PTSD may also experience a loss of sustaining faith or a sense of despair.

B. Assessment

a.   Risk factors: Although anyone can experience traumatic stress, there are factors that can increase risk: experiencing intense or long-lasting trauma; history of prior trauma; history of mental health problems; family history of mental health problems; and lack of a good support system. In a meta-analysis, Trickey and colleagues (2012) examined 25 risk factors for PTSD in children and adolescents and found: a small effect size for race and younger age, a medium-sized effect for female gender, low intelligence, low socioeconomic status, pre- and posttrauma events, pretrauma low self-esteem, posttrauma parental psychological problems, bereavement, time post-trauma (an inverse relationship), trauma severity, and exposure to the event by media; while a large effect was observed for low social support, peri-trauma fear, perceived life threat, social withdrawal, comorbid psychological problems, poor family functioning, distraction, and thought suppression. The authors note that only six of the 25 variables were investigated in 10 or more studies, and emphasize the need for future research, especially some very rudimentary potential risk factors (e.g., low intelligence, race, perceived life threat, low social support).

b. Short-term distress is expected after a traumatic event. Children may experience sadness, anger, irritability, new fears, separation anxiety (young children), sleep problems (including nightmares), reduced concentration, decline in school work, loss of interest in normal activities, and somatic complaints, as well as dysfunction within the family, peer group, or school. However, most children are resilient and return to their previous level of functioning.

c. PTSD symptoms vary greatly among children and adolescents, depending upon the traumatic event itself, its severity, duration, and the child's developmental age at the time of the trauma. The way a child reexperiences and shows his or her feelings of distress related to a traumatic event is also likely to change with age.

- Young children (under age 5) may reenact their trauma through play and drawings. Their play themes may relate directly to the trauma or they may be nonspecific. Thus, one child who was victimized by violence may act out the violence on a doll or stuffed animals, while another victimized by the same type of trauma may playact that he or she is killing a monster. Young children may not experience flashbacks the way older children and adults do, but may instead experience them in a way that mimics a psychotic disorder.

- School-age children (ages 5–12) may not have flashbacks, or problems remembering parts of the trauma, the way adults do. However, children might place the trauma events in the wrong order, and they might think there were signs that the trauma was going to happen. Thus, they think that they will see these signs again before another traumatic event happens, believing that if they pay attention, they can avoid future traumas. Some school-age children may act out the trauma in their play; others may fit it into their daily lives by doing things such as carrying a gun to class.

- Adolescents (ages 13 to 18) may show the same signs as adults, which include invasive images (that they may not talk about), restlessness, aggression, difficulty sleeping, and difficulty concentrating, as well as loss of interest in previously enjoyed activities, withdrawal from family and peers, and changes in significant life attitudes. The onset of PTSD during adolescence can have a particularly damaging impact since it may impair the acquisition of life skills needed for independence and self-sufficiency. Mastery of these skills occurs within a limited time. These skills must be accomplished in order to meet the demands of the adult world, because if they are not achieved before the onset of adulthood, the impairment can last throughout life. Teens who suffer with chronic PTSD triggered by repeated or prolonged trauma may suffer primarily from dissociative symptoms, numbing, sadness, restricted affect, detachment, self-injury, substance abuse, and aggressive outburst.

C. Diagnosis

Traumatic stress disorders underwent changes in the *Diagnostic and Statistical Manual of Mental Disorders,* 5th edition (*DSM-5*; American Psychiatric Association [APA], 2013), the first of which was their shift from the category of anxiety disorders to the new category of trauma and stressor-related disorders. The heterogeneous nature of the disorders is recognized, as is the difference in symptomatology between preschoolers and those who are older.

a.   Acute stress disorder is most often diagnosed when an individual has been exposed to a traumatic event within the month prior to the onset of symptoms. The youth may experience negative mood, recurrent and unwanted dreams/memories/ flashbacks (intrusion symptoms), an inability to remember features of the trauma or a feeling of altered reality (dissociative symptoms), and hypervigilance or an exaggerated startle response (arousal symptoms; APA, 2013). The presence of acute stress disorder does not necessarily predict the occurrence of PTSD.

b.   PTSD is a potentially debilitating illness that occurs when a person is exposed to a traumatic stressor. PTSD symptoms usually appear within 3 months after the stressor, but may not occur for as long as a year after it. The person experiences the same intrusive, dissociative and arousal symptoms as in acute stress disorder, as well as emotional numbing, relationship difficulties, lack of interest in pleasurable activities, self-destructive behaviors, and difficulty sleeping and/or concentrating. Children under age 6 may act out their trauma in their play, regress to earlier developmental behavior, have difficulty with physical contact, and socially withdraw. They may also act out aggressively without awareness that the behavior is connected to the trauma (usually abuse; APA, 2013; Lubit, 2014b).

Screening tools for PTSD include:

- Child and Adolescent Psychiatric Assessment: Life Events Section and PTSD Module (CAPA-PTSD) is a 33-item PTSD scale for youths aged 8 to 18 years that measures the frequency and intensity of symptoms, as well as their impact (Angold, Cox, Prendergast, Rutter, & Simonoff, 2008).

- The Children's PTSD Inventory (CPTSD-I) is a structured interview for children ages 6 to 18 to assess PTSD symptoms, diagnoses, qualifying event, and current functioning (Saigh, 2004).

- The Child PTSD Symptom Scale (CPSS) is a child version of an adult scale. This is a 17-item, self-report measure that assesses the frequency of PTSD symptoms (Nixon et al., 2013).

c.   PTSD in children may mimic other childhood mental health disorders. These include: acute stress disorder, adjustment disorder, attention deficit hyperactivity disorder (ADHD) and other disruptive disorders, depression, other anxiety disorders, and sleep disorders. Symptoms may overlap, and some children suffer from more than one mental health disorder.

d.   Children and adolescents may also demonstrate impulsivity and inattentiveness, which frequently negatively affects their academic achievement, and they may isolate themselves from others and withdraw from their peers. They may also demonstrate regressive behaviors such as enuresis, encopresis, and thumb-sucking. As with adults, PTSD can have comorbid problems, and is associated with mood disorders, conduct disorder, substance abuse, risk-taking that poses considerable danger, disruptive behavior disorders, eating disorders, sexual acting out, other risk-taking activities, depression, the full range of anxiety disorders, dissociation, mood lability, violence, and difficulty concentrating.

D. Levels of Prevention/Intervention

a.   Primary

- There is minimal research on the primary, pretrauma prevention of PTSD, and a systematic review of seven studies by Skeffington, Reese, and Kane (2013) showed there is no solid body of evidence on the primary prevention of PTSD to justify or guide interventions.

- Zohar et al. (2011) note that typical practices in the aftermath of trauma such as event debriefing and benzodiazepines require careful consideration in view of their potential harm to the spontaneous recovery process and the trajectory of PTSD.

- Noting that systematic reviews suggested that single session debriefing may be harmful, the World Health Organization (WHO, 2012) strongly recommends that psychological debriefing not be used for people recently exposed to a traumatic event to reduce posttraumatic stress.

b.   Secondary

- The goal of secondary prevention is to assist youth who have experienced a traumatic event in order to minimize or prevent the occurrence of a stress disorder. This can best be accomplished through crisis intervention after traumatic incidents; encouraging family, peer, and school support; and providing a brief course of therapy, if needed. Built on the concept of human resilience, psychological first aid (PFA) helps survivors in the immediate aftermath of a traumatic event. PFA can help everyone from children to adults to families. This therapy reduces the initial distress caused by the event and acknowledges the seriousness of the experience of danger and the increased feelings of vulnerability that often follow. PFA fosters long- and short-term adaptability, basic functioning, and coping skills, and can be used in schools and traditional settings. PFA involves providing comfort and support and letting children know their reactions are normal, and teaches calming and problem-solving skills. It also helps caregivers deal with changes in the child's feelings and behavior. While beneficial for many children, those with more severe symptoms may be referred for added treatment.

- Youth may also find strength through their faith. Primary care providers can also assist children and their families in understanding about trauma reactions, reestablishing their routines, and respecting their readiness and willingness for treatment (APA, 2013).

- Traumatic events can lead to other stressors and traumas, such as criminal justice interventions; funerals; disruption of and displacement from home, school, and other routines; loss of possessions, friends, and pets; and financial stress. Primary care providers can help families with these challenges with referrals to victim resource and social service agencies (APA, 2013).

c. Tertiary

- Treatment of children with acute stress disorder involves the basic principles of trauma intervention: ensure the child is safe and that immediate needs are met; reduce stress; engage support systems; promote coping; and help children reframe cognitive distortions (Lubit, 2014a).

- For some children, the symptoms of PTSD go away on their own after a few months, while for others, the symptoms last for years without treatment. Since PTSD symptoms can greatly disrupt a child's development and since some children with PTSD also have other disorders, all children should be evaluated by an appropriate mental health care professional.

- As with adults, there are multiple treatment options for children with PTSD. These include psychotherapies, medications, and alternative treatments. Treatment should focus on the multiple emotional and behavioral problems that can arise, such as depression, anxiety, impulsive behavior, substance abuse, aggression, eating disorders, sexual acting out, labile mood, rage, panic attacks, and dissociation. Treatment of these problems may involve medication, psychotherapy, or a combination of these, as well as supportive treatments. Specific treatment depends on the child's development and symptoms, as well as on the nature of the trauma.

- The first step is helping the child gain a sense of mastery over the trauma and helping the child to feel safe again. For older children, gaining a sense of mastery includes the ability to recall and talk about the trauma without dissociating or feeling overwhelmed. Meditation and relaxation training may help the child to do this.

- Play helps younger children work through the trauma, but the play often breaks down in PTSD, and may turn into repetitive reenactment that is not enjoyable and that may require other interventions to allow the child to feel safe again and avoid the fear of scary thoughts returning.

- It is important that you destigmatize the child's symptoms. Families need to understand that the repeated recollections, numbing, and hyperarousal are natural responses to trauma and not signs of serious mental illness or weakness. Parents should avoid burdening their child with their own painful feelings and verbalizing fears that the child is permanently damaged.

  - Psychotherapy: There are different types of psychotherapy for PTSD, and three are outlined here. Cognitive behavioral therapy (CBT) techniques have been shown to be effective in treating children and adolescents with PTSD. CBT can reduce serious trauma reactions, other anxiety and depressive symptoms, and behavioral problems. One type of CBT is called trauma-focused CBT (TF-CBT), during which the child may talk about his or her memory of the trauma. TF-CBT also includes techniques that help lower worry and stress and that help teach the child how to assert himself or herself. The therapy may involve learning to change incorrect thoughts or beliefs about the trauma, such as that the world is not a safe place. The child can be taught to remember scary memories at his or her own pace and to relax while thinking about the trauma. That way, the child learns that he or she does not have to be afraid of the child's memories. CBT often uses training for parents and caregivers, too, and it is important for caregivers to understand the effects of PTSD and to learn coping skills that will help them help their child. Eye movement desensitization and reprocessing (EMDR) combines elements of behavioral and client-centered approaches. The client concentrates intensely on the most distressing segment of a traumatic memory while moving the eyes rapidly from side to side (by following the therapist's fingers moving across the visual field). Following the initial focus on the memory segment, after each "set" of eye movements (of about 30 seconds), the client is asked to report anything that "came up," whether an image, thought, emotion, or physical sensation (all are common). The focus of the next set is determined by the client's changing status. Play therapy can help young children with PTSD who are unable to deal with the trauma more directly. Play therapists use games, drawings, and other methods to help children process their traumatic memories.

- Medication: There are no large-scale randomized clinical trials that guide choices for the pharmacological treatment of PTSD in children. Clinical experience suggests that selective serotonin reuptake inhibitors (SSRIs), which are proven for PTSD in adults, are helpful but are off-label and warrant informed consent regarding the Food and Drug Administration (FDA) black box warning concerning the risk for suicidality in children. SSRIs are used for managing anxiety, depression, avoidance behavior, and intrusive recollections. Other medications have also been used, even though the evidence supporting their use is not as robust as for antidepressants (in adults). Beta-blockers and alpha-adrenergic agonists help to reduce arousal, decrease forced reexperiencing of the trauma, and avoid the neurophysiological kindling that can contribute to chronic illness. These medications are most helpful if used very soon after the onset of symptoms. Mood stabilizers can help deal with increased arousal, and impulsivity; carbamazepine can help reexperience symptoms, while valproic acid can help avoidance symptoms—the two are not interchangeable. Antipsychotics are used only for children who are unresponsive to other medications or when marked agitation or psychosis is present (Lubit, 2014b).

E. Parenting Tips

a.   Some children withstand an onslaught of stressors. No matter what happens, they bounce back in the face of stressful events and situations. These children tend to have specific characteristics:

- They have a loving relationship with at least one adult, and connections with adults outside the family.
- They believe in their own effectiveness, and that they are lovable and worthwhile.
- They can solve problems effectively.
- They believe that they have the ability to make things better for themselves.
- They have spiritual resources.

b.   Your child is at increased risk for suicide if he or she fits any of the following risk factors. If any of these apply to your child, talk to your child's health care provider:

- Previous suicide attempts (risk is greater if happened in past 3 months)
- Psychiatric disorder
- Family member with mood disorder or suicide attempt or success
- Child or family member has substance abuse problem
- Family discord
- Impulsiveness
- Hostility
- Poor social skills
- School problems, including truancy
- Romantic breakup
- Homosexual or bisexual preference

c. Bring him or her to an emergency facility immediately for any of these:

- Stating he or she wants to hurt or kill himself or herself
- Any suicide plan
- Irrational speech
- Sudden alienation from family
- Sudden interest or loss of interest in religion
- Taking unnecessary risks
- Hears voices or sees visions
- Drug and alcohol abuse
- Giving away his or her possessions
- Writing notes or poems about death
- Preoccupation with death-themed music, movies, art, or video games
- Feelings of hopelessness
- Statements like "You won't have to worry about me anymore"

Resources

American Academy of Child & Adolescent Psychiatry: Posttraumatic Stress Disorder: www.aacap.org/AACAP/Families_and_Youth/Facts_for_Families/Facts_for_Families_Pages/Posttraumatic_Stress_Disorder_70.aspx

Kidshealth: Post-Traumatic Stress Disorder: http://kidshealth.org/parent/positive/talk/ptsd.html

A Look at Acute Stress Disorder and PTSD: www.childmind.org/en/posts/articles/2012-11-14-acute-stress-disorder-and-ptsd-exploring-traumatic

MedlinePlus: Posttraumatic Stress Disorder: www.nlm.nih.gov/medlineplus/posttraumaticstressdisorder.html

National Center for PTSD: www.ptsd.va.gov

References

American Psychiatric Association. (2013). *Diagnostic and statistical manual of mental disorders* (5th ed.). Washington, DC: Author.

American Psychological Association. (2008). *Children and trauma*. Washington, DC: Author. Retrieved from www.apa.org/pi/families/resources/children-trauma-update.aspx

Angold, A., Cox, A., Prendergast, M., Rutter, M. Simonoff, E. (2008). The child and adolescent psychiatric assessment. Retrieved from http://devepi.duhs.duke.edu/eMeasures/Child%20Life%20Events%20 (for%20review%20only).pdf

Lubit, R. (2014a). Acute stress disorder. *Medscape emedicine.* Retrieved from http://emedicine .medscape.com/article/2192581-overview

Lubit, R. (2014b). Posttraumatic stress disorder in children: Treatment and management. *Medscape emedicine.* Retrieved from http://emedicine.medscape.com/article/918844-treatment#d9

National Child Traumatic Stress Network. (n.d.). *Types of traumatic stress.* Retrieved from http:// nctsnet.org/trauma-types

Nixon, R. D., Meiser-Stedman, R., Dalgleish, T., Yule, W., Clark, D. M., Perrin, S., & Smith, P. (2013). The Child PTSD Symptom Scale: An update and replication of its psychometric properties. *Psychological Assessment, 25*(3), 1025–1031.

Saigh, P. A. (2004). *A structured interview for diagnosing Posttraumatic Stress Disorder: Children's PTSD Inventory.* San Antonio, TX: PsychCorp.

Skeffington, P., Reese, C., & Kane, R. (2013). The primary prevention of PTSD: A systematic review. *Journal of Trauma & Dissociation: The Official Journal of the Society for the Study of Dissociation (ISSD), 14*(4), 404–422.

Trickey, D., Siddaway, A. P., Meiser-Stedman, R., Serpell, L., & Field, A. P. (2012). A meta-analysis of risk factors for posttraumatic stress disorder in children and adolescents. *Clinical Psychology Review, 32*(2), 122–138. doi:10.1016/j.cpr.2011.12.001

World Health Organization. (2012). *Psychological debriefing in people exposed to a recent traumatic event.* Author. Retrieved from www.who.int/mental_health/mhgap/evidence/resource/other_comp laints_q5.pdf?ua=1

Zohar, J., Juven-Wetzler, A., Sonnino, R., Cwikel-Hamzany, S., Balaban, E., & Cohen, H. (2011). New insights into secondary prevention in post-traumatic stress disorder. *Dialogues in Clinical Neuroscience, 13*(3), 301–309.

APPENDICES

APPENDIX A

Developmental Milestones Chart

AGE	INFANTS			
	SOCIAL/COGNITIVE	LANGUAGE	FINE MOTOR	GROSS MOTOR
2 weeks	• Observes mother's face when talking • Reflexive sensorimotor	• Cries to express displeasure	• Grasp	• Lifts head when prone
2 months	• Social smile • Primary circular reactions	• Differentiated crying • Coos	• Holds rattle briefly	• Lifts chest when prone
4 months	• Starts to discriminate strangers by 5 months • Demands attention • Becomes bored when left alone • Begins to show memory	• Coos, babbles, laughs • Vocalizes when smiling • "Talks" when spoken to • Makes consonant sounds (b, g, k, n, p)	• Carries object to mouth • Holds 2 objects (4–5 months)	• Rolls over • Sits with support
6 months	• Begins to fear strangers • Has likes and dislikes • Recognizes parents • Begins to imitate • Briefly searches for dropped object	• Imitates sounds • Ma, mu, da • Vocalizes to mirror images	• Transfers hand to hand (5 months) • Secures cube on sight	• Sits without support (5–7½ months)

(continued)

INFANTS				
AGE	SOCIAL/COGNITIVE	LANGUAGE	FINE MOTOR	GROSS MOTOR
9 months	• Holds arms out to be picked up (7–8 months) • Exhibits aggression by biting (7–8 months) • Begins to show fear of being alone • Puts arm in front of face to avoid washing • Shows interest in pleasing parent	• Makes sound (d, t, w) • Listens to familiar words • Combines syllables (mama) • Responds to simple verbal commands • Understands "no-no"	• Reaches for toy • Bangs spoon • Searches for dropped toy within hand reach • Pincer grasp	• Pulls to stand • Stands with support • Cruises
12 months	• Shows emotions • Clingy; fearful of strange situations • Increasing determination to practice locomotor skills • Searches for object where it was last seen	• Recognizes objects by name • Comprehends several words • Says 5–10 words • Imitates speech and animal sounds	• Puts three or more objects in container	• Stands alone • Walks alone (11½–14 months

AGE	SOCIAL/COGNITIVE	LANGUAGE	FINE MOTOR	GROSS MOTOR
15 months	• Tolerates some separation from parents • Stranger fear less likely • Kisses and hugs • Tantrums • Uses "no" even when in agreement	• Jargon • Asks for objects by pointing • Uses "no"	• Persistently tosses objects to floor • Builds 2-cube tower • Scribbles	• Walks without help • Assumes standing position without support • Creeps upstairs
18 months	• Imitates • Manages spoon • Transitional object important • Peak age for thumb sucking • Tantrums more evident • Understands "my"	• Says more than 10 words • Points to 2 or 3 body parts	• Builds 3–4-cube tower • Turns book pages 2–3 at a time	• Runs but clumsy • Pushes and pulls toys • Climbs stairs one at a time with hand held • Throws ball overhand without falling
24 months	• Parallel play begins • Starting attention span • Tantrums decrease • Increased independence	• Has 300-word vocabulary • Uses 2–3 word phrases ("me go") • Uses pronouns • Knows first name • Verbalizes basic needs • Talks constantly	• Builds 6–7-cube tower • Turns book pages one at a time • Imitates vertical and circular strokes	• Climbs stairs one at a time without holding hand
30 months	• Separates more easily from mother • Knows own sex • May be toilet-trained except for wiping	• Knows first and surname • Uses appropriate pronoun for self • Uses plurals • Names a color	• Builds 8-cube tower; adds chimney to cubes • Good hand–finger coordination • Imitates vertical and horizontal strokes	• Jumps on two feet • Stands on one foot for brief period

TODDLERS

AGE	SOCIAL/COGNITIVE	LANGUAGE	FINE MOTOR	GROSS MOTOR
3 years	• Egocentric • Begins to understand time; pretends to tell time • Attempts to please parents and conform • Separates easier from parents • Aware of gender role functions	• Has 900-word vocabulary • Uses 3-4-word complete sentences • Constant talker • Asks questions • Starts to sing	• Builds 9-10-cube tower • Copies circle and cross	• Rides tricycle • Stands on one foot for few seconds • Alternates feet going up steps • Tries to dance
4 years	• Takes aggression out on siblings and parents • Sibling rivalry • May "run away" from home • Identifies with parent of opposite sex • Very imaginative • Understands simple analogies • Judges everything in one dimension • Counts but does not understand numbers	• 1,500-word vocabulary • Questioning peaks • Starts to understand prepositions • Names more colors	• Uses scissors • Can lace shoes • Copies square and diamond	• Skips and hops on one foot • Can catch ball • Walks down steps alternating feet
5 years	• Gets along with parents • Identifies with parent of same sex ("mommy's girl," "daddy's boy") • Questions parents' thinking • Begins to understand numbers • Increasingly understands time	• 2,100-word vocabulary • Uses all parts of speech • Names coins • Knows days of week, months • Can follow three commands in succession	• Adapt with pencil • Copies triangle • Adds 7-9 parts to stick figure	• Skips, alternating feet • Jumps rope • Skates • Balances on alternate feet while closing eyes

SCHOOLAGERS

AGE	SOCIAL/COGNITIVE	FINE MOTOR	GROSS MOTOR
6 years	• Shares and cooperates better • Cheats to win • Mimics adults • Boasts • Jealous; rough • Likes table games • Reads from memory • Difficulty taking responsibility for misbehavior • Brushes teeth and hair • Enjoys oral spelling games	• Uses utensils • Shows gradual increase in dexterity • Likes to draw, color	• Very active • Can walk straight line
7 years	• Becoming "family member" • Group play, but likes to spend time alone (loner) • Prefers members of same sex • May steal • Can read clock	• Can cut meat with knife • Needs no help to brush teeth and hair	• Repeats performances to master them
8–9 years	• Dramatic • Likes rewards • Concept of reversibility; concepts of space; cause and effect; and conservation • Describes common objects in detail • More aware of time • Can understand parts and wholes	• Cursive writing • Increased speed and smoothness in fine motor control	• More limber • Movements more fluid • Likes to overdo • Crouches on toes
10–12 years	• Friends important; choosey about friends • Beginning to develop interest in opposite sex • Likes family; respects parents • Writes stories and letters • Uses telephone • Reads for information and enjoyment	• Continues to develop fine motor skills	• Posture more like adults' • Catches ball with one hand (9–11 years)

ADOLESCENTS	
AGE	**BEHAVIOR**
12–14 years	• Mood swings • Prefer to spend time with friends over family • Body conscious • Concerned about being normal • Abstract thinking • Asks "dumb questions" (pseudo-stupidity) • Imaginary audience • Personal fable • Can solve math and logic problems
15–16 years	• Parental conflict peaks • Being attractive becomes very important • Defies limits of bodies with excessive physical activity, resulting in periods of lethargy • Essence of adolescent subculture • Peer involvement is intense • Sexual drive emerges • Feelings of omnipotence • Experimentation
17–21 years	• Plans for the future • Preparing for college, military, marriage, workforce • Makes decisions on how to contribute to society • Usually relates to family as adults • Adult-level reasoning skills • Most have established sexuality and entered into intimate relationship • Adolescents who enter workforce tend to consolidate their identities earlier than those who enter college.

Resources

Ball, J., Bindler, R. M., & Cowen, K. J. (2012). *Principles of pediatric nursing: Caring for children* (5th ed.). Boston, MA: Pearson.

Birth to 5: Watch Me Thrive! A Primary Care Provider's Guide for Developmental and Behavioral Screening: www.acf.hhs.gov/sites/default/files/ecd/pcp_screening_guide_march2014.pdf

Centers for Disease Control and Prevention: Child Development: www.cdc.gov/ncbddd/child development/index.html

Centers for Disease Control and Prevention: Parenting Tips: www.cdc.gov/ncbddd/childdevelopment/positiveparenting/index.html

Centers for Disease Control and Prevention. (2015). *Developmental milestones.* Retrieved from www.cdc.gov/ncbddd/actearly/milestones/index.html

Hockenberry, M. J., & Wilson, D. (2012). *Wong's essentials of pediatric nursing* (9th ed.). St. Louis, MO: Mosby.

APPENDIX B

Pediatric Symptom Checklist-17

Scoring the PSC-17

The Pediatric Symptom Checklist-17 (PSC-17) is a psychosocial screen designed to facilitate the recognition of cognitive, emotional, and behavioral problems so that appropriate interventions can be initiated as early as possible. The PSC-17 consists of 17 items that are rated as "never," "sometimes," or "often" present. A value of 0 is assigned to "never," 1 to "sometimes," and 2 to "often." The total score is calculated by adding together the scores for each of the 17 items. Items that are left blank are simply ignored (i.e., score equals 0). If four or more items are left blank, the questionnaire is considered invalid. A PSC-17 score of 15 or higher suggests the presence of significant behavioral or emotional problems, and a need for further evaluation. Both false positives and false negatives occur, and only an experienced clinician should interpret a positive PSC score as anything other than a suggestion that further evaluation may be helpful. All forms of the PSC are scored in this same way. To determine what kinds of mental health problems are present, determine the three factor scores on the PSC:

- Attention Problems Subscale:
  - Fidgety, unable to sit still
  - Daydreams too much
  - Distracted easily
  - Has trouble concentrating
  - Acts as if driven by a motor

AT RISK—Children with scores of 7 or higher on this subscale usually have significant impairments in attention.

©1988, M.S. Jellinek and J.M. Murphy, Massachusetts General Hospital.

- Internalizing Problems Subscale:
  - Feels sad, unhappy
  - Feels hopeless
  - Is down on himself or herself
  - Worries a lot
  - Seems to be having less fun

AT RISK—Children with scores of 5 or higher on this subscale usually have significant impairments with anxiety and/or depression.

- Externalizing Problems Subscale:
  - Fights with others
  - Does not listen to rules
  - Does not understand other people's feelings
  - Teases others
  - Blames others for his or her troubles
  - Takes things that do not belong to him or her
  - Refuses to share

AT RISK—Children with scores of 7 or higher on this subscale usually have significant problems with conduct.

Pediatric Symptom Checklist (PSC-17)

Please mark under the heading that best describes your child:

	(0)	(1)	(2)
	NEVER	SOMETIMES	OFTEN
1. Feels sad, unhappy	⊙	⊙	⊙
2. Feels hopeless	⊙	⊙	⊙
3. Is down on self	⊙	⊙	⊙
4. Worries a lot	⊙	⊙	⊙
5. Seems to be having less fun	⊙	⊙	⊙
6. Fidgety, unable to sit still	⊙	⊙	⊙
7. Daydreams too much	⊙	⊙	⊙
8. Distracted easily	⊙	⊙	⊙
9. Has trouble concentrating	⊙	⊙	⊙
10. Acts as if driven by a motor	⊙	⊙	⊙
11. Fights with other children	⊙	⊙	⊙
12. Does not listen to rules	⊙	⊙	⊙
13. Does not understand other people's feelings	⊙	⊙	⊙
14. Teases others	⊙	⊙	⊙
15. Blames others for his or her troubles	⊙	⊙	⊙
16. Refuses to share	⊙	⊙	⊙
17. Takes things that do not belong to him or her	⊙	⊙	⊙
Does your child have any emotional or behavioral problems for which he or she needs help?		No	Yes

YOUTH PEDIATRIC SYMPTOM CHECKLIST-17 (Y PSC-17)

Name: _____   Record #: _____

Date of Birth: _____   Today's Date: _____

Please mark under the heading that best fits you:		NEVER	SOMETIMES	OFTEN
◆	Fidgety, unable to sit still	◆	0	1	2
✳	Feel sad, unhappy	✳	0	1	2
◆	Daydream too much	◆	0	1	2
❏	Refuse to share	❏	0	1	2
❏	Do not understand other people's feelings	❏	0	1	2
✳	Feel hopeless	✳	0	1	2
◆	Have trouble concentrating	◆	0	1	2
❏	Fight with other children	❏	0	1	2
✳	Down on yourself	✳	0	1	2
❏	Blame others for your troubles	❏	0	1	2
✳	Seem to be having less fun	✳	0	1	2
❏	Do not listen to rules	❏	0	1	2
◆	Act as if driven by a motor	◆	0	1	2
❏	Tease others	❏	0	1	2
✳	Worry a lot	✳	0	1	2
❏	Take things that do not belong to you	❏	0	1	2
◆	Distract easily	◆	0	1	2

OFFICE USE ONLY

Total ◆ _____ Total ❏ _____ Total ✳ _____ Grand Total ◆+❏+✳ _____

Form adapted with permission for *Feelings Need Check Ups Too*, 2004

©1988, M. Jellinek & J.M. Murphy, Massachusetts General Hospital (PSC-17 created by W. Gardner & K. Kelleher) and Bright Futures in Practice: Mental Health, 2002

APPENDIX C

Crisis Intervention: A Quick Guide for Health Care Professionals

- Remain calm at all times.
- Follow a step-by-step approach to crisis management (Kavan, Guck, & Barone, 2006):
  - **STEP 1.** Provide reassurance through validation of the problem and active listening.
  - **STEP 2.** Evaluate the severity of the crisis by conducting a rapid, focused assessment that includes suicide and violence evaluation and mental status exam. Obtain information from collateral sources (records, family members, emergency personnel), as needed.
  - **STEP 3.** Ensure the safety of the patient and others, securing close monitoring by family and friends; hospitalization may be required if the patient is dangerous to self or others.
  - **STEP 4.** Stabilize the patient's emotional status, explore options for managing the crisis, develop a specific written action plan, and obtain commitment from the patient to follow through. Help the patient focus on strengths and on how these and other coping mechanisms were used successfully in the past. Utilize family and community support systems.
  - **STEP 5.** Follow up with the patient to provide ongoing support and to reinforce appropriate action planning.
- Utilize Suicide Assessment and Five-Step Evaluation Triage (SAFE-T; Education Development Center, INC and Screening for Mental Health, INC, 2009).
  - Recognize and assess the risk including history of suicide attempts, psychiatric history, current symptoms, family history, causative events, and access to weapons.
  - Identify mechanisms of coping that have worked in the past and any responsibility the patient may have in his or her life.
  - Investigate suicidal ideation including thoughts, plan, and intent, and identify details of each.

- Assess level of risk from low, medium, and high suicidality.
- Provide accurate documentation.
- Intervention
- Ensure the safety of the patient: Provide a safe room as well as monitoring of patient at all times.
- Utilizing clinical judgment, separate the patient for an individual interview providing the clinician and patient are safe.
- Utilize active listening to validate patient's feelings as well as creating a sense of safety and understanding for the patient (Bryant, 2009).
- Be open and nonjudgmental.
- Suicidal risk:
  - High risk: Refer to emergency department or call 911.
  - Moderate risk: Assess possibility of hospital admission, or create an emergency plan including a contract for safety, parental monitoring at all times, and outpatient referral for mental health services.
  - Low risk: Contract for safety, create an emergency plan, ensure outside supports, and refer to outpatient mental health services (Education Development Center, INC and Screening for Mental Health, INC, 2009).

Resources

Crisis Prevention Institute: www.crisisprevention.com/

Knoll, J. The Psychiatric ER Survival Guide: www.psychiatrictimes.com/all/editorial/psychiatrictimes/pdfs/psych-survival2.pdf

References

Bryant, L. (2009). The art of active listening. *Practice Nurse, 37*(6), 49–52.

Education Development Center, INC and Screening for Mental Health, INC. (2009). Suicide assessment and five-step evaluation and triage for mental health professionals. In Substance Abuse and Mental Health Administration. Retrieved from www.integration.samhsa.gov/images/res/SAFE_T.pdf

Kavan, M. G., Guck, T. P., & Barone, E. J. (2006). A practical guide to crisis management. *American Family Physician, 74*(7), 1158–1164.

APPENDIX D

Motivational Interviewing

Originated by Miller and Rollnick (2008) for the treatment of problem drinkers, motivational interviewing (MI) is client-centered counseling that guides clients through the process of making a change through the exploration and resolving of ambivalence. Although first used with adults, MI is easily adaptable to the pediatric population. It is especially applicable during adolescence for problems such as weight loss, drug abuse, obsessive compulsive disorder (OCD), tobacco use, and alcohol use.

The basic approaches of MI are:

O—Open-ended questions avoid yes and no answers. Opening dialogue begins the encounter with phrases such as "Tell me what you would like to discuss," or "Tell me what you think." This allows the youth to feel as if he or she has some control over the topic.

A—Affirmations build rapport. Authentic use of statements like "that sounds like a great idea," or "I appreciate what you are saying" helps promote youths' strengths and enables them to feel supported. The affirmations should be congruent and supportive; insincerity can destroy trust.

R—Reflective listening uses the language of the youth by seeking more information through clarification and leading comments to expand on what the youth is trying to communicate. This demonstrates that you have a genuine understanding. Listen carefully, but guide the youth.

UTILIZING THE ABOVE FORMAT OF OARS WITH THE PRINCIPLE OF	CONCEPTS TO AVOID
Expressing empathy	Displaying authority over the client
Developing discrepancy	Coercion for change
Avoiding arguing	Argumentation
Rolling with resistance	Justification of the problem
Supporting self-efficacy	Voicing expert opinion

S—Summaries pull the essential information together for a better mutual understanding. This serves as a conclusion or transition to shift the focus or to conclude the encounter. (Erickson, Gerstle, & Feldstein, 2005; Miller & Rollnick, 2008)

Application of MI is appropriate when the individual is committed to wanting a change Gold & Kokotailo, 2007; Jackman, 2012):

Step 1   Engage the youth, develop a trusting relationship.

Step 2   Focus on what the youth wants to change (listen to his or her cues).

Step 3   Assist the youth to self-identify the change needed by utilizing OARS.

Step 4   Guide the youth in developing a plan to implement the change, utilizing OARS.

Resources

Enhancing Motivation for Change in Substance Abuse Treatment: www.ncbi.nlm.nih.gov/books/NBK64967/pdf/Bookshelf_NBK64967.pdf

Motivational Interviewing: http://motivationalinterviewing.org/

Motivational Interviewing SAMHSA: www.integration.samhsa.gov/clinical-practice/motivational-interviewing

References

Gold, M., & Kokotailo, P. (2007). Motivational interviewing strategies to facilitate adolescent behavior change. *American Academy of Pediatrics, 20*(1), 1–6.

Erickson, S., Gestle, M., & Feldstein, S. (2005). Brief interventions and motivational interviewing with children, adolescents and their parents in pediatric health care settings. *Journal of Pediatric Adolescent Medicine, 159*(12), 1173–1180.

Jackman, K. (2012). Motivational interviewing with adolescents: An advanced practice nursing intervention for psychiatric settings. *Journal of Child and Adolescent Psychiatric Nursing, 25*(1), 4–8.

Miller, W., & Rollnick, S. (2008). *Motivational interviewing: Preparing people for change* (2nd ed.). New York, NY: Guilford Press.

APPENDIX E

Cognitive Behavioral Therapy Mini-Guide

Cognitive behavioral therapy (CBT) teaches the client to be aware of the connection between his or her thoughts, emotions, and actions. When a clinician and a client collaborate to understand, identify, and change the dysfunctional pattern, a healthy model of behavior is the result.

CBT is delivered to the individual and operates on the premise that the clinician assists the person in restructuring his or her maladaptive way of thinking and destructive pattern of behaviors. This is achieved by identifying the interplay between the client and his or her thoughts, feelings, and behaviors that is the basis for the client's psychopathology (Wheeler, 2015, p. 314). It is important to note that CBT is a process of guiding the client in discovering his or her maladaptive cognition instead of directly confronting or challenging the client, which will facilitate the client's ability to formulate his or her own behavioral solutions to his or her difficulties (Wheeler, 2015, p. 339). CBT is a proven, effective therapy for addressing depression, anxiety, post-traumatic stress disorder (PTSD), self-harm, and personality disorders (Cully & Teton, 2008, p. 7).

CBT is a structured process with a definitive time frame, with assigned homework to be accomplished between sessions. Homework (action plans) is a key component of CBT, which serves the purpose of continuing the work from the session in a real-life situation and allows the reinforcement of the concepts learned in the session (Knight, 2015).

CBT Approach

1. Guide the client to begin to notice when he or she is experiencing negative emotions.
2. Have the client begin a journal to record when he or she is having negative thoughts, what triggers those thoughts, and the client's instinctive reaction to those thoughts.

3. Educate the client on exploring the connections between his or her maladaptive thoughts and the resulting behaviors.

4. Explore the possible reasons for the maladaptive thought process, that is, "Why this thought, why not think about it differently?"

5. Objectively explore alternative reasons for the behavior.

6. Begin to exchange negative thoughts for positive reality-based thoughts.

7. Experiment with this change of thought process, and record the result in a personal journal to share with the clinician at the next session.

8. This process will undoubtedly uncover maladaptive thought processes that can then be changed to create a new, healthy method of cognition (Cully & Teton, 2008).

CBT Process

First, it must be determined that the client is a suitable candidate for the therapy, committed to change and able to complete the homework assigned between sessions. The clinician and the client should have a genuine rapport and mutual respect for each other, and the client must be willing to truly explore and examine his or her thought process (Cully & Teton, 2008). CBT can be a short-term therapy, and the focus is on the client becoming, in essence, his or her own therapist by creating his or her own solutions via exploration of their behavior and thoughts (Beck & Beck, 2011). The benefit of CBT is that it can be a time-limited intervention as brief as 6 to 12 sessions for uncomplicated anxiety or depression, with treatment extending to 6 months to 1 year for more complicated psychopathologies. Clients may also need occasional visits after treatment concludes to continue to fine-tune the process and address any lingering issues (Beck Institute of Cognitive Therapy, 2015).

First CBT Session Agenda

1. Validate the client and begin the process of establishing therapeutic rapport.

2. Create a problem-solving list from most distressing to least.

3. Educate the client about the psychotherapeutic process, CBT framework, and concepts.

4. Discuss a general overview of the treatment course: agendas, homework, journaling, number of sessions, expectations, and so forth.

5. Be sure to impress upon the client the crucial aspects of being self-aware and homework.

6. Explore the client's feelings and reactions to the sessions.

Subsequent Sessions

1. Explore the client's current mental status, and create session agenda.
2. Review homework (techniques and thought journaling), and address issues with not doing homework assignments.
3. Focus on the particular problem to explore for that session: dysfunctional thinking patterns, negativity. Explore strategies and alternatives for problem solving.
4. Other components for subsequent sessions can include teaching relaxation methods, thought stopping, examining cognitive distortions, problem-solving strategies, helping the client to schedule "worry time," assertiveness training, role-playing.
5. Discuss homework assignment for upcoming week.
6. Explore the client's feelings and reaction to the session at completion.
7. Discuss a possible agenda for the next session, assess mental status.
8. Wrap up session (Cully & Teton, 2008).

Some Examples of Cognitive Distortions

1. All-or-nothing thinking: Things are black or white, the client sees himself or herself as a success or failure, or views people/situations as either good or bad.
2. Catastrophizing: Expecting the worst case scenario to be the only outcome.
3. Overgeneralizing: A negative event becomes the pattern for future events.
4. Mind reading: The client assumes he or she knows what someone else is thinking about him or her (something negative) without any real evidence for the assumption.
5. Comparing: The client automatically assumes that he or she is not as good/competent/smart/accomplished as another person.
6. Emotional reasoning: The client believes that because he or she feels incompetent, it must, therefore, be true.
7. Personalization: The client views himself or herself as the cause of some negative external event for which he or she was not primarily responsible (Wheeler, 2015).

Websites for specific disorders, providing brief overviews, manuals, and treatments:

Anxiety:	https://socialanxietyinstitute.org/why-cbt-works-social-anxiety-disorder
	www.anxietynetwork.com
Depression:	www.psychologyinfo.com/depression/cognitive.htm
Obsessive compulsive disorder:	www.ocdonline/definecbt.php

Addiction:	www.nida.nih.gov/Tmanuals/CBT/CBT1.html
Child sexual abuse:	www.childwelfare.gov/pubPDFs/trauma.pdf
Eating disorders:	http://eatingdisorder.org/treatment-and-support/therapeutic-modalities/cognitive-behavioral-therapy/
PTSD	www.med.upenn.edu/ctsa/ptsd_treatment.html

Resources

Academy of Cognitive Therapy: www.academyofct.org

Association for Behavioral and Cognitive Therapies: www.findcbt.org/xFAT/

Beck Institute for Cognitive Behavior Therapy, Resources for Lay People and Professionals Alike: www.beckinstitute.org/

References

Beck, J. & Beck, A. (2011). *Cognitive behavioral therapy.* New York, NY: Guilford Press.

Cully, J., & Teton, A. (2008). *A therapist's brief guide to cognitive behavioral therapy.* Retrieved from Department of Veterans Affairs South Central MIRECC website: www.mirecc.va.gov/visn16/docs/therapists_guide_to_brief_cbtmanual.pdf

Knight, C. (2015). Humanistic-existential and solution-focused approaches to psychotherapy. In K. Wheeler (Ed.) *Psychotherapy for the advanced practice psychiatric nurse: A how-to guide for evidence-based practice* (2nd ed., pp. 369-406). New York, NY: Springer Publishing Company.

INDEX

Printed in the United States
By Bookmasters